Allergy Free
naturally

Allergy Free
naturally

1,000
Nondrug Solutions
for More Than
50 Allergy-Related
Problems

RICK ANSORGE, ERIC METCALF
and the Editors of
PREVENTION
Health Books

RODALE

"The Traditional Healthy Asian Diet Pyramid" on page 137 is © 2000 by Oldways Preservation and Exchange Trust. Reprinted with permission.

The "Do You Need EFA Supplements?" quiz on page 156 is from *The Four Pillars of Healing* by Leo Galland, © 1997 by Renaissance Workshops Ltd. Used by permission of Random House, Inc.

The "Are You Allergic?" quiz on page 207 is adapted from "The Quick and Easy Allergy Screening Quiz," which originally appeared on the Web site www.tamingallergies.com. Used by permission of Eddie L. Gaines, M.D.

Library of Congress Cataloging-in-Publication Data

Ansorge, Rick, date.
    Allergy free naturally : 1,000 nondrug solutions for more than 50 allergy-related problems / Rick Ansorge, Eric Metcalf, and the Editors of Prevention Health Books.
        p.   cm.
    Includes index.
    ISBN 1–57954–327–8   hardcover
    ISBN 1–57954–392–8   paperback
    1. Allergy—Popular works.   I. Metcalf, Eric.   II. Prevention Health Books.   III. Title.
RC585 .A575   2001
616.97—dc21

            2001002695

Distributed to the book trade by St. Martin's Press

2 4 6 8 10 9 7 5 3 1   hardcover
2 4 6 8 10 9 7 5 3   paperback

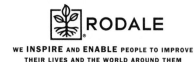

WE **INSPIRE** AND **ENABLE** PEOPLE TO IMPROVE
THEIR LIVES AND THE WORLD AROUND THEM

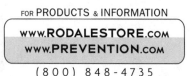

FOR PRODUCTS & INFORMATION

WWW.RODALESTORE.COM
WWW.PREVENTION.COM

(800) 848-4735

About *PREVENTION* Health Books

The editors of *Prevention* Health Books are dedicated to providing you with authoritative, trustworthy, and innovative advice for a healthy, active lifestyle. In all of our books, our goal is to keep you thoroughly informed about the latest breakthroughs in natural healing, medical research, alternative health, herbs, nutrition, fitness, and weight loss. We cut through the confusion of today's conflicting health reports to deliver clear, concise, and definitive health information that you can trust. And we explain in practical terms what each new breakthrough means to you, so you can take immediate, practical steps to improve your health and well-being.

Every recommendation in *Prevention* Health Books is based upon reliable sources, including interviews with qualified health authorities. In addition, we retain top-level health practitioners who serve on the Rodale Books Board of Advisors. *Prevention* Health Books are thoroughly fact-checked for accuracy, and we make every effort to verify recommendations, dosages, and cautions.

The advice in this book will help keep you well-informed about your personal choices in health care—to help you lead a happier, healthier, and longer life.

NOTICE

Allergy Free Naturally Staff

EDITOR: Roslyn Siegel

WRITERS: Rick Ansorge, Eric Metcalf

CONTRIBUTING WRITERS: Jennifer Bright, Doug Dollemore, Bryon Laursen, David Levine, Wyatt Myers, Jacques Picard

INTERIOR DESIGNERS: Leanne Coppola, Richard Kershner

COVER DESIGNER: Carol Angstadt

PHOTO EDITOR: Robin Hepler

ILLUSTRATOR: Molly Borman-Babich

ASSISTANT RESEARCH MANAGER: Sandra Salera Lloyd

PRIMARY RESEARCH EDITOR: Anita C. Small

RESEARCH EDITOR: Jennifer Bright

LEAD RESEARCHER: Teresa A. Yeykal

EDITORIAL RESEARCHERS: Molly Donaldson Brown, Christine Dreisbach, Jennifer Goldsmith, Carrie Havranek, Lois Guarino Hazel, Janice McLeod, Josh Popichak, Holly Swanson, Rebecca Theodore, Barbara Thomas-Fexa, Lucille Uhlman, Lisa Vroman, Dorothy A. West

DEVELOPMENTAL EDITOR: Amy Fisher Kovalski

SENIOR COPY EDITOR: Karen Neely

COPY EDITOR: Jennifer Kearney Strouse

EDITORIAL PRODUCTION MANAGER: Marilyn Hauptly

LAYOUT DESIGNER: Bethany Bodder

PRODUCT SPECIALIST: Brenda Miller

Rodale Women's Health Books Group

VICE PRESIDENT, EDITORIAL DIRECTOR: Elizabeth Crow

EDITOR-IN-CHIEF: Tammerly Booth

SENIOR PRODUCT MARKETING DIRECTOR: Denyse Corelli-Nuccio

WRITING DIRECTOR: Jack Croft

RESEARCH DIRECTOR: Ann Gossy Yermish

MANAGING EDITOR: Madeleine Adams

ART DIRECTOR: Darlene Schneck

OFFICE STAFF: Julie Kehs Minnix, Catherine E. Strouse

Acknowledgments

We wish to thank the more than 150 experts from various disciplines who contributed to this project. We would especially like to extend our gratitude to the following, who provided in-depth information for certain portions of this book. The book in its entirety does not reflect the opinions of the individual contributors.

Leonard Bielory, M.D., director of the division of allergy and immunology at UMDNJ–New Jersey Medical School in Newark

Renata Engler, M.D., chief of the allergy and immunology department at the Walter Reed Army Medical Center in Washington, D.C.

Marianne Frieri, M.D., Ph.D., professor of medicine and pathology at the State University of New York at Stony Brook and director of the allergy/immunology training program at the Nassau University Medical Center/North Shore University Hospital in East Meadow and Manhasset, New York

Robert Rountree, M.D., a holistic physician in Boulder, Colorado, and co-author of *Immunotics*

CONTENTS

Introduction xi

Part One: The Allergy Epidemic

The Emerging Allergic Majority 3
The Case for a New, Self-Help Approach to Allergies 12
The Conventional View of Allergies 14
The Conventional Approach to Diagnosing and
    Treating Allergies 24
The Environmental-Medicine View of Allergies 33
The Alternative View of Allergies 47
Finding the Best Treatment 56

Part Two: The Allergy-Free Environment

Outwit Allergy Triggers Wherever You Are 71
The Allergy-Free Home 73
The Allergy-Free Yard 98
The Allergy-Free Workplace 111
Allergy-Free Travel 122

Part Three: The Allergy-Free Lifestyle

Learn How to Lower Your Allergic Response 133
The Allergy-Free Diet 135
The Allergy-Free Supplementation Schedule 149
The Allergy-Free Exercise Plan 159
Allergy-Free Stress Busters 173
The Allergy-Free Child 185

Part Four: Allergy-Free Action Plans

Are You Allergic? (quiz) 207
Learn to Dodge Allergic Woes from Head to Toes 209
Anaphylaxis 211
Asthma 222
Drug Allergies 261

Dust Mites, Roaches, and Other Insect Allergies 268
Food Allergies and Intolerances 278
Hay Fever 307
Latex Allergy. 327
Mold Allergy 340
Nickel Allergy 349
Pet Allergy 356
Physical Allergy 367
Poison Plant Allergy. 373
Sinusitis 381
Stinging and Biting Insect Allergies. 393

**Part Five: Common Allergic Symptoms:
Causes and Treatments**

Symptom Solvers 405
Symptom Solver: Skin Problems 411
Symptom Solver: Eye Problems. 426
Symptom Solver: Ear Problems 434

Part Six: The Hidden Allergy Connection

Unearth the Causes of Some Mysterious Conditions 443
Attention-Deficit Hyperactivity Disorder 445
Candidiasis 450
Chronic Fatigue Syndrome 456
Depression. 465
Headaches. 468
Inflammatory Bowel Disease. 475
Multiple Chemical Sensitivity 480

Resource Guide 497

**Guidelines for Safe Use of Herbs, Essential Oils,
    and Supplements** 501

Index 509

INTRODUCTION

WE ARE PROUD to bring you the very best, most comprehensive book on preventing and treating your allergies that exists anywhere.

We know how much you need help with the sneezing, wheezing, runny noses, teary eyes, stuffed-up ears, stomachaches, rashes, and all the other unpleasant symptoms that drive you nuts. We know, because many of the writers, editors, and doctors who worked on this book have allergies, too. In fact, so many people have allergies that doctors call it "The Silent Epidemic." A new survey conducted by the American College of Allergy, Asthma, and Immunology has found that an estimated 100 million Americans suffer from allergies. That's 36 percent of the population, and the estimate of people with undiagnosed allergies is much higher. Many people are still unaware that their symptoms, from headache to fatigue, could be traced to an allergic trigger. The bad news is that there are hidden causes of allergies lurking everywhere. The good news is that once the triggers are identified, most people who have allergies can improve the quality of their lives enormously.

We promise that this book will help you feel better. For the past 2 years, we have studied hundreds of scientific papers and consulted more than 150 doctors—conventional, environmental, and alternative—to bring you scientifically valid information and potential treatment options. Within the covers of this book you will find crucial information on a surprising number of hidden allergic triggers that you can now easily avoid. You'll read about dozens of simple lifestyle strategies and avoidance tactics that can help prevent symptoms. You'll discover hundreds of gentle nondrug, alternative techniques that may help you cut down on your conventional medications (look for the 🌿 denoting "natural"), and you'll find self-treatment plans for dozens of different allergic conditions, because if you have one allergy, there's a good chance you have others. You'll be armed with a unique series of Symptom Solver charts to track down your triggers. And you'll be provided with the latest scientific information to empower you to make informed choices when you discuss action plans with your doctor. But best of all, you will find immediate, safe relief from many of your allergic symptoms for a greatly improved quality of life.

—Rick Ansorge, Eric Metcalf, and the Editors of *Prevention* Health Books

PART ONE

The Allergy EPIDEMIC

The
Emerging Allergic
MAJORITY

AFTER THE FALL of the Berlin Wall, researchers from the Robert Koch Institute in Berlin saw a golden opportunity to study the effects of lifestyle on allergies. Reunited Germany made an ideal laboratory.

Since World War II, the country had been divided into capitalist West Germany and communist East Germany. For 45 years, Cold War tensions, concrete walls, and barbed-wire fences kept the two Germanys apart. Essentially, the West Germans and East Germans were one people living on separate and unequal planets.

Thanks to their postwar "economic miracle," West Germans enjoyed one of the world's highest standards of living. Many lived in luxurious homes, cruised the autobahn in gleaming Mercedes-Benzes, and ate whatever they pleased.

Not all was perfect in this capitalist utopia, however. Universal car ownership polluted the atmosphere with excessive levels of nitrogen dioxide. In fact, the West German government's indifference to environmental concerns gave rise to a new political party, the Greens.

Still, living conditions were far worse in East Germany. Intent on industrialization, the nation's communist rulers ignored the nation's infrastructure, allowing roads, railways, and buildings to deteriorate. Living standards were abysmally low, with housing and consumer goods in extremely short supply. The typical East German had to wait years in order to buy a shoddily built East German automobile.

In this low-rent "workers' paradise," environmental protection was an oxymoron. Industrial areas were plagued with excessively high levels of air pollution, especially sulfur dioxide and particulate matter.

Growing citizen discontent led to the fall of the Berlin Wall in 1989 and the reunification of Germany in 1990.

From 1991 to 1992, the Robert Koch Institute tested more than 5,300 West Germans and more than 2,600 former East Germans for allergies. Guess which ones were most likely to be sneezing and wheezing? Those from the impoverished, polluted East?

Nope.

Researchers found that allergies were far more common among Germans from the affluent West, especially those who were born after World War II. In fact, West German baby boomers were up to 83 percent more likely than their East German counterparts to have allergic rhinitis (also known as hay fever) and asthma. Since no such differences in allergy rates were found in Germans born *before* World War II, researchers suspected that West Germany's postwar lifestyle had somehow sensitized its children to pollen, mold, dust mites, and other types of allergens.

Why should we care about a bunch of wheezy West German baby boomers?

Because as goes West Germany, so goes the Western world.

The incidence of allergy and asthma has been rising in every country in the Western world since about 1980.

Most alarming is the increase in asthma. In the United States alone, more than 15 million people, including 5 million children, have this life-threatening disease. Each year, asthma accounts for nearly 2 million emergency room visits, 500,000 hospitalizations, and more than 5,000 deaths.

The annual cost to American society: a staggering $4.5 billion.

Although experts can't agree on the exact causes behind the epidemic, this much seems clear: We're literally choking to death on our own abundance.

The High Cost of the Good Life

Is giving up our worldly goods, heading for the hills, and taking up subsistence farming our only hope of beating allergies?

Not at all. As the German study suggests, the allergy epidemic isn't caused by factors that are beyond our control, such as air pollution. If pollution were the culprit, then asthma would have run rampant in East Germany.

Nor is the allergy epidemic some kind of genetic curse. Until recently, most experts believed that allergy resulted from having the wrong parents. If you have allergies, you probably already know the score. If both of your parents have allergies, your odds of developing them are 40 to 60 percent. If one of your parents has allergies, your odds are 20 to 40 percent.

If allergies were solely dependent on genetics, though, countries as homogeneous as East and West Germany would have nearly identical allergy rates. "Genetic differences cannot explain the increased allergies in the West compared to the former East Germany," the German researchers say.

"This implies that environmental exposure or living conditions (lifestyle) are factors causing the differences in sensitization rates in East and West Germany."

Throughout the world, examples of the "German paradox" abound. In Great Britain, high social class is associated with higher rates of eczema. In the Zimbabwean capital of Harare, the wealthiest residents have the highest rates of asthma. In Asia, allergies are more common in Japan than in China.

"These are people who are of common genetic descent," says Donald Leung, M.D., head of pediatric allergy and immunology at the National Jewish Medical and Research Center in Denver and editor of the *Journal of Allergy and Clinical Immunology*. "Although heredity is very important, the environment has become even more important in the rise of allergies."

If Dr. Leung is right, that opens up a world of possibilities. For if allergies are a consequence of the Western lifestyle, we should be able to reduce or even eliminate our allergy symptoms by changing our lifestyle. We should be able to lead the "good" life with a clear conscience—and clearer sinuses, lungs, and skin.

Indeed, the wide disparity in allergy rates from country to country is forcing even the most conservative doctors to rethink their stand on the nature-versus-nurture debate. In a world of haves and have-nots, the haves definitely have more allergies—up to 15 times more.

When researchers from the International Study of Asthma and Allergies asked 13- and 14-year-olds if they had experienced asthma symptoms during the previous year, positive responses ranged from 29 to 32.2 percent in such countries as Australia, New Zealand, the Republic of Ireland, and the United Kingdom, to only 2.1 to 4.4 percent in such countries as Russia, China, Indonesia, and Greece.

As further proof of the role of the Western lifestyle in increasing allergy rates, experts point out that the Western-born children of parents from developing countries are just as likely to develop allergies as Western kids.

In the United States, which practically invented the Western lifestyle, the allergy rate is spinning out of control. A recent study by the American College of Allergy, Asthma, and Immunology shows that approximately 38 percent of Americans have at least one kind of allergy.

That's over 100 million people.

Allergies: The Next Generation

Across the board, allergies are becoming more prevalent. And not just the most common ones either. In addition to increased cases of asthma, allergic rhinitis, eczema, and chronic sinusitis, Americans are developing allergies that were almost unheard of a generation ago, to substances as diverse as latex, nickel, and peanuts.

Since such substances are found in thousands of products, they can be hidden sources of misery to people who don't even suspect they have allergies. Latex proteins, for instance, can be transferred from food handlers' gloves to the foods they serve. Nickel can be found in even the most expensive gold jewelry. And peanuts? They're nearly impossible to avoid. Have you ever seen a food label that reads: "May or may not contain peanuts"?

That's because the food-processing industry uses peanuts and may not be aware if its equipment is contaminated with peanut residue, according to Marianne Frieri, M.D., professor of medicine and pathology at the State University of New York at Stony Brook and director of the allergy/immunology training program at Nassau University Medical Center/North Shore University Hospital in East Meadow and Manhasset, New York.

Add to this the millions of Americans who have become sensitive to things such as chemicals, cosmetics, smoke, and pollutants—in some cases so sensitive that they've chosen to live in porcelain-lined trailers—and you have the makings of an "allergic majority."

If the allergy epidemic continues unabated, more than 50 percent of Americans will soon have some kind of allergy or sensitivity. The cost of treating these conditions will make today's $18-billion-a-year tab seem like, well, peanuts.

The Environmental Factors behind Increasing Allergy Rates

Our immune systems aren't supposed to be hypersensitive. They're supposed to behave like smart bombs, destroying hostile invaders such as viruses, bacteria, and parasites. But Western immune systems are more like dumb bombs. They've become so oversensitized that they explode in the presence of such seemingly benign substances as pollen grains, mold spores, animal dander, and food.

Let's look at some of the environmental factors that might be responsible for all this mayhem.

Outdoor pollution. First, let's clear up a common misperception. As noxious as air pollution is, it doesn't cause allergies. "No one is allergic to ozone," confirms Gary Gross, M.D., an allergist and clinical professor of medicine at Southwestern Medical School in Dallas.

Another common misperception is that air pollution is getting worse. "Air quality has actually been improving in both the United States and Europe during the last two decades," says Harold Nelson, M.D., senior staff physician at the National Jewish Medical and Research Center in Denver.

That said, there's no question that air pollution can set off underlying allergies and make existing allergies worse. "There's some evidence that chronic ozone exposure may be a risk factor for developing asthma," Dr. Nelson adds.

That could be one reason why African-Americans—who tend to live in heavily polluted urban areas—are three times as likely to die of asthma as are other racial groups.

Increasing truck traffic may be contributing to asthma problems, says Robert Nathan, M.D., associate clinical professor of medicine at the University of Colorado Health Sciences Center in Denver and an allergy practitioner in Colorado Springs. Trucks spew diesel exhaust, an irritant that causes airway inflammation. They also scatter tire debris, not just onto the highway but also into the atmosphere. "As latex particles become airborne, they may be triggering an increasing immune response," Dr. Nathan says.

Indoor pollution. Experts say it's no accident that the allergy epidemic began shortly after the oil crisis in the 1970s. Remember the mad rush to make our homes more energy-efficient? In our zeal to defeat OPEC (Organization of the Petroleum Exporting Countries), we insulated and sealed up our homes.

Unfortunately, by sealing out cold air, we inadvertently sealed in a host of allergens and irritants, including mold, dust mites, cockroaches, animal dander, cigarette smoke, wood smoke, and formaldehyde. And let's not forget the fumes emanating from the toxic-waste dumps in our workshops and under our kitchen sinks. Without good ventilation, these bad guys were free to concentrate, circulate, and contaminate.

We even gave them a cushy hideout, right under our feet. Allergy experts now

Over the Barrel

To visualize how lifestyle affects allergies, think of your body as working like a rain barrel, says Steven Bock, M.D., cofounder and codirector of the Rhinebeck Health Center in Rhinebeck, New York, and the Center for Progressive Medicine in Albany and coauthor of *Natural Relief for Your Child's Asthma*.

Your genetic predisposition to allergies is one of the factors that can raise the water in the barrel to a certain level, and then the environment comes into play. Outdoor pollution, indoor pollution, toxic exposure, infections, lack of exercise, a poor diet, the stress of modern living—all of these may elevate the water level in the rain barrel until symptoms are the overflow that are manifested in sneezing and wheezing.

"Allergy can be multifactorial," Dr. Bock says. "The immune system can become hypersensitive and start a cascade of reactivity."

know that wall-to-wall carpeting conceals a multitude of allergens.

By the mid-1980s, rising drug-related crime in some cities was forcing us to flee our parks, streets, and sidewalks and spend even more time in our contaminated homes. In some neighborhoods, opening a window to let in fresh air was tantamount to waving a banner reading "Rob Me." Even in relatively crime-free areas, many of us got caught up in indoor activities such as playing video games, spending time on computers, and increased television watching. As we cocooned with our families and friends, we blissfully thought we were creating an oasis of calm.

At the same time, our homes were getting older and more decrepit. No matter how hard we tried to maintain them, we often fought a losing battle against planned obsolescence.

"The housing in this country was built to last a certain amount of time, around 50 years, let's say," says Jay Portnoy, M.D., chief of allergy, asthma, and immunology at Children's Mercy Hospitals and Clinics in Kansas City, Missouri. "At the end of 50 years, though, people don't leave their homes and build new ones. They just continue to live in them as they fall apart." Many of the homes Dr. Portnoy has inspected in metropolitan Kansas City, Missouri, are so moldy that no amount of remediation can save them. "We'd be better off just tearing them down," he says.

Lack of exercise. Since we're spending so much more time in our homes, is it any wonder we're out of shape?

"The consequences of sitting for 3 or more hours per day—in front of a television, video, or computer—are decreased activity, increased obesity, and increased exposure to indoor allergens," says Thomas Platts-Mills, M.D., an epidemiologist and professor at the University of Virginia in Charlottesville. "Prolonged sitting may also influence lung mechanics and predispose children to asthma."

For people with allergies, a sedentary lifestyle can set in motion a vicious cycle of weight gain and worsening symptoms. The heavier they get, the lousier they feel, and the less likely they are to get up and get moving.

But as tempting as it might be to abandon exercise, it's a self-defeating strategy. Since their cardiovascular systems are already under stress, people with allergies need all the aerobic exercise they can get. "People who are in shape do better," Dr. Portnoy says. "They have more heart-lung capacity, so they can do more before they run into problems."

They also feel better. "Exercise stimulates endorphins, so it always has a modulating effect on the immune system," explains Steven Bock, M.D., cofounder and co-director of the Rhinebeck Health Center in Rhinebeck, New York, and the Center for Progressive Medicine in Albany and coauthor of *Natural Relief for Your Child's Asthma.*

Further, even those people with exercise-induced asthma probably aren't as allergic to exercise as they think. Many are pleasantly surprised to find that swimming burns calories and builds strength in a warm, humid environment that's good for twitchy lungs.

If you need proof, look no further than Olympic swimmer Amy Van Dyken. Despite having asthma, she won four gold medals at the 1996 Summer Games in Atlanta. Then, at the 2000 Olympic Games in Sydney, Australia, she won yet another gold medal with her teammates in the 4 × 100 freestyle relay.

Other notable athletes with asthma include track star Jackie Joyner-Kersee, baseball Hall-of-Famer Jim "Catfish" Hunter, and football player Jerome "The Bus" Bettis.

Poor diet. Our allergy woes often begin with our first swallow of non-mother's milk. Since infant formulas contain such allergens as cow's milk and soy, overreliance on them is strongly associated with childhood allergies and intolerances.

The more you breastfeed, the less likely it is that your children will have allergies. If they do have them, it's possible they'll be less severe.

Even more important is delaying the introduction of foods that can cause a lifetime of misery. Besides cow's milk and soy, the most notorious offenders include wheat, seafood, eggs, and peanuts.

As we get older, life in the fast-food lane makes allergies even worse. Eating fatty foods promotes inflammation, which is the common denominator of allergies and asthma.

Since the typical American diet is high in fat and woefully short of vitamins, minerals, and nutrients, many of us are seemingly robust but seriously undernourished. Fatty foods will promote inflammation and possibly cause asthma flare-ups. A more recent diagnosis on the allergy scene is termed *leaky-gut syndrome.* Some doctors say this occurs when allergies to food and other substances in the gastrointestinal tract create irritation, inflammation, and permeability of the intestinal wall, allowing certain molecules to pass through the wall and sensitize the immune system.

When you add in stress—which depletes the body of its natural allergy-fighting hormones, epinephrine and cortisone—you have the perfect recipe for an allergic assault.

The hygiene hypothesis. In recent years, experts have theorized that we've become more susceptible to allergies because we're too squeaky clean. Compared to people in developing countries, we're far more likely to sanitize our homes and offices with antiseptics. We're also more likely to sanitize ourselves with antibiotics, including the broad-spectrum varieties that were introduced around 1960.

"It may be that our immune systems are not being exposed to as many infectious diseases, so they respond to outside exposures in an abnormal 'allergic' manner," Dr. Portnoy says.

The German researchers found that most West German preschoolers stayed at home, so they had little contact with other children and little exposure to routine childhood respiratory infections. Most East German preschoolers, by contrast, attended day care, so they got their full quota of daily germs.

According to proponents of the hygiene hypothesis, young children need certain challenges in order for their immune systems to develop normally. "The unifying theme is probably bacterial stimulation," Dr. Nelson says. "That's why early antibiotics are bad."

While no one is suggesting that we ought to live like our long-ago ancestors, in conditions of filth and squalor, the message is clear: Maybe we've become *too* obsessed with cleanliness.

The Next Step in Allergy Treatment

If you belong to the emerging allergic majority, you might believe that life isn't even worth living without Benadryl.

Not so. The picture isn't nearly as grim as it seems.

In recent years, there has been an explosion of research done on allergies. More treatment options—conventional, alternative, and self-care—are available than ever before. So stop thinking of yourself as a hapless victim of circumstance who picked the wrong parents. There's much you can do *on your own* to reverse the curse.

Sometimes, even a minor lifestyle adjustment is enough. It can be as simple as buying the right cover for your pillow. For less than $10, you'll get 3 years of protection from house dust.

More often than not, though, managing allergies isn't simple. If you have allergies, you know just how difficult it can be simply to *identify* the source of your misery, let alone determine your best treatment options.

In succeeding chapters, we'll help you take the guesswork out of this process. First, you'll learn to go after your allergies like a dogged detective. You'll become adept at identifying both the usual and the more unusual suspects, and become familiar with all of their hideouts.

As we take you "undercover" to show you what's behind your allergies, you'll learn the many ways that "covert" substances can make you sick. Once you understand these hidden connections, you can take steps to either banish these substances from your life or, if that's not possible, find the path to peaceful coexistence.

Since we favor a natural, nondrug approach, we'll show you how to allergy-proof your home as well as yourself. Our detailed Action Plans for the most common allergic conditions will show you hundreds of natural self-help strategies that will put an end to your sneezing and wheezing.

If these chapters don't provide enough clues to get to the bottom of your allergies, we've also included chapters about unusual conditions that might be allergy-related.

Since allergies can be serious, and even life-threatening, we realize that a strictly natural approach isn't always advisable. So if the best option for a certain condition is conventional medical care, we'll say so. Even then, however, we'll show you how natural strategies in the areas of diet, exercise, and self-help can reduce your dependence on conventional drugs.

Our goal is to transform you into an allergy sleuth and an allergy enforcer.

Keep reading to see how you can become allergy-free naturally.

The Case for a New,
Self-Help Approach to
ALLERGIES

WITH A WAVE of his staff, King Menes of Egypt could command mighty armies and force thousands of people to build pyramids—without even thinking to offer them a decent health insurance plan. But in the end, Menes was brought down by a bug.

After being stung by a wasp in 2641 B.C., he collapsed and died. His demise was recorded on a wall painting in his tomb, which shows him all dressed up in his mummy suit and ready to go to the hereafter. In the painting's foreground is his nemesis—the wasp. Apparently, it would have been impolitic of the painter to show the wasp's true size, so he enlarged it to roughly the size of a Rottweiler.

Since this is history's first account of a fatal allergic reaction, it's appropriate that the wasp is larger than life. If you have allergies, the sources of your misery probably loom large in your mind, too.

If you have hay fever, you might think of pollen grains as fiery projectiles that make your nose red and your eyes burn.

If you have asthma, you might think of mold spores as voracious blobs that absorb all of the air in your lungs.

If you have dust mite allergy, you don't have to resort to any such flights of fancy. All you have to do is look at a blown-up photograph of a dust mite to know that you're messing with a monster that makes Godzilla look like a gecko lizard.

But you don't need anyone to tell you that allergies are the bane of your existence. Even when they don't threaten your life, they usually threaten your life*style*, affecting everything from your work and play to your sex life.

Still, count yourself lucky that you live in 21st-century America, for you have more allergy-fighting options than anyone in history. You can choose from among the following approaches.

• Conventional medicine, which offers environmental control, drugs, and allergy shots

• Environmental medicine, which focuses on environmental control and its own forms of allergy shots

• Alternative medicine, which recommends herbs and mind-body therapies

If Menes were alive today, he'd probably get some form of professional care, but he'd probably also practice aggressive self-help. After all, if there's one thing that unites conventional, environmental, and alternative medicine, it's the conviction that patients need to take charge of their allergies.

So Menes would know he was allergic to wasps, and he'd learn how to avoid them. At company picnics at the pyramids, he'd always be the guy sitting the farthest away from the garbage cans.

He also might get conventional allergy shots to desensitize himself to wasp venom. This form of therapy is now so effective that doctors have all but declared it a cure for wasp-sting allergy.

When Menes invaded a neighboring country—Canada, say—he'd probably carry a prescription epinephrine injector such as an EpiPen Auto-Injector. That way, if he were stung by a wasp during the Battle of Winnipeg, he'd just stick his thigh with his EpiPen and keep on fighting.

Since he was obviously allergy-prone, he might also have hay fever, asthma, and eczema. Even if he were taking conventional drugs for these conditions, chances are still almost one in four that allergies would cramp his style.

If so, Menes would probably also explore environmental and alternative medicine. That's where he'd find some of the most practical, do-it-yourself advice for controlling his environment and improving his diet. Although he'd certainly keep his EpiPen handy, he'd probably learn dozens of natural, nondrug strategies that could reduce his reliance on other allergy medications and vastly improve his quality of life.

The purpose of this book is to take the best of the three approaches—conventional, environmental, and alternative—and fuse them into a new self-help approach that offers more choices and promises more relief than any one alone.

First, however, we'd like to show you where this approach came from. So in the next chapters, we'll explain the basics of conventional medicine, environmental medicine, and alternative medicine. We'll also explain how each of these disciplines understands, diagnoses, and treats allergies. Finally, drawing from these disparate and often conflicting schools of thought, we'll show how using the best that each has to offer will speed you to your goal: an allergy-free life.

The Conventional
VIEW OF ALLERGIES

SINCE ANCIENT TIMES, doctors have known that supposedly harmless substances can cause serious problems. Among these doctors was Hippocrates, the father of modern medicine. In the 4th century B.C., Hippocrates noted that milk gave some people hives and that shellfish sent some people into shock.

Since ancient and medieval doctors had more pressing concerns, such as the Black Death, they didn't give these reactions much thought. For centuries, such reactions were filed under the heading of "medical curiosities."

That changed in the late 18th century, during the Industrial Revolution. As Western countries switched from a farm-based to a factory-based economy, there was a sudden surge of people reacting to pollen, mold, dust mites, animal dander, and the ominous brown clouds that enveloped industrial centers.

Doctors knew an epidemic when they saw one. They also knew that a nebulous term like *hay fever*, which has nothing to do with either hay or fever, couldn't begin to describe what they were observing.

In 1906, Austrian pediatrician Clemens von Pirquet and a colleague, Dr. Bela Schick, were horrified to see that some patients were dropping dead after being immunized against diphtheria. Since most people could easily tolerate the immunizations, they knew these deaths weren't caused by a toxic reaction.

The doctors suspected that another kind of reaction was to blame, one that didn't yet have a name. So they coined one, combining the Greek words *allos* (meaning "other") and *ergon* ("work") into one word—*allergy*—which they defined as "altered reaction." The new term quickly caught on and became a catchall diagnosis for almost any abnormal reaction affecting the eyes, nose, lungs, skin, and gastrointestinal tract.

From the start, scientists suspected that an overactive immune system was to blame for allergies. But they didn't understand how the immune system made people miserable.

One breakthrough came in 1910, when British scientist Sir Henry Dale isolated one of the immune system's worst troublemakers: histamine, a chemical that causes watery eyes, a runny nose, and wheezy breathing. This discovery led to the development of antidotes called antihistamines.

The biggest breakthrough, though, came in 1966 at the Children's Asthma Research Institute in Denver, where husband and wife researchers Kimishige and Teruko Ishizaka discovered the so-called allergy antibody: immunoglobulin E, or IgE.

IgE—which looks like "Iggy" in print but is actually pronounced "I-G-E"—is responsible for many allergic reactions. People with allergies have 10 times as much of it in their bloodstreams as people who are unaffected by allergies.

When IgE comes in contact with an allergen—the scientific name for the foreign substances that cause allergies—it triggers the release of such chemicals as histamine, prostaglandins, and leukotrienes. It's these chemicals, not the allergens themselves, that cause the sneezing, wheezing, and other symptoms that most people recognize as allergy.

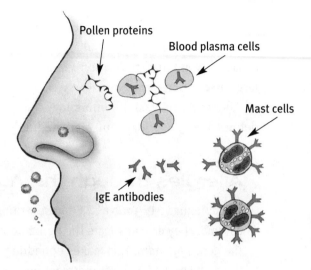

1. When the body first comes into contact with an allergen, such as pollen, blood plasma cells create a type of antibody called IgE.

2. The IgE antibodies then attach themselves to mast cells.

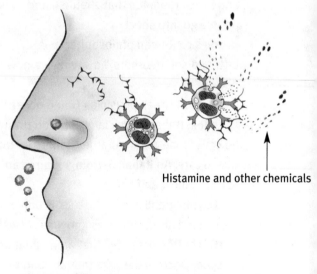

3. When the same type of pollen or other allergen enters the body again, its proteins attach to the waiting IgE.

4. The IgE triggers the mast cells to release chemicals such as histamine, prostaglandins, and leukotrienes. It's these chemicals that cause sneezing, wheezing, and itchy eyes.

Before the discovery of IgE, conventional medicine defined allergy quite broadly. Even today, the nation's largest allergy association—the American Academy of Allergy, Asthma, and Immunology—still defines allergy as a "harmful, increased susceptibility to a specific substance."

For all practical purposes, though, allergy and IgE are now inseparable. "In common usage, an allergic reaction *is* a reaction involving the IgE antibody," says Gary Gross, M.D., an allergist and clinical professor of

Allergies through the Ages

Approximately 3000 B.C.: Chinese writings describe the disease we now know as asthma. They also advocate the herbal remedy ma huang, from the bark of trees of the genus *Ephedra*. This makes ephedrine, a drug still used in some asthma medications, the earliest known treatment for any allergic disease.

2641 B.C.: Egyptian pharaoh Menes dies after being stung by a wasp. A wall painting of a giant wasp menacing Menes is believed to be the first recorded description of a fatal anaphylactic reaction.

400 B.C.: Greek physician Hippocrates observes that milk can cause stomach upset and hives. He notes that shellfish and nuts can cause similar problems or even make people go into shock.

100 B.C.: Roman philosopher/poet Lucretius writes, "What is food to some may be bitter poison to others," a saying we now know as "One man's meat is another man's poison."

A.D. 200: Greek physician Galen observes that poison ivy can cause skin reactions.

1500s: Italian physician Leonardo Botallo describes an asthmalike condition that he calls "rose cold." Another Italian doctor describes a patient who's unusually sensitive to cats. An Italian astrologer cures an archbishop's asthma by taking away his feather pillow and bed.

1819: England's John Bostock is one of the first doctors to describe hay fever, which for a short time was known as "Bostock's summer catarrh."

1860s: Doctors prove that animal dander and pollen can cause allergic reactions.

1900: Doctors theorize that antibodies are somehow responsible for allergic reactions.

1902: Charles Richet and Paul Portier coin the term *anaphylaxis* to describe the most dangerous allergic reactions.

1906: Pediatricians and Bela Schick Clemens von Pirquet coin the term *allergy*.

medicine at Southwestern Medical School in Dallas. So dominant is the IgE definition, in fact, that even alternative-minded doctors—many of whom believe that other antibodies also play a role in allergy—have grudgingly come to accept it.

"The definition of allergy was placed on the IgE mechanism. So if that's allergy and nothing else can be, then we have to call everything else sensitivities," says Charles Hinshaw, M.D., an environmental-medicine doctor in Wichita, Kansas, and past presi-

1910: English scientist Sir Henry Dale identifies histamine, a body chemical responsible for many allergic reactions.

1911–1914: Leonard Noon and John Freeman introduce immunotherapy against hay fever.

1916: Robert Cook and Albert Vanderveer demonstrate the role of heredity in allergic disease.

1920s: Storm van Leeuwen demonstrates the role of environment in allergic disease by removing asthma patients from their homes and watching their symptoms improve.

1937: David Bovet synthesizes the first antihistamine.

1938: One of the first bronchodilators, theophylline, is introduced.

1942: American College of Allergy, Asthma, and Immunology is founded.

1943: American Academy of Allergy, Asthma, and Immunology is founded.

1948: Steroid drugs are first used to control asthma.

1965: Dr. Theron Randolph, who believes that chemicals and foods are responsible for many allergic symptoms, breaks with conventional allergists and forms the Society for Clinical Ecology. The group later changed its name to the American Academy of Environmental Medicine.

1966: Denver-based researchers Kimishige and Teruko Ishizaka discover the allergy antibody: immunoglobulin E, or IgE.

1970s: Inhaled beta$_2$-agonists such as albuterol are introduced for asthma treatment.

1979: Professor Bengt Samuelsson receives the Nobel Prize for identifying leukotrienes, chemicals released by the body during asthma attacks.

1996: The first leukotriene-modifying drug, zafirlukast, is introduced.

2000: The first anti-IgE drug, rhuMAb-E25, is approved by the FDA.

dent of the alternative-minded American Academy of Environmental Medicine.

Some conventional allergists, however, believe that the pendulum may be swinging back. "Some allergists are still really short-sighted in that they look just at IgE," says Jay Portnoy, M.D., chief of allergy, asthma, and immunology at Children's Mercy Hospitals and Clinics in Kansas City, Missouri. "They don't think about other mechanisms. The other mechanisms are there, and they're very important, and we need to spend more resources looking at them."

The Most Common Allergy-Related Conditions

Conventional allergists treat conditions that are universally accepted as either allergies or allergy-related. Major ones include:

Allergic rhinitis. An estimated 40 million Americans have this upper respiratory disease, which is also known as hay fever. It's often associated with asthma and otitis media (see below). It not only causes itchy eyes and a runny nose but also may contribute to sleep disorders and temporary deafness.

Asthma. This serious lung disease strikes more than 15 million Americans, 78 percent of whom also have nasal symptoms. Severity ranges from mild to life-threatening. More than 5,000 Americans die each year of asthma.

Rhinosinusitis. This inflammatory disease of the sinuses affects 14.7 percent of the population. It commonly occurs with rhinitis and asthma, so it's sometimes called asthma of the sinuses. Doctors believe it must be treated first to get asthma under control.

The Atopic March

Although allergy can strike at any age, most frequently it begins in infancy or early childhood. The first sign of trouble is often a food allergy, usually to cow's milk. Such children often go on to develop eczema, allergic rhinitis, and asthma. This is known as the atopic march.

Some of the children who wheeze during their preschool and kindergarten years will eventually "outgrow" their asthma. Others, especially if they have a family history of allergies, may continue to have respiratory problems. Unfortunately, about 40 percent of them will develop asthma again later in their lives.

Since untreated lung inflammation can cause permanent damage, conventional allergists believe it's essential to start children on an aggressive regimen that often includes antihistamines and inhaled or nasal corticosteroids.

Eczema. Also known as atopic dermatitis, this itchy skin disease afflicts 10 to 15 percent of children and 3 percent of the general population.

Otitis media. This inflammation of the middle ear is often associated with allergic rhinitis. It's the most common childhood disease requiring physician care.

Food reactions. Unlike alternative practitioners, conventional allergists don't believe that food allergies are responsible for scores of physical and mental problems. But they've changed their thinking on prevalence. They now believe food allergies affect as many as 2.5 percent of adults, and they recognize them as the second leading cause of anaphylactic shock, the most serious allergic reaction.

Anaphylactic shock. This condition can attack the entire body, causing swelling of body tissues (including those in the throat), vomiting, cramps, and a sudden drop in blood pressure. It often occurs in persons who are particularly sensitive to penicillin, stinging insects, and shellfish or nuts.

Conventional allergists also treat many other conditions, including bronchitis, conjunctivitis, drug allergy, dust mite allergy, exercise-induced asthma, hives (urticaria) and swelling (angioedema), insect bite/sting allergy, latex allergy, mastocytosis, mold allergy, nickel allergy, pet allergy, poison plant allergy, and rodent allergy.

The Ins and Outs of Allergens

If you have allergies, you might think of pollen, mold, and other allergens as your mortal enemies. There's no question that they're invaders. They get into your body any way they can, usually through your respiratory or gastrointestinal tract, but also sometimes through your skin.

Surprisingly, then, allergens are relatively few in number. Out of the vast variety of substances we inhale, eat, and touch every day, only a handful are associated with allergies. Most of them are just tiny specks of protein that can easily penetrate mucous membranes. Cat dander, for instance, is a mixture of dried saliva and skin flakes that can stay airborne for as long as 6 months after you've removed a cat from your house.

Unlike viruses and bacteria, however, these little specks aren't intent on making you sick. They just happen to be floating on the breeze in search of a friendly landing strip, and you just happen to make a pretty good airport.

If you don't have allergies, these accidental tourists won't give you any grief. They simply camp out in your mucous membranes until your body's janitorial antibodies uneventfully sweep them away.

If you do have allergies, though, your body's reaction to them is anything but uneventful.

Remember from your history books how World War I got started? A lone terrorist as-

The 10 Most Wanted Allergy Triggers

According to a survey conducted by the Marist Institute for Public Opinion in Poughkeepsie, New York, 36 percent of Americans have allergies. Here's what the respondents identified as the worst allergy triggers.

- Pollen grains: 27 percent
- Drugs and medications: 19 percent
- House dust/dust mites: 17 percent
- Mold: 15 percent
- Chemical fumes and gases: 12 percent
- Indoor air pollution: 12 percent
- Perfumes: 12 percent
- Animals: 11 percent
- Foods: 10 percent
- Stinging insects: 10 percent

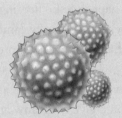
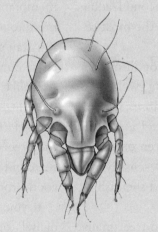
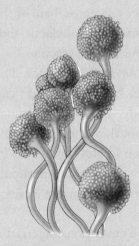

Pollen grains can be found anywhere there are trees, grasses, or weeds. They are the culprits in numerous hay fever and asthma attacks.

A relative of the spider measuring just $\frac{1}{100}$ of an inch long, dust mites consume sloughed-off human skin. Their feces can trigger asthma attacks. They're abundant in mattresses, pillows, down comforters, carpets, and Oriental rugs.

Mold is a primitive plant that releases allergenic spores and can cause hay fever, asthma, and even toxic reactions. Its hiding spots include carpets, books, bedding, foam rubber, houseplants, and in and under refrigerators.

sassinated an Austrian nobleman, prompting the Great Powers to freak out and declare war on each other. The terrorist wasn't responsible for causing the war, only for triggering it.

Your allergies follow exactly the same pattern. A foreign substance tickles your mucous membranes, prompting another Great Power—your immune system—to freak out and declare war on you. The allergen isn't actually responsible for the war, only for triggering it. This is an important distinction to make, because once you understand that the real troublemaker is your own overactive immune system, you can take steps to tame it and, in so doing, ease your allergies.

Why does the immune system overreact? Theories abound, but one of the most intriguing ones is that the immune system originally unleashed IgE antibodies to attack intestinal worms and insect larvae. Since such internal parasites no longer exist in most Western countries, it's believed that the IgE antibodies attack allergens because they have nothing better to do.

Allergy Risk Factors

Conventional allergists once thought of allergy as an accident of birth. They believed that if one or both of your parents slipped you some "allergic" genes, it was like drawing the Monopoly card that says, "Go directly to jail." You were doomed by heredity to spend the rest of your life in a kind of allergic prison.

If your parents didn't give you those genes, you were home-free. You got to pass "Go" and collect $200 that you otherwise would have spent on facial tissues.

As the incidence of allergies started rising in the 1970s, that theory crumbled. Genetics alone could no longer explain the spectacular increases in allergic rhinitis, asthma, and other allergic conditions.

Today, researchers believe that in addition to genetics, the environment also plays a critical role in determining who will and who won't develop allergies. Since allergies are strongly associated with the Western lifestyle, researchers have begun to suspect that a multitude of lifestyle factors are involved.

Although scientists haven't yet found all the pieces to the puzzle, their message is empowering. For if allergy is even partly a consequence of making the wrong lifestyle choices, then it should be possible to reduce or even eliminate allergic woes by making the right lifestyle choices.

"You can't change an inherited predisposition to allergy, but you can adjust your lifestyle and modify your environment to influence immunity in the right direction," says Andrew Weil, M.D., director of the program in integrative medicine and clinical professor of medicine at the University of Arizona College of Medicine in Tucson. "Allergy is a learned response of the immune system, and anything learned by this system can be unlearned."

Here's a brief description of how genetics, environment, and lifestyle place you at risk for developing allergies.

• Genetics

Interleukin-4 is one of the key proteins that play an essential role in allergic reactions.

It increases production of the IgE antibody, which is what makes you sick. Scientists theorize that high occurrences of a gene that promotes interleukin-4 production may be the reason why African-Americans have higher rates of allergies and asthma. Studies show that African-Americans have very high levels of interleukin-4, probably because their ancestors needed it to fight off tropical parasites. Since the immune system is not happy unless it has something to fight, it's possible that African-Americans' immune systems have switched targets from harmful parasites to harmless allergens.

• Environment

Over and over again, researchers have found that people of similar racial backgrounds have radically different rates of allergy if they live in different environments.

For the most part, the world's "haves" have much greater incidences of allergy than the "have-nots." The pattern holds true in Asia, where the urbanized Japanese are more allergic than the rural Chinese. It also holds true in Africa, where metropolitan residents are more allergic than people living in the countryside.

One of the most telling studies was conducted immediately after East and West Germany were reunified. It found that affluent West Germans were far more allergic than their relatively impoverished East German counterparts. This study blew the lid off the theory that industrial pollution—which was notoriously high in the former East Germany—was responsible for the allergy epidemic.

"I'm sure their original hypothesis was that they'd find more asthma in East Germany than in West," says Harold Nelson, M.D., senior staff physician at the National Jewish Medical and Research Center in Denver. "Everybody wants to blame air pollution for the increase in asthma."

It simply isn't so. Although there's strong evidence that indoor tobacco smoke increases children's risk of developing asthma, there's little proof that such outdoor pollutants as sulfur dioxide, particulate matter, and ozone increase anybody's risk of developing allergies.

There is a strong association, however, between allergies and other environmental factors, such as socioeconomic status, family size, early-childhood infections, and diet. Exactly how these factors combine with heredity to produce allergy is an area that still needs more research.

If you have any doubt that environment is a driving force in allergy, consider what happened in the former East Germany within 10 years of reunification with West Germany. As billions of marks were spent bringing the one-time socialist state into the capitalist fold, living standards in the East rose dramatically. But so, regrettably, did its allergy woes.

Today, all of Germany is plagued with shockingly high allergy rates.

• Lifestyle

When scientists first identified allergy as a disease of Western living, they thought the explanation was simple: Western homes have more of everything, including indoor pollution, pets, and processed foods.

"We first thought that the increasing prevalence of asthma was related to the decreasing quality of the indoor environment because of increased insulation, warmer homes, tighter homes, more moisture, and all that," Dr. Nelson says. "There's no question that indoor air quality of homes has deteriorated with Westernization. Everybody thought that was the whole answer. Then we started seeing situations where it didn't fit."

As proof, Dr. Nelson cites European studies showing that infants exposed to dogs or cats at home have only half as many allergies as children coming from petless homes. "That's where the hygiene hypothesis comes in," he says.

The hygiene hypothesis states that our oversanitized Western lifestyle keeps our immune systems confused, off balance, and unable to distinguish friend from foe. Researchers believe that much of this confusion begins in infancy. Increasing evidence shows that a baby's immature immune system can't develop properly unless it's exposed to such things as the bacteria found in fermented foods. "You want the right stimulus down in your gut when you're an infant," Dr. Nelson says.

Early exposure to antibiotics, however, seems to create the wrong stimulus by disrupting the balance of friendly and unfriendly bacteria. The result is an increased risk of allergy.

The challenge facing scientists in the 21st century is to figure out just how the oversanitized Western lifestyle, genetics, and environment combine to create allergy. But since two of these three factors are controllable, there's great hope that one day a life interrupted by allergies will be a thing of the past.

The Conventional Approach to Diagnosing and Treating ALLERGIES

THE LAST TIME you were sneezing, wheezing, and generally feeling miserable because of your allergies, did you think, "There ought to be a vaccine for this!"? Well, for some allergies, there is. Though it's not a one-time-and-you're-cured sort of thing, allergy vaccination—or allergen immunotherapy—can be effective for such things as allergic rhinitis (also known as hay fever) and allergies to certain stinging insects.

Allergen immunotherapy is just one strategy in the three-pronged approach used by conventional-medicine doctors to treat allergies. Read on to learn more about this approach—and how conventional medicine diagnoses allergies in the first place.

How Are Allergies Diagnosed?

If you suspect that you have allergies and you visit a conventional allergist, the first thing you'll probably be asked to do is to sit down and chat. That's because the first step a conventional allergist usually takes to determine whether or not people have allergies is to take their history.

Your doctor will ask you about such things as regular coughing, noisy breathing, poor sleeping, and exercise intolerance. He also will look for such clues as dark circles under your eyes, skin rashes, and a runny nose. It's important to know when and how the symptoms developed and if they're associated with certain seasons, damp weather, physical activity, and diet.

The doctor will want to know about your occupation, hobbies, and personal habits, such as smoking. He will inquire about your home environment and whether or not you have fitted carpets and indoor pets, among other allergen havens.

You might also be asked about your use of cosmetics. A favorite cologne or perfume can be the cause of nasal symptoms, while a soap may be the cause of chronic eczema.

For some people, history alone may be enough to make a diagnosis. "The easiest patients to diagnose are those who have symptoms only during specific seasons and have had them for several years in a row," says Robert Nathan, M.D., associate clinical professor of medicine at the University of Colorado Health Sciences Center in Denver and an allergy practitioner in Colorado Springs. "The only thing that causes seasonal symptoms year after year are pollen allergies."

If your doctor suspects that you have allergies, the next step will be to use any of a number of conventional testing methods to determine which allergens cause your body to react and which do not. After all, if you don't know what substances you're allergic to, you can't take the proper steps to avoid them.

Because allergies can be extremely difficult to identify, patients aren't always the best judges of what's bugging them. For example, when Mayo Clinic researchers asked 100 patients to predict which substances they were allergic to before getting a skin test, most of them flunked. Eighty-eight percent of them incorrectly guessed they were allergic to mold, and more than 70 percent of them incorrectly guessed they were allergic to dust mites and tree, grass, and weed pollen. The message is clear: Get tested, even if you're "sure" that you know your enemy.

Here are the tests most commonly used by conventional allergists.

Skin tests. Drops of suspected allergens are either placed onto or injected into your skin. If you're allergic to the substance, a round wheal or flare will form on your skin after 15 to 20 minutes.

Blood tests. These tests measure either the total amount of immunoglobulin E, or IgE, in your bloodstream or the IgE that's specific to certain allergens, such as ragweed pollen. When IgE comes in contact with an allergen, it releases chemicals such as histamine, prostaglandins, and leukotrienes. These chemicals cause the symptoms of allergies.

Pulmonary function tests. To measure your airflow, you blow into a device called a spirometer. Then a reading is taken. If asthma is suspected, you are given a bronchodilator and are then tested again. If your airflow improves, it's a good indication that asthma is present.

Patch tests. A piece of blotting paper is soaked with the suspected allergen, then it is taped to your skin for 24 to 48 hours. If a rash develops on the site, it's a sign of eczema.

Provocation tests. Performed only if specific allergy testing is not available, these tests require you to inhale or swallow a very small amount of the suspected allergen so that your reaction to it can be observed. Because of the risk of serious reactions, these tests must be done only under a doctor's supervision.

How Are Allergies Treated?

Conventional allergists rely on three major forms of treatment: avoidance, drugs, and allergy shots (allergen immunotherapy).

As conventional doctors go, allergists are relatively holistic. "Allergists treat allergy as a systemic disease: one body, one disease," says Donald Leung, M.D., head of pediatric allergy and immunology at the National Jewish Medical and Research Center in Denver and editor of the *Journal of Allergy and Clinical Immunology*. "The allergist looks at the environment of the individual and asks about things that trigger symptoms."

Yet unlike holistic doctors, who often customize a treatment plan to the specific patient, allergists are not inclined to experiment with individualized treatments. Since they believe in treatments that have repeatedly proven successful in large-scale studies, they unabashedly favor more of an evidence-based, cookie-cutter approach.

When to See an Allergist

Although you can use the natural self-help strategies in this book for most allergies, there are certain conditions that are best treated by an allergist. You should see an allergist if:

- Your asthma or allergies are interfering with your ability to carry on day-to-day activities.
- You are experiencing warning signs of asthma, such as having to struggle to catch your breath; wheezing or coughing often, especially at night or after exercise; or being frequently short of breath or feeling tightness in your chest.
- You have been previously diagnosed with asthma, but despite treatment you have frequent acute asthma attacks.
- Your allergies are causing secondary symptoms such as chronic sinus infections, nasal congestion, or difficulty breathing.
- You experience allergic rhinitis (hay fever) or other allergy symptoms several months of the year.
- Antihistamines and other over-the-counter medications do not control your allergy symptoms, or they create unacceptable side effects, such as drowsiness.
- You cough up mucus that is gray, yellow, green, brown, or bloody.
- You cough up mucus as small strings or plugs. (This is a sign that it's overstayed its welcome in your airways.)
- You have persistent sinus pain or chronic postnasal drip.

"I'm a big fan of cookbook medicine," says Jay Portnoy, M.D., chief of allergy, asthma, and immunology at Children's Mercy Hospitals and Clinics in Kansas City, Missouri. "In our clinic, all patients are treated exactly the same way. If you treat every patient differently, ad hoc, then you can't measure outcomes because you don't know what procedure the outcome is measuring."

Most of the time, conventional strategies work. "Allergies and asthma are very con-trollable diseases, and people with them should be able to live normal lives," says Martha White, M.D., director of research at the Institute for Asthma and Allergy in Washington, D.C. "They should not have symptoms all that often if they're under good care."

As with any chronic disease, however, there are intractable cases. When symptoms show no sign of abating, doctors often prescribe oral steroids in addition to the asthma medicine. Unfortunately, these multiple

(continued on page 30)

- You experience persistent headaches.
- Your eyes are constantly itchy, you have red eyes without itching, or your eyes have any kind of discharge.
- You experience ear pain or hearing loss.
- You have eczema that becomes thick or scaly.
- You have an itchy rash on your eyelids that doesn't respond to antihistamines.
- You get a rash after using a new drug. Some prime offenders are penicillin and sulfa drugs.
- You notice a rash that seems to be caused by eating certain foods.

Note: If you have chronic conditions such as emphysema, diabetes, heart disease, or kidney disease, don't treat yourself with over-the-counter allergy remedies. They could adversely interact with your prescription medications.

In addition, be aware that hives normally disappear within 6 to 10 hours, so you should see your doctor if you develop a case of hives that lasts longer than several days.

Also note that hives can be the first sign of anaphylaxis, which is a medical emergency. Get help immediately if hives appear suddenly and are associated with rapid swelling of the throat, tongue, lips, or fingers and an overall feeling of sickness.

Finally, schedule an appointment with your pediatrician if your infant or toddler develops a rash. So-called diaper rash can be a sign of milk allergy.

The Pros and Cons of Allergy Drugs

There are numerous allergy drugs on the market that are effective at relieving symptoms. Unfortunately, as with most drugs, many of these allergy medications have side effects. Below is a list of the specific benefits and drawbacks of the most commonly used allergy drugs.

Class of Allergy Drug	Example of Drug	Benefits
Antihistamines	Diphenhydramine (Benadryl)	Relieve sneezing and itching in the nose, throat, and eyes; reduce nasal swelling and drainage
Anti-inflammatory inhalants	Cromolyn (Intal)	Reduces inflammation in the airways
Bronchodilators	Theophylline (Asmalix)	Long-acting bronchodilators prevent asthma attacks; short-acting "rescue" bronchodilators relieve them by opening up the bronchial tubes so more air can flow through.
Decongestants	Pseudoephedrine and ibuprofen (Advil Cold and Sinus)	Relieve nasal congestion by shrinking blood vessels, which decreases the amount of fluid that leaks out
Inhaled corticosteroids	Flunisolide (AeroBid)	Decrease airway swelling in the bronchial tubes, reduce mucus production by the cells lining the bronchial tubes, and decrease the chain of overreaction in the airways
Leukotriene modifiers	Zafirlukast (Accolate)	Leukotrienes are body chemicals that cause contraction of the smooth muscle in the airway, leakage of fluid from blood vessels in the lung, and inflammation. Anti-leukotriene medications neutralize these inflammatory chemicals.
Oral corticosteroids	Prednisolone (Prelone)	Relieve severe asthma that won't respond to any other treatment
Topical nasal steroids	Fluticasone (Cutivate)	Relieve allergic rhinitis by reducing the number of mast cells in the nose, mucus secretion, and nasal swelling (often used in combination with antihistamines)

Drawbacks

Over-the-counter antihistamines cause drowsiness. So-called nonsedating antihistamines may actually be sedating if taken with certain drugs. Be sure to tell your doctor about any medications you may be taking. Other common side effects of antihistamines include dry mouth, difficulty urinating, and constipation. Children may experience nightmares, unusual jumpiness, or nervousness, restlessness, and irritability.

Almost none

Side effects include rapid heartbeat, anxiety, insomnia, and headache. Elderly patients and children may be more sensitive to the side effects of bronchodilators.

Side effects include nervousness, sleeplessness, and elevation in blood pressure. When used for a prolonged period, over-the-counter decongestants can cause "rebound rhinitis," actually increasing nasal congestion. Prescription nasal sprays and drops don't have this effect and can be used for longer periods of time.

Can cause hoarseness and thrush, a fungal infection of the mouth and throat. Such problems can be minimized by mouth-rinsing and using a spacer device that can reduce the amount of medication residue in the mouth and throat. Some studies show that these drugs may cause slower-than-normal growth in children. Several case reports suggest that psychiatric disturbances such as mania, depression, and mood disturbances may occasionally occur.

Can make some drugs stay in the system longer, and its actions are altered when it is taken with aspirin or theophylline (a bronchodilator). Side effects include headache, infection, and nausea.

Short-term use can cause slight weight gain, increased appetite, menstrual irregularities and cramps, and heartburn or indigestion. Withdrawal symptoms include loss of energy, poor appetite, severe muscle aches, and joint pains. Long-term use can cause ulcers, weight gain, cataracts, weakened bones and skin, high blood pressure, elevated blood sugar, easy bruising, decreased growth in children, depression, mania, and mood disturbances.

Mostly the same as for inhaled corticosteroids, as well as an increased risk of nasal irritation and bleeding

medications often have side effects, Dr. Leung says. "For these people, there's an unmet need. We need to find out more about what's going on in the immune system and how we can intervene."

And for other people, taking medications for a lifetime can be an expensive, inconvenient, and possibly unsafe undertaking.

• The Avoidance Strategy: The Most Elegant Natural Control

Avoidance is based on a simple concept: Stay away from substances that bother you, and you'll be okay. By making changes and lowering your exposure, you can reduce symptoms without medication. It's a non-invasive, anti-inflammatory, and entirely natural approach.

For this strategy to work, the allergist must become a detective, pointing patients to the obvious and not-so-obvious sources of their problems, especially in bedrooms. "Do what you can to cut down on the dust collectors in your bedroom," Dr. Nathan instructs. "The boxes, the stuffed animals, the small items that people never clean. Those things are putting off dust that you're inhaling all night long. That's why it's not uncommon for people to be at their very worst when they wake up in the morning."

Although some allergy professionals say it's enough to create a bedroom "oasis," others practice tough love, urging patients to rid their homes of allergenic triggers, including plants, pets, and treasured family heirlooms. "If you already have moldy furnishings, you need to discard them or move them to an area in the home where you spend little time, even if it breaks your heart," emphasizes Mary Lou Hayden, R.N., a family nurse practitioner at Virginia Adult and Pediatric Allergy and Asthma in Richmond.

• Allergy and Asthma Drugs: Effective but Not without Side Effects

Ever notice how blissed-out everyone looks in allergy-drug advertisements?

They can dash through a field of daisies, swat a golf ball from a sand trap, and pucker up to kiss a puppy. Yet their eyes never water, their noses never run, and their faces never have that deer-in-the-headlights expression of someone who's about to let loose with a window-rattling sneeze.

The message is enticingly clear: If you want to frolic with the flower children, just ask your doctor to send you to Planet Zyrtec. Or Planet Allegra. Or Planet Claritin.

Despite such hype, it's true that allergy medications are much safer and more effective than they used to be. "In the 1960s, we had some drugs that had three or four different things in them. It wasn't considered terribly scientific because you couldn't adjust the dose of each," says Betty Wray, M.D., interim dean of the Medical College of Georgia School of Medicine in Augusta and past president of the American College of Allergy, Asthma, and Immunology.

Since patients were exposed to multiple drugs, they often experienced multiple side effects. Further, some of the older asthma medications contained phenobarbital, a depressant drug that's often fatal when mixed with alcohol.

"We have such good medications now that if you're a compliant patient, it's very unlikely you'll have a problem," Dr. Nathan says. "Certainly there are exceptions, but we're talking about a couple percent of patients."

For asthma, especially, the approach to treatment has changed significantly. Until recently, the thinking was that asthma was caused by bronchospasm—a contraction of the bronchial tubes. As a result, bronchodilating drugs were the treatment of choice. Today, however, doctors believe that the underlying problem in asthma is inflammation, so inhaled corticosteroid drugs have become the new gold standard. Most bronchodilators are now usually reserved for use as rescue medications during asthma flare-ups or when other drugs aren't working.

Among many patients, the shift to corticosteroids has created some apprehension. Some people confuse inhaled corticosteroids with oral corticosteroids such as prednisone or the anabolic steroids illegally used by some athletes to pump up their physiques.

Although inhaled corticosteroids carry some risks, they're much safer than either the oral or anabolic variety. "Remember, these are special steroids," Dr. Leung says. "They've been chemically modified from the steroids that ordinarily occur in our bodies. When used at FDA-approved doses, they are not absorbed into the bloodstream at sufficient enough levels to cause serious side effects. And if they get absorbed by the gastrointestinal tract, they're rapidly cleared by the liver."

It's important to note, however, that oral corticosteroids can still cause nasty side effects, among them osteoporosis, cataracts, and a decrease in the adrenal gland's ability to produce its own cortisol. Although recent studies have had difficulty confirming this finding, some research shows that children who use corticosteroids may grow at a slower rate, although the jury is still out on whether or not the drugs affect their final adult height.

Since drugs treat the allergy symptoms instead of the underlying cause, perhaps their biggest drawback is that they must be taken for life. "My objection to all these drugs is that they suppress or block the allergic process and in doing so only perpetuate the disease by frustrating it," says Andrew Weil, M.D., director of the program in integrative medicine and clinical professor of medicine at the University of Arizona College of Medicine in Tucson. "I've had intense ragweed allergy all my life, and I know that it's possible to make things better by changing your lifestyle and attitude."

• Immunotherapy: A "Cure" for Allergies?

Immunotherapy is a century-old therapy that is based on the theory that a little "hair of the dog that bit you" can relieve your allergies. Commonly known as allergy shots, immunotherapy is the closest thing to a cure for allergic rhinitis, asthma caused by allergy to pollens and dust mites, and stinging-insect allergy.

After testing positive for certain allergens, you begin receiving injections containing weak concentrations of those allergens. Over a period of weeks or months, the concentration is gradually increased so that you build up a tolerance to the allergens in your environment.

"The only way you can really alter your allergic response is to take allergy shots, which can create blocking antibodies that compete with allergic antibodies," Dr. Nathan says. "After a number of years, you also get an actual decrease in the allergic antibodies."

Allergists have long believed that immunotherapy is effective, but until recently there was little scientific proof. Today, Dr. Nathan notices that allergy shots relieve allergic rhinitis in up to 90 percent of his cases.

Don't be surprised, though, if your doctor refers to this therapy as vaccination. It seems that allergists have battled public confusion over the term *immunotherapy* for decades. "When you tell people they can be vaccinated against allergies, they understand," says Dr. Wray. "But when you say immunotherapy, they think you're talking about a cancer treatment."

In addition to some P.R. problems with terminology, there are also some medical drawbacks that you should be aware of before beginning immunotherapy.

• Risk of adverse reactions. Some patients develop swelling at the site of the injections. This reaction can be resolved by taking oral antihistamines, using ice packs, and adjusting the dose or vaccine. Rarely, a person may experience asthma symptoms or anaphylaxis.

• Inconvenience. Immunotherapy requires patience and a substantial time commitment. After each injection, you must remain in the clinic for at least 20 minutes so staffers can monitor you for adverse reactions.

• Limited applications. Immunotherapy won't work for nonallergic rhinitis. In addition, researchers have yet to develop safe and effective immunotherapies for food and latex allergies.

The
Environmental-Medicine
VIEW OF ALLERGIES

THE CONVENTIONAL VIEW and treatment of allergy are based on worldwide scientific research. In the United States, the two largest organizations that represent board-certified allergists are the American Academy of Allergy, Asthma, and Immunology (AAAAI), which has 6,000 members, and the American College of Allergy, Asthma, and Immunology (ACAAI), which has 4,000 members. Although they have their differences, these groups, which were both founded in the 1940s, mostly agree on what constitutes proper allergy testing, treatment, and management.

Outside the mainstream, however, is a third "party": the American Academy of Environmental Medicine (AAEM). This organization, which was founded in 1965 by maverick allergists and has 400 members, advocates its own theories, tests, and procedures.

Although environmental medicine is not an officially recognized medical specialty, those who adhere to it do share some common ground with their conventional counterparts, especially where the area of environmental control is concerned. "Avoidance always works if your avoidance is good enough," notes Charles Hinshaw, M.D., an environmental-medicine doctor in Wichita, Kansas, and past president of the AAEM.

Beyond that, however, environmental-medicine doctors hold radically different views on how allergy should be defined, diagnosed, and treated. Compared to conventional allergists, they are far less likely to believe that the immunoglobulin E, or IgE, antibody is the major source of allergic trouble and are far more likely to advocate nondrug treatments. These include several different forms of allergy shots, which they claim are more effective than conventional immunotherapy.

The Father of Environmental Medicine

Although a number of alternative-minded allergists were responsible for splitting the medical treatment of allergy into separate camps, the best known is the late Theron Randolph, M.D. Considered to be the father of environmental medicine, Dr. Randolph spent more than a half-century advocating beliefs that conventional allergists consider heretical.

Among the beliefs forwarded by Dr. Randolph is the notion that food allergy is widespread and that it's the cause of many different physical and emotional disorders. When Dr. Randolph was on the faculty of the Northwestern University Medical School in Chicago, his suggestion that food allergy causes mental illness was greeted with such derision that the university terminated his tenure, alleging that he was "a pernicious influence for medical students."

But Dr. Randolph persevered, publishing nearly 400 articles in scientific journals before his death in 1995. His research demonstrated that allergy plays a role in migraine headaches, seizure disorders, alcoholism, myalgia, psychosis, arthritis, and fatigue.

Dr. Randolph's greatest achievement, however, was the idea that chemical exposure is responsible for many allergic and nonallergic disorders. Born and raised on a Michigan farm, he got his first taste of chemical contamination while passing by a malodorous Dow Chemical Company plant during a cattle drive. Eventually, his ideas gave rise to such controversial diagnoses as multiple chemical sensitivity.

His theory on the link between chemical exposure and allergies and other disorders was the primary reason he broke with conventional allergists in 1965 to found the Society for Clinical Ecology, which later changed its name to the American Academy of Environmental Medicine.

True to its name, the AAEM believes that exposures to substances in the environment—including chemicals and foods—are responsible for a host of adverse reactions. "There are 70,000 chemicals that are in our environment that weren't there before World War II," says AAEM president-elect George Miller, M.D., an obstetrician in Lewisburg, Pennsylvania. "The things we eat, touch, and smell impinge upon our wellness."

Since most insurers won't cover the tests and treatments used by environmental-medicine doctors, patients usually pay for such services out of pocket. Still, many patients are willing to bear the burden because they haven't been helped by conventional medicine.

Allergy Redefined: The Environmental View

Like conventional allergists, environmental-medicine doctors define allergy as an abnormal response to substances that your system recognizes as foreign instead of familiar. But their list of those offending substances goes beyond pollen, dander, mold, dust, and foods. It also includes chemicals, drugs, air pollution, and perfumes.

Environmental doctors also believe that allergies affect more than the respiratory tract, the gastrointestinal system, and the skin. In their view, allergy can produce symptoms in almost every organ of the body—including the brain, bladder, and vagina—while masquerading as other diseases.

Choosing an Environmental-Medicine Doctor

Environmental-medicine doctors are medical doctors, and some are board-certified allergists. They're more likely, however, to be certified in family practice, ob-gyn, internal medicine, or some other specialty. What unites them is the belief that allergy and "environmental illness" are often one and the same.

Environmental-medicine doctors are not "certified" in the usual sense. But they must complete a core curriculum in order to be considered a "referable" physician by the American Academy of Environmental Medicine (AAEM). This four-course curriculum gives them an intensive grounding in the basic theories and practices of environmental medicine.

With the exception of immunotherapy for food allergies, which can cause anaphylaxis, conventional allergists do not consider any of the AAEM's major techniques to be dangerous. The American Academy of Allergy, Asthma, and Immunology (AAAAI) does, however, consider most environmental tests and treatments to be "controversial and unproven."

The AAAAI's position statement on environmental medicine states: "It is time-consuming and places severe restrictions on the individual's lifestyle. Individuals who are being treated in this manner should be fully informed of its experimental nature."

If you're considering environmental medicine, take these precautions.

- Be certain the practitioner is a medical doctor.
- Check to see if the practitioner is AAEM-"referable." That means he has taken the AAEM's required instructional courses.
- Beware of practitioners who rely exclusively on such controversial diagnostic procedures as cytotoxic testing. Even within the AAEM, such tests are considered outside the bounds of standard practice.
- Tell your conventional doctor or allergist about any new treatments that you're considering.

Unlike conventional allergists, environmental-medicine doctors don't believe that the IgE antibody is the root of all evil. In their view, other antibodies also play a significant role, among them IgG, IgA, and IgM. "The broadest definition of allergy is an abnormal reaction to an environmental exposure," Dr. Hinshaw says. "That can involve a number of immune mechanisms."

Delayed reactions, for example, are mediated by the IgG mechanism. "Since that involves a lot of food allergies, I think it's very important to deal with IgG immune responses," Dr. Hinshaw says.

Since environmental-medicine doctors embrace such an expansive definition of allergy, they believe that many allergic reactions may originate outside the immune system. Their primary suspect is the autonomic nervous system, which regulates breathing, heartbeat, and digestion.

They even admit that some allergic reactions are of unknown origin. "We probably don't know the action mechanism of many of these reactions," says Allan Lieberman, M.D., an environmental-medicine doctor in North Charleston, South Carolina. "One thing we do know is that it is not always IgE-mediated."

So pervasive is the influence of the main-

The Basics of Environmental Medicine

Conventional allergists tend to think of allergy in terms of *specific* stress. For example, when you're exposed to a specific allergen such as cat dander, your immune system reacts in a specific way, and you experience specific symptoms such as watery eyes, a runny nose, and asthma.

In contrast, environmental-medicine doctors tend to think of allergy in terms of *cumulative* stress. The way they see it, all the stressors in your life—emotional as well as physical—interact cumulatively to disrupt your body's control systems and cause or worsen your allergies. They've developed several theories to explain how this process works. These include:

Total load. Adherents believe that chronic stress—emotional as well as physical—accumulates like drops of water in a rain barrel. Eventually, the rain barrel becomes so full that it overflows, resulting in diseases such as allergies. In theory, then, reducing your total load should make you less susceptible to allergic reactions.

Individual susceptibility. Adherents believe that your susceptibility to allergies is largely determined by your "turf." That includes your heredity, gender, and physical, emotional, and nutritional condition. In short, all the things that make you you, says Allan Lieberman, M.D., an environmental-medicine doctor in North Charleston, South Carolina.

stream allergy associations that environmental-medicine doctors are loathe to label any non-IgE reaction as a "true" allergy. So they call all other reactions sensitivities.

"The allergists tend to say that only IgE-mediated reactions are 'true' allergies, and I don't really quarrel with that, because it's semantics," Dr. Hinshaw says. "It's an artificial separation that's been promoted by the allergists."

From a patient's point of view, however, the difference between an "allergy" and a "sensitivity" is purely academic. "Who cares?" Dr. Hinshaw asks. "It's still an abnormal reaction."

The Causes of Allergies

Like conventional allergists, environmental-medicine doctors say that heredity determines whether or not you're susceptible to allergies. If several of your family members have allergies, especially severe allergies, you're probably more likely to start sneezing and wheezing early in life.

Gender plays a role, too. In childhood, more boys than girls have allergies. But in adulthood, the balance shifts. Women tend to have more allergies than men until they reach menopause. Then everything evens out. Among seniors, the incidence of allergy is about the same for both women and men.

Unlike conventional allergists, however, environmental-medicine doctors say that

it's mostly the environment that determines whether or not you actually *develop* allergies. Here are some environmental factors that can increase your risk.

• Infection. A severe infection—viral, bacterial, or fungal—can trigger the onset of allergic sensitivities.

• Chemical exposure. The most notorious allergy-provoking chemicals include pesticides and other petrochemicals.

• Stress. Increased stress, whether it's emotional or physical, can exacerbate allergy. This is true even for so-called happy stressors, like marriages and births.

• Nutrition. Just as a poor diet sets you up for other chronic diseases, it increases your chances of developing allergies.

How Common Are Allergies?

Although conventional allergists believe that the allergy epidemic is serious and getting worse, their highest estimate of the number of Americans who have allergies is 38 percent. This figure is based on a representative sample of 1,004 American adults.

Environmental-medicine doctors, however, suspect that the actual percentage might be much higher. "My first law is that everybody is allergic to something," Dr. Hinshaw says. "The second is that there's nothing in the world that someone isn't allergic to. That's a little bit facetious, but it's pretty close to true."

THE HIDDEN CONNECTION

"Mystery" Substances Can Spell Misery

If you sneeze and wheeze every fall, chances are that you blame the ragweed that floats invisibly on the breeze. But the real problem might be as plain as the dessert on your plate.

Fall allergies are frequently made worse by a coexisting allergy to a food that just happens to be in season during the fall. This is especially the case with certain fruits. Among the most notorious offenders are melons.

If you suspect that a coexisting food allergy might be making you feel worse, try to avoid eating fruit or other suspect foods when pollen counts are high, advises Charles Hinshaw, M.D., an environmental-medicine doctor in Wichita, Kansas, and past president of the American Academy of Environmental Medicine. If you find that your symptoms subside, chances are you have what environmental-medicine doctors call a concomitant food allergy.

Fortunately, you now have a strategy that can help you sail through the fall allergy season.

Environmental-medicine doctors base this belief on the assumption—not shared by their conventional-medicine colleagues—that food allergy is much more widespread than is commonly believed. "I think at least 25 percent of the population has food allergies, and the percentage could be much higher," Dr. Hinshaw says. On the other hand, conventional allergists believe that the incidence of food allergy is as low as 2.5 percent.

"Conventional doctors use a skin-prick test for food allergies," Dr. Hinshaw says. "That is not a good way to test for food allergies. They miss them all the time."

Environmental-medicine doctors use tests including extracts administered via injection or sublingual drops to ferret out food allergies. Often, they say, conventional allergists assume that allergic or nonallergic rhinitis is the cause of a person's problems when in fact the real culprit is a hidden food allergy.

For example, some people develop itchy noses, throats, and eyes in August and stay miserable until the first hard frost. These are the hallmarks of ragweed allergy, yet such patients test negative to ragweed. That's when environmental-medicine doctors put on their Sherlock Holmes hats and start looking for other causes.

"Chances are, it's a concomitant food allergy," Dr. Hinshaw says. "It's a combination of a pollen and a food that causes the reaction."

Your Dinner Could Be Stressing Your Body

Consider the amount of food that you eat for breakfast, lunch, dinner, and snacks. Where do all these munchies go?

Straight into your gut, or alimentary tract, the largest surface area in your entire body. From your mouth to your anus, your alimentary tract measures a whopping 540 square meters. By comparison, the surface area of your lungs is just 80 square meters, and the surface area of your skin is a scant 1 square meter.

Stress has been defined as the number of molecules to which the body is exposed, says Dr. Lieberman. When you consider how many millions of molecules you pour into your gut every day, it's easy to see why environmental-medicine doctors consider food to be the single greatest stress on the human body.

"Many years ago, doctors said that disease begins in the bowel," Dr. Lieberman says. "The reason they said that is because the gastrointestinal tract has so many important functions. There are actually more nerve fibers in the intestine than there are in the brain. Further, there's probably more immunologic tissue in the gastrointestinal tract than there is in the rest of the immune system." And food can have a major direct effect on these regulatory systems.

When environmental-medicine doctors investigate food allergy, they don't just look for immediate, IgE-mediated reactions such as stomach cramping, diarrhea, skin rashes, hives, swelling, wheezing, and the most-dreaded complication of all: anaphylactic shock. They also look for the more subtle signs of delayed-onset food allergies. In their view, these reactions are usually mediated by the IgG antibody and appear anywhere from 2 hours to 7 days after eating a suspect food.

Delayed-onset food allergies can affect the brain, joints, muscles, hormone-producing glands, lungs, kidneys, and nervous system. Environmental-medicine doctors believe such allergies are associated with more than 100 different medical conditions, including migraine headaches.

• Leaky-Gut Syndrome

How can something as innocuous as food be the source of so much trouble?

Environmental-medicine doctors say that it's not so much the food itself as it is the combination of poor digestion, contamination of food by pesticides and herbicides, and overuse of antibiotics and other medications, as well as changes in the friendly bacteria in our gastrointestinal tracts.

The result: a condition called leaky-gut syndrome.

As its name implies, leaky-gut syndrome affects the ability of the intestines to contain its contents. Like a water balloon with thousands of tiny pinholes, the intestines become more and more porous, allowing incompletely digested food and other harmful molecules to pass through the intestinal wall into the bloodstream. It's a vicious cycle as the leaky gut causes allergy and allergy causes a leaky gut.

"When those larger molecules enter the bloodstream, the immune system sees them like a B-52 on a radar screen," Dr. Hinshaw says. "They're seen as foreign material, so you get an allergic reaction."

What to Expect When You Visit an Environmental-Medicine Doctor

Patients often turn to environmental medicine because they've been tested for allergens X, Y, and Z and been told the results are zip, zip, and zip. Still desperate for relief, they don't mind paying out of pocket for services that conventional medicine deems "experimental."

"One of the beauties of environmental medicine is that we offer services, both diagnostic and treatment, that are very effective when other methods of diagnosis and treatment don't work," Dr. Hinshaw says.

Read on to learn how the process works.

• Your Medical History

Like conventional allergists, environmental-medicine doctors start by taking a detailed medical history. In fact, you can expect to spend an hour or two telling an environmental-medicine doctor your life story.

During the initial stage of the interview,

You Can Be Allergic to Allergy Tests

Sometimes, allergens show up where you least suspect them. For example, Charles Hinshaw, M.D., an environmental-medicine doctor in Wichita, Kansas, and past president of the American Academy of Environmental Medicine, once ran a blood test on a patient who had gone into shock after being skin-tested for wasp-venom allergy at another doctor's office.

To his surprise, the blood test showed that the patient was only mildly allergic to wasp venom.

Dr. Hinshaw eventually determined that the patient actually was allergic to the glycerin used as a preservative in skin-test extracts.

"I've had a lot of patients who are allergic to glycerin," notes Dr. Hinshaw. "It's a very common allergy."

you'll do most of the talking. The doctor's job is simply to listen to your story in a non-judgmental manner.

Dr. Randolph, the father of environmental medicine, practiced a technique called poker-faced medicine. As patients spoke, he dispassionately recorded their comments on a typewriter. Today's environmental-medicine doctors are more likely to use a tape recorder.

Once you've had your say, the doctor will ask, "Is there anything else you want to tell me?" If not, he will begin the formal part of the interview.

"Basically, we start back at conception," Dr. Hinshaw says. "Some of us ask questions about the health of your parents at the time of conception and how your mother's pregnancy went."

Your childhood history is extremely important. The doctor will want to know if you experienced any of the following conditions.

- Allergic rhinitis (hay fever)
- Asthma
- Attention deficit disorder (ADD) or attention deficit hyperactivity disorder (ADHD)
- Bed-wetting
- Eczema
- Frequent colds or other upper-respiratory infections
- Nocturnal leg cramps
- Recurrent ear infections (otitis media)
- Recurrent sore throats or tonsillitis

The doctor will want to know if these conditions improved or worsened after you reached puberty. He also will ask whether you had a bad reaction to any of your childhood vaccinations.

As you might expect, environmental-medicine doctors will ask detailed questions about any adverse environmental exposures you experienced as a youngster. "Early exposures are part of the total load," Dr. Hinshaw says. "A lot of chemicals are retained in the body because they're soluble in fat."

Sometimes, history alone is enough to make a diagnosis. "You pick up food allergies right away," Dr. Hinshaw says. "Patients will tell you something like, 'I was really healthy the first 3 months when I was breastfed, but then they put me on cow's milk, and I started having all these bad ear infections. I had shots, was given antibiotics, and had my tonsils out.' The reason they got the infections was the food allergy."

• Diagnostic Tests

Unlike conventional allergists, environmental-medicine doctors don't use skin-prick testing. The gold standard of food allergy testing is the deliberate feeding challenge test, says Dr. Lieberman.

In addition, environmental-medicine doctors use a blood test known as a radioallergosorbent test (RAST) to look for the presence of several different antibodies, not just IgE. "You can identify IgE antibodies against offending chemicals in some chemically sensitive patients," Dr. Hinshaw says. "You can also identify IgG and IgM antibodies."

Here are the most commonly used tests in environmental-medicine practices.

Intracutaneous one-to-five serial dilution titration. A small amount of allergen is in-

jected into your skin, where it forms a wheal the size of a mosquito bite. If you are allergic to the substance, the wheal's size will increase within 10 minutes.

Clinical titration. Suspect foods or chemicals are either injected into your arm or administered as drops under your tongue to

Two Controversial Tests

When environmental-medicine doctors can't identify the source of your trouble with their usual tests, they'll sometimes turn to procedures such as cytotoxic testing and the antigen leukocyte cellular antibody test (ALCAT). These tests are so controversial, however, that the mention of their names is enough to make conventional allergists cross themselves and reach for their blood pressure medications. Environmental-medicine doctors regard them as highly controversial gold-*plated* standards because it's difficult to interpret the results.

During cytotoxic testing, living blood cells are exposed to a suspect substance and observed under a microscope. Sometimes the white blood cells show changes in the movement of little granules inside their membranes. Other times the red blood cells and platelets clump and swell. "Sometimes the cells even swell enough that they actually burst," reports Charles Hinshaw, M.D., an environmental-medicine doctor in Wichita, Kansas, and past president of the American Academy of Environmental Medicine.

ALCAT, done on a blood sample by computerized equipment, measures a change in the normal cell volume distribution caused by chemicals, foods, pollen, and so on.

"Neither of these tests is recognized within the practice standards of environmental medicine," Dr. Hinshaw says. "The problem is that we don't have a very clear understanding of the mechanism that's causing the changes in the cells. We don't know whether we're dealing with IgE, IgM, IgA, or something entirely different."

Still, cytotoxic testing and ALCAT may provide important clues. "Sometimes you're backed into a corner," Dr. Hinshaw says. "You may have a patient whom you think is reacting to chemicals, but you can't get any IgE or IgG antibodies against him. You do an ALCAT, and you can show there is a cellular response. That's pretty good evidence that a patient needs to stay away from that substance."

provoke allergic reactions, which are measured to determine the degree of sensitivity.

Individual deliberate feeding tests, elimination diets, and rotary-diversified diets. You abstain from eating certain foods for 3 to 5 days. Then foods are reintroduced so that the doctor can measure the reaction.

Comprehensive environmental control program. With this test, you are placed in a controlled environment, usually a hospital, where substances are introduced one at a time as reactions are recorded.

As an alternative to hospitalization, a few environmental-medicine practices use a double-blind procedure called booth testing. You are seated inside a glass-walled booth, then exposed to either a harmless substance or a suspect substance, usually a chemical. Neither you nor the doctor knows which is which, and the chemical is so diluted that it can't be smelled. The doctor measures your pulse and breathing, and periodically asks how you are feeling.

Treating Allergies with Environmental Medicine

Like conventional allergists, environmental-medicine doctors place a premium on environmental control. "We preach having at least your bedroom as an oasis," Dr. Hinshaw says. "You want a place where you can get a good night's sleep because that'll often be enough to give you good health through the day when you're exposed to those things you react to. You have to reduce the total load."

Like conventional allergists, environmental-medicine doctors also use drugs and immunotherapy. However, for them, the balance is heavily tipped on the side of immunotherapy.

"With immunotherapy, we can get better control of the symptoms and often have permanent response over a period of a couple of years, so we think it's treating the patients better," Dr. Hinshaw says. "Drugs have some benefits, but they also carry the baggage of side effects."

Still, drugs are sometimes a necessary evil, especially when the pollen is so thick that you can barely see out of your car windshield. "On those kinds of days, anyone who's pollen-sensitive is going to have symptoms," Dr. Miller says. "That's why you need oral medications or inhalers. Thank goodness you can get symptomatic relief from these medications."

• Immunotherapy

Environmental medicine's approach to allergy shots is similar to that of conventional medicine. By taking a little "hair of the dog that bit you," you gradually retrain your immune system to tolerate substances that set it off. If you're lucky, the effect is permanent and you're essentially "cured."

The difference is that environmental-medicine doctors are able to use higher starting concentrations of the offending substance, which have been shown to bring more immediate and long-lasting symptom relief. Unlike conventional allergists, they also use allergy shots to treat food and chemical sensitivities.

Although conventional doctors do not claim that these higher concentrations are necessarily harmful, they believe that allergy shots are primarily useful for inhalant allergies—such as pollen and mold—and can be dangerous when used to treat food allergies.

Here are a couple of environmental medicine's forms of immunotherapy.

Enzyme-potentiated desensitization. This form of immunotherapy is used to desensitize patients to an entire category of allergens. For example, the aeroallergens category would include pollen, mold, and animal dander. Tiny injections of these allergens are given several weeks apart. Since doses are much weaker than other allergy shots, an enzyme called beta-glucuronidase is added to increase, or "potentiate," the effect.

Optimal-dose immunotherapy. The "optimal" dose is just short of the dose that produces symptoms. By starting with higher concentrations, environmental-medicine doctors have shown that patients can complete a course of immunotherapy in as little as 2 years.

• Additional Allergy Treatments

In addition to immunotherapy, the following treatments may also be used by en-vironmental-medicine doctors.

Dietary changes. Great emphasis is placed on finding and eliminating foods in the diet that cross-react with other allergens, especially pollens. One example is eggs, which sometimes cause a double reaction in patients who are allergic to oak tree pollen. Practitioners often counsel their patients to cut back on or eliminate sugar, refined wheat, and dairy products, and they encourage eating a varied, organic diet.

Exercise. "Most of us simply don't move enough," says Russell Roby, M.D., director of the Texan Allergy Center in Austin and founder of the Online Allergy Center. "Probably 50 percent of all the symptoms in the patients I see are caused by insufficient physical movement. Most patients will achieve about half of the relief that is available to them simply by adding an hour of appropriate physical movement into their daily routine—even walking whenever possible."

Sauna therapy. Also known as heat depuration therapy, sauna therapy is often used to treat multiple chemical sensitivity, based on the knowledge that sweating releases toxins stored in fat. When supervised by a doctor, patients in the sauna are generally given vitamin, mineral, and fluid replacements.

Stress reduction. Since emotional upheaval can make allergies worse, environmental-medicine doctors often recommend supplemental mind and body therapies such as psychotherapy and massage. "Getting rid of stress helps the whole system," says Steven Bock, M.D., cofounder and co-director of the Rhinebeck Health Center in Rhinebeck, New York, and the Center for Progressive Medicine in Albany. If they follow a stress program that lowers the level of cumulative stresses, patients often get better, even without any additional lifestyle changes, he adds.

Supplements. The number of vitamin, mineral, and herbal supplements that can be used for allergy is almost limitless. But some supplements come up over and over again in the medical literature. Among them are vitamin C, vitamin B_6, zinc, and magnesium.

Could Allergies Be Linked to Other Medical Conditions?

Environmental-medicine doctors believe that allergies might trigger much more than a rash or runny nose. Though further investigation is needed, they theorize that the following conditions may have an allergy link.

Addictions. Decades ago, Dr. Randolph wrote that alcoholism may be the "pinnacle" of the food-addiction pyramid. "He taught us that allergy is addiction and addiction is allergy," Dr. Lieberman says. "That is, you're often addicted to what you're allergic to. The alcoholic is not addicted, per se, to alcohol. He's addicted to the source of

the alcohol, which in most cases are cereal grains and yeasts."

Attention deficit hyperactivity disorder. Environmental-medicine doctors buck conventional wisdom by asserting that ADHD, autism, and other behavioral disorders are sometimes a consequence of food or other environmental allergy. A prime suspect is corn. "I've had my share of children with ADHD," Dr. Hinshaw says. "Their level of unfocused activity decreases right before your eyes when you eliminate suspected allergens."

Candidiasis. Many environmental-medicine doctors believe that the typical Western diet favors an overgrowth of yeast in the gastrointestinal tract of susceptible individuals and that this is one cause of leaky-gut syndrome. To correct the imbalance, they often prescribe probiotics, which are supplements containing *Lactobacillus acidophilus* and other "friendly" bacteria, as well as antifungal drugs such as nystatin (Mycostatin). "Often I will try to treat the candidiasis before I tackle the allergies," Dr. Miller says. "I won't do the dust, mold, trees, grass, and weed pollen skin tests until the patient has been on nystatin for a month." This reduces the total load and makes testing easier.

Chronic fatigue immune dysfunction syndrome. There is a clear connection between this illness and environmental illness. This is true with any chronic disease, however, because anything that increases the total stress load will exacerbate the disease process. "In these patients, seasonal patterns are common because pollen increases the total stress load, as do food, chemicals, infections, and especially yeast," says Dr. Lieberman. Treatment consists of dietary changes, nutritional supplements, and oral medications.

Depression. Although conventional doctors blame depression on a chemical imbalance in the brain, environmental-medicine doctors believe the imbalance can be triggered by any environmental stress, including pollen and mold. Dr. Lieberman recalls a university president who became depressed every fall. As it turned out, the culprit wasn't anxiety over the start of a new school year but an allergy to ragweed.

Headaches. Call it a quirk of the alphabet, but environmental-medicine doctors blame many headaches, including migraines, on foods that start with the letter C. "It usually comes down to the Four Cs: cane (as in sugar), corn, cola, and chocolate," Dr. Lieberman says.

Inflammatory bowel disease. Environmental-medicine doctors have long noted that intestinal flare-ups are more likely to occur on high-pollen days. Dr. Lieberman says that he instantly relieved one patient's agonizing abdominal distress by giving her a neutralizing dose of mountain cedar pollen.

Multiple chemical sensitivity. Although this condition is defined as a disability under the 1991 Americans with Disabilities Act, it continues to be highly controversial. To environmental-medicine doctors, conditions such as multiple chemical sensitivity and sick-building syndrome are core diagnoses. In their view, chemical exposure causes a multitude of illnesses, including allergy. In a review of several thousand cases of chemical sensitivity, more than 50 percent were caused by exposure to pesticides.

Detractors of multiple chemical sensitivity say that the symptoms—including headaches, loss of consciousness, poor memory, palpitations, shortness of breath, dizziness, joint pain, and fatigue—are too broad to be blamed on a single illness. Some even say it's a "hysterical" (that is, psychological) epidemic. More research is needed.

Rheumatoid arthritis. Environmental-medicine doctors believe that allergy is strongly associated with rheumatoid arthritis and other autoimmune diseases. Dr. Hinshaw recalls a young tennis instructor who was referred for evaluation of rheumatoid arthritis symptoms. The pain improved after she received neutralization therapy for beef and corn allergy. (With neutralization therapy, the patient is treated with a dose of allergen too small to produce a reaction but large enough to prevent one.)

The Alternative
VIEW OF ALLERGIES

"ALTERNATIVE-MEDICINE USERS are well-educated persons with higher incomes who want to take charge of their health care. They're looking beyond soulless technology for some kind of complete feeling that includes spirit, soul, and healing touch. Alternative practitioners tend to spend time with their patients. So people feel very good about the experience, in contrast to the way they feel about the managed-care model of 'run 'em through quickly.'"

If these words sound like those of a typical alternative practitioner—an herbalist, say, or a naturopathic physician—think again.

They were actually voiced by a mainstream allergist, Renata Engler, M.D., chief of the allergy and immunology department at the Walter Reed Army Medical Center in Washington, D.C., during a national conference of the mainstream American Academy of Allergy, Asthma, and Immunology.

Dr. Engler is one of a growing number of allergists who not only acknowledge the increasing popularity of alternative medicine but also support responsible research to assess the effectiveness of alternative-medicine treatments. "There are some things the alternative-medicine community is doing right," she says. "We should learn from that and reincorporate it into our practices."

Does that mean she has abandoned conventional pills, inhalers, and allergy shots in favor of herbs, aromatherapy, and homeopathic remedies? Emphatically not. Still, the fact that she can even discuss such things before an audience of medical doctors without getting hooted off the stage is proof that alternative medicine for the treatment of allergies and asthma is getting a more respectful hearing.

Worldwide, only 10 to 30 percent of the population receives care from conventional, biomedically oriented practitioners. Everyone else relies upon self-care; community-based care from family, friends, and neighbors; and professionalized health care from alternative-medicine systems such as Traditional Chinese Medicine, acupuncture, and homeopathy.

In the United States, studies show that 40 percent of the population use some form of alternative medicine. And among people with allergies and asthma, some experts believe that the number who experiment with alternative and complementary medicine might be as high as 75 percent.

According to a 65-page article, "Herbal Interventions in Asthma and Allergy," published in the *Journal of Asthma*, alternative therapies for asthma are widely used in Western as well as non-Western cultures.

In Western nations, such therapies include acupuncture, acupressure, homeopathy, chiropractic, osteopathy, herbs, hypnotherapy, biofeedback, aromatherapy, neuropathy, massage, reflexology, iridology, magnetic therapy, shamanism, and Buteyko (a breathing technique developed in the former Soviet Union).

All of the above-mentioned therapies are practiced in the United States. Alternative practitioners here often recommend supplements including vitamins, magnesium, selenium, acetylcysteine, omega-3 fatty acids, ginkgolides, and herbs.

Although conventional doctors emphasize that more research needs to be done,

those who have studied alternative therapies believe that some herbal remedies can be just as effective as conventional drugs. If research proves that such herbs are beneficial, doctors see no reason why they shouldn't become part of the allergists' armamentarium.

Allergy Redefined: The Alternative View

Unlike conventional medicine and its off-shoot, environmental medicine, alternative medicine has no universally agreed upon definition of allergy.

Although some alternative practitioners speak of immunoglobulin E (IgE) antibodies, mast cells, and chemical "mediators" of allergy, they're more likely to think of allergy as they think of other diseases: a disturbance in the patient's natural equilibrium. Traditional oriental-medicine doctors, for instance, look for imbalances of the patient's *chi*, or vital energy, while Ayurvedic practitioners look for imbalances or stresses in the patient's consciousness.

Devi S. Nambudripad, Ph.D., an acupuncturist, chiropractor, kinesiologist, and registered nurse in Buena Park, California, is the originator of Nambudripad's Allergy Elimination Technique (NAET). Her understanding of allergy's cause is deeply rooted in Eastern thought: "Allergy is defined in terms of what a substance does to the energy flow in the body," says Dr. Nambudripad. Allergies are the result of energy imbalances in the body, leading to a diminished state of health in one or more organ systems.

"When contact is made with an allergen, it causes blockages in the energy pathways, called meridians," she says. "Thought about in another way, it disrupts the normal flow of energy through the body's electrical circuits. This energy blockage causes interference in communication between the brain and body via the nervous system. This blocked energy flow is the first step in a chain of events that can develop into an allergic response."

Robert Rountree, M.D., a holistic physician in Boulder, Colorado, and coauthor of *Immunotics*, also views allergy as an "imbalance" in the immune system, likening it to a bad cold that won't go away. "It's as if the eyes, nose, and lungs are 'on fire,'" he says.

Like most alternative practitioners, Dr. Rountree is concerned that conventional allergy treatments, especially drugs, only suppress the symptoms of allergy rather than treat the underlying disease. "While this may help a lot of people, it can also create a sense of frustration and helplessness," he says. "Wouldn't it be preferable to examine the problem more holistically? We can't change our genetic framework, but mounting evidence suggests that the right combination of dietary factors, including herbs and nutritional supplements, can strongly influence the way our genes are ex-

pressed. The more we understand what causes the symptoms, the better able we are to design a comprehensive, nontoxic approach to treatment."

How Do Alternative Practitioners Diagnose Allergies?

Like conventional- and environmental-medicine doctors, alternative-medicine practitioners start by taking your history and conducting a physical examination. During this exam, they look not only for the obvious symptoms of allergic rhinitis (hay fever) and asthma, such as sneezing and wheezing, but also for clues of hidden food allergy.

These clues can be very general symptoms, such as a runny nose, dark circles under your eyes, digestive upset, or skin rashes, explains Mark Stengler, N.D., a naturopathic and homeopathic physician in La Jolla, California.

Often, Dr. Stengler says, people who think that they're allergic to microscopic particles, such as pollen, mold, and animal dander, are actually allergic to the macroscopic particles they push into their mouths with a spoon and fork. "I'm not saying they don't have sensitivities to things like ragweed pollen," he says. "But in quite a few cases, food sensitivities are causing some of their symptoms."

Like environmental-medicine doctors,

many alternative-medicine practitioners believe that multiple chemical sensitivity is a real illness. "A lot of medical doctors argue it's psychological, but that hasn't been my experience," notes Dr. Stengler. "My patients come in with environmental allergies, allergies to chemicals and perfumes. When I detoxify them, they get better."

Dr. Stengler argues that conventional allergy tests, especially skin-prick tests, are useless for diagnosing food sensitivities, which he considers to be a much more widespread problem than classic food allergies. "When someone has a food allergy to something like peanuts, it's very obvious. The throat closes off," he says. "Food sensitivities are milder. You get mucus forming in the lungs, nose, and throat, with congestion and wheezing."

In the natural-health field, there are three main types of allergy tests.

Electro-dermal testing. For this test, the practitioner attaches an electrode to one of your acupuncture points. A wire from the electrode leads to a machine with a test tube containing a suspect substance, often a food. To complete the circuit, you hold a ground wire. The doctor then sends a small amount of electrical current through the circuit and measures the resistance level of your skin. If the reading is low, it's a sign that you are allergic or sensitive to the food or substance.

Blood tests. Unlike most conventional blood tests, these measure various anti-bodies and antibody subclasses, such as IgG4.

Elimination diets. In these tests, you abstain from eating a suspect food for a period of time, and then it is reintroduced. If your allergy symptoms reappear, it's evidence that you are allergic or sensitive to the food.

In addition to these three main types of tests, alternative-medicine practitioners use many of the same tests that are used by environmental-medicine doctors (see The Environmental-Medicine View of Allergies on page 33). They also use such procedures as kinesiology testing, during which your muscle strength is measured before and after holding a suspect substance. If muscle strength decreases while you are gripping a particular substance, it's a sign of an allergy or sensitivity.

How Do Alternative Practitioners Treat Allergies?

Although the range of allergy treatments used by alternative practitioners is practically limitless, the goal is usually the same: nondrug relief.

At the La Jolla Whole Health Medical Clinic, which Dr. Stengler codirects, the vast majority of patients with asthma come in on inhalers before he places them on a natural protocol. "In almost every case, we're able to either dramatically reduce the medications or get the patients off them totally,"

Dr. Stengler says. "I find I'm especially able to get children off the medications totally."

In general, alternative-medicine advocates believe that conventional treatments carry more risks than benefits. "Conventional treatments for allergy are not very good," says Andrew Weil, M.D., director of the program in integrative medicine and clinical professor of medicine at the University of Arizona College of Medicine in Tucson. "Antihistamines often reduce symptoms, but they can also make you drowsy and lethargic. I consider them toxic drugs that often perpetuate an allergy by suppressing it rather than changing it. This is also true of steroid inhalers, which can be very effective at relieving symptoms but may also weaken immunity."

Despite their antagonism toward conventional drugs, alternative-medicine practitioners, including Dr. Weil, do not categorically rule them out, especially for people with moderate-to-severe asthma. Since asthma demands a two-pronged attack—one aimed at managing acute attacks, the other at controlling inflammation—Dr. Weil sometimes recommends prescription inhalers. Among the ones he likes best is the brand AeroBid, a prescription inhaler containing a synthetic steroid (flunisolide) that generally stays where it belongs—in the lungs.

For people with allergic rhinitis, Dr. Weil sometimes recommends NasalCrom, an over-the-counter drug that contains cromolyn sodium. NasalCrom prevents the mast cells in your nose and elsewhere from releasing their toxic loads of histamine and other chemicals. "It seems to have fewer side effects than any other allergy medication," he notes.

Like most alternative-medicine practitioners, however, Dr. Weil strongly advises patients to pursue natural therapies—including dietary modifications, vitamin/mineral supplements, and herbs—before going pharmacological.

If there's one thing that practitioners from the most conventional to the most alternative agree on, it's the need to rid your home of allergens and irritants. By definition, such strategies are natural because they include vacuuming floors, washing curtains and other dust collectors, banishing furry pets from bedrooms, and clearing the air with HEPA (high-efficiency particulate air) filters.

Some alternative practitioners, however, suggest that it might be even more "natural" to filter the air with plants that have been shown to absorb indoor pollutants. These include spider plants, English ivy, Chinese evergreen potted mums, Brazilian palms, wide-leaved wandering Jews, and marigolds.

A note of caution: Some pollen-sensitive people are allergic to certain varieties of houseplants. In addition, don't overwater your plants, since damp soil may encourage allergy-inducing molds.

The following list shows you the range of alternative therapies used to treat allergies and asthma. Please think of it solely as a general overview. We'll recommend specific therapies in the chapters about individual allergies and allergy-related conditions.

Acupuncture. Practiced for at least 2,500 years in China, acupuncture is based on the idea that illness results from an imbalance or blockage of energy (*chi*) that flows within and without all beings. To improve the flow, acupuncturists insert extremely thin needles into specific points on your body called meridians.

Aromatherapy. Essential oils are concentrated plant extracts containing hormones, vitamins, natural antibiotics, and antiseptics. Many allergy remedies contain eucalyptus oil, which is believed to work as an antiseptic, antispasmodic, and expectorant. During an asthma or allergy attack, the oil can be massaged on your chest and back. Inhaling its fragrance is believed to help clear the sinuses and relieve chest congestion. Other oils used to treat respiratory disorders include fir, hyssop, lavender, pine, frankincense, rosemary, and cajeput. Oils used to relieve the stress associated with allergies include neroli, lavender, marjoram, rose, and ylang-ylang.

Ayurveda. Practiced for more than 5,000 years in India, Ayurveda also is based on the idea that illness results from energy imbalances. Its treatments include dietary modifications, herbs, meditation, and yoga.

Breathing exercises. Alternative practitioners often recommend breathing exercises for people with allergies, especially those with asthma. Among the many different kinds of exercises are deep diaphragmatic breathing, which teaches patients to exhale more completely; specific inspiratory muscle training, which aims to reduce the feelings of breathlessness; and Buteyko, a Russian method that teaches patients to take slow, shallow breaths. Dr. Weil promotes his "4-7-8 Breath," a reference to the number of counts that patients are supposed to make while inhaling, holding the breath, and exhaling.

Chiropractic. This century-old American system emphasizes the connection between illness and maladjustments in the spine. Chiropractors believe that certain corrections may relax the nervous system and prevent asthma attacks, particularly those whose triggers have not been identified. A related treatment, NAET, diagnoses allergies by using kinesiology muscle-response testing and then treats them with chiropractic, acupressure, acupuncture, and dietary modifications.

Cranial therapy. A part of traditional osteopathic medicine, it involves the manipulation of the patient's head and is sometimes used to treat asthma.

Detoxification. In the treatment of allergies and asthma—especially those in which chemical contamination is believed to play a role—sauna therapy is often recommended as a way to "sweat out" toxins stored in fat cells. Before starting patients on such therapy, however, alternative practitioners prefer to bolster their antioxidant status with vitamins, herbs, and other supplements. Some practitioners believe that hot baths can serve the same purpose.

Dietary changes. Even if your allergies aren't food-related, dietary modifications can help tame a hyperactive immune system. General dietary advice includes reducing consumption of dairy products, protein, and sugar, and increasing consumption of fruits, vegetables, and whole grains. The carotenoids and flavonoids in fruits and vegetables help to reduce inflammation, as do the essential fatty acids in flaxseed oil, deep-sea fish, evening primrose oil, borage oil, and black currant oil. Intestinal function is enhanced by the fiber in whole grains, nuts, and seeds. Some people with asthma have obtained relief by adopting a strict vegetarian diet. In addition, drinking the recommended 8 to 10 glasses of water a day appears to loosen phlegm and flush toxins from the body.

Homeopathy. A favorite of naturopathic physicians, homeopathy is a century-old European system based on the principle that like cures like. Allergy and asthma patients are prescribed homeopathic remedies containing infinitesimal amounts of the substances that bother them. For example, some homeopathic remedies for allergic rhinitis contain a mixture of pollens while others contain a mixture of molds. Concentrations are so low that the remedies can be used in conjunction with conventional therapies. Advocates believe that homeopathy, like conventional allergy shots, can retrain the immune system on a cellular level.

Manipulative work. Many different kinds of bodywork besides chiropractic are used to help relieve the symptoms and stress of allergies and asthma. Treatments that usually require professional care include traditional massage, acupressure, osteopathic manipulation of the chest, reflexology, and Rolfing (a form of deep-tissue massage). Self-treatments include facial massages from qigong, a branch of Traditional Chinese Medicine.

Mind-body techniques. Since allergic reactions straddle the mind-body border, alternative practitioners use treatments such as hypnosis, guided imagery, meditation, yoga, and scientific healing affirmations with their allergy clients. The latter requires patients to write a first-person, present-tense statement affirming that a desired goal has already been met. A simple example: "I am allergy-free."

Sinus irrigation. As one of the few instant-relief remedies available for nasal congestion, sinus irrigation floods the nose with a saline solution, flushing away pollen, mold, dust, and excess mucus. An irrigation can be performed using a squeeze bottle, an Ayurvedic neti pot, or a mechanical sprayer similar to a Waterpik.

Steam inhalation. Steam therapy is used to break up accumulated phlegm in the sinuses and lungs. Some advocates recommend adding 1 or 2 drops of an essential oil such as eucalyptus to the water to enhance the decongestive effect. Do not use eucalyptus essential oil for more than 2 weeks without the guidance of a qualified practitioner, however, and do not use it at the same time as homeopathic remedies.

The Use of Supplements in Alternative Medicine

In addition to using therapies such as acupuncture, homeopathy, and aromatherapy, alternative practitioners advocate all kinds of vitamins, minerals, herbs, and other dietary supplements for treating allergies and asthma. Still, no superstar supplements for allergies and asthma have emerged in the same way that St. John's wort has emerged as a treatment for mild-to-moderate depression or saw palmetto has emerged as a treatment for benign prostate enlargement.

Within alternative circles, some of the best-known supplements are the herb stinging nettle and the bioflavonoid quercetin for allergic rhinitis, and the herbs ephedra (ma huang) and lobelia (Indian tobacco) for asthma.

Allergy supplements can be problematic. Since 1996, the FDA has received more than 800 reports of people suffering adverse reactions to ephedra alone.

Still, allergy supplements do have some interesting properties. Herbalist Douglas Schar, Dip.Phyt. (diploma in phytotherapy), M.C.P.P. (member of the College of Practitioners of Phytotherapy), M.N.I.M.H. (member of the National Institute of Medical Herbalists), of London likes to use a class of herbs called adaptogens, which have immune-stimulating as well as immune-depressing properties. Examples include licorice root and gotu kola. "The freaky thing is that the body seems to pick up the part it needs," he says. "These herbs can be used for all allergic reactions."

Even among alternative practitioners, however, there's disagreement about which supplements are best. An herb that one practitioner rates near the top might be an herb that another practitioner ranks near the bottom. One natural-health book might tout a supplement that another book completely ignores.

The reality that is no one herb works for all people. It's a trial-and-error procedure to find the allergy herb that is best for you. Try one herb at a time for at least 2 months before judging its effects. If after 2 months you are no better, move on.

That said, there *are* some supplements that appear repeatedly in alternative-medicine literature. Listed below are some supplements that are often recommended for people with allergies and asthma. Please consider this list as an overview only, not as a treatment plan. We'll make specific recommendations about supplements, including dosages deemed safest and most effective, in the Action Plans of chapters devoted to individual allergies and allergy-related conditions.

Vitamins and minerals. This group includes vitamin C, vitamin B_6, tocopherol (vitamin E) complex, carotenoid complex, selenium, zinc, magnesium, and calcium.

Bioflavonoids. The bioflavonoid quercetin can be used to inhibit the release of histamine. It's often taken with bromelain, an anti-inflammatory enzyme, to enhance absorption.

Herbs and dietary supplements. Alternative practitioners have a large number of dietary supplements at their disposal to help treat allergies, including stinging nettle, ephedra, lobelia, licorice, ginkgo biloba, ginseng, cayenne pepper, pine bark extract, mullein leaf, green tea, ginger, curcumin (from turmeric), proanthocyanidin (grape seed extract), EPA (eicosapentaenoic acid from fish oil), GLA (gamma-linolenic acid from borage or black currant seed oil), caffeinated beverages (coffee, tea, and so on), probiotic supplements containing *Lactobacillus acidophilus*, and methylsulfonylmethane (MSM), which is believed to enhance the action of cortisol, the body's natural inflammation fighter.

Hormonal supplements. These include DHEA and pregnenolone. Hormonal supplements are usually recommended only if blood levels are low.

Combination remedies. Many alternative practitioners recommend combination remedies. Among such remedies are Aller-Max (an oral remedy with quercetin, N-acetyl cysteine, bromelain, L-histidine, vitamin A, vitamin C, pantothenic acid, zinc, pycnogenol, stinging nettle, and cayenne); Raja's Cup (an Ayurvedic tea with clearing nut, kasmard, licorice, and winter cherry); and Olbas Analgesic Oil (a massage oil with menthol, cajeput, clove, wintergreen, and eucalyptus).

Finding the Best
TREATMENT

SOMETIMES, THE TOTAL really can be greater than the sum of its parts. In the preceding chapters, we've explained three different approaches to allergy: conventional, environmental, and alternative.

In this chapter, we'll discuss combining the best elements of all three. In fact, for the first time in any book about allergies, you'll get all the best possible treatment options—both drug and nondrug. Our philosophy is that it's better to give you as many good options as possible to relieve your symptoms.

We interviewed the most eminent experts and examined the most reputable studies, all with the goal of synthesizing the best advice into our allergy management plan.

The Three Disciplines: Closer Than You Might Think

Take a close look at conventional, environmental, and alternative medicine, and you'll find that these three disciplines have more in common than you might imagine.

For starters, they're united in the belief that allergy is a complex condition that demands a complex approach. All sides say that there are no magic bullets. They believe that the first step to quality care is prevention. The second step is to use conventional medications to control the symptoms.

They also agree on a core strategy that should be used by everyone who has allergies and asthma: avoidance, or environmental control. If you're allergic to pollen, for example, they'll tell you to use air conditioners and air filters. If you're allergic to mold, they'll tell you to seal water leaks in your house or apartment. If you're allergic to your cat, they'll tell you to either banish it from your bedroom or find it another home.

Conventional, environmental, and alternative practitioners also advocate some form of therapy aimed at "desensitizing" patients to bothersome substances. They agree that desensitization—also known as immunotherapy and vaccination—is the closest thing to a "cure" for allergies.

To desensitize their patients, traditional allergists promote conventional allergy shots, while environmental-medicine doctors promote variations such as enzyme-potentiated desensitization. On the other hand, alternative practitioners promote homeopathic remedies. Although the means are different, the goal is the same: to gradually tame an overactive immune system.

Obviously, the beliefs of conventional, environmental, and alternative practitioners diverge the most when it comes to drugs. In general, conventional allergists are pro-drug, while environmental and alternative practitioners are antidrug.

Even in this arena, however, there are some similarities. Consider, for example, some of these parallel strategies.

• Allergic rhinitis (hay fever) control. Conventional remedies include synthetic antihistamines such as loratadine (Claritin), while alternative remedies include natural antihistamines such as stinging nettle.

• Asthma prevention. Conventional remedies include inhaled corticosteroids such as fluticasone (Flovent), whereas alternative remedies include steroid-containing herbs such as licorice root.

• Asthma relief. Conventional remedies include ephedrine, while alternative remedies

A Hands-On Approach That Combines the Best of Two Worlds

In Boulder, Colorado, Robert Rountree, M.D., practices an integrated allergy treatment plan that combines elements of conventional and alternative medicine. Among his techniques is prescribing licorice root to asthma patients who are using oral or injected corticosteroids.

In doses only slightly above standard, licorice root can cause high blood pressure, whereas corticosteroids can cause a multitude of problems, including blood sugar elevation.

By using a little of each, Dr. Rountree finds that he can minimize such side effects while still achieving the desired result: reduced inflammation.

"Instead of fearing an interaction, why not take advantage of the overlapping actions of these two substances?" he asks. "In essence, this is true integrative medicine. We may find that the blending of these two approaches produces a kind of medicine that is more effective—and less toxic—than either one alone."

include the herb from which ephedrine is derived: ephedra (also known as ma huang).

Collaboration Is Key to Better Medicine

Of course, there are some fundamental differences among the practitioners of the three disciplines. In fact, despite some common threads, they can't even stitch together a mutually satisfactory definition of the word *allergy*.

A large part of the problem is that they're locked into ideologies that keep them apart. They're trained to think of each other as combatants instead of collaborators.

Fortunately, not all conventional, environmental, and alternative practitioners avoid each other as scrupulously as they tell

What Conventional Docs Can Learn from Alternative Medicine

Not so long ago, conventional doctors dismissed any kind of alternative medicine with a haughty "just say no."

"I remember the 1980s and the scoffing that our traditional doctors directed at anything related to vitamin supplementation," says Renata Engler, M.D., chief of the allergy and immunology department at the Walter Reed Army Medical Center in Washington, D.C.

Now that so many people are using vitamins, herbs, and other alternative therapies, today's doctors can no longer afford to be so condescending. So the more enlightened of them are encouraging patients to tell them which supplements they're taking, and doing so in as neutral a manner as possible. "It's important to avoid judgmental labels and to make patients comfortable enough to reveal an interest in or use of complementary and alternative medicine," Dr. Engler says.

Indeed, conventional doctors are increasingly realizing that they can learn a thing or two from their alternative counterparts. Among the major areas for improvement are:

Establishing rapport with their patients. "Women tend to go to the alternative arena more than men," Dr. Engler says. "They do it for their children and their spouses. Even though there's a long cultural tradition of women as healers in the home, the traditional medical system frequently disenfranchises women

their patients to avoid pollen, mold, and animal dander. Some of them do believe that they should stop butting heads and start sharing ideas. And détente-minded doctors have started speaking out in public, even in such orthodox forums as national allergy conventions.

Some of these experts believe that a free exchange of information between the conventional and alternative medical worlds is in the best interest of patients. "Both sides have a lot to learn from each other," says Renata Engler, M.D., chief of the allergy and immunology department at the Walter Reed Army Medical Center in Washington, D.C. "We need cooperative efforts between physicians, nurses, and complementary-medicine practitioners. We must define what's useful and what's harmful. We need to send the message that if you have a good

and women's issues. So alternative medicine challenges us to reach out and take better care of women and make them feel as though they have a place in traditional medical care."

For example, by asking about any vitamin supplements their patients might be taking, conventional doctors not only learn whether the supplements are helping or hindering treatment but also begin to establish the kind of rapport that most alternative practitioners have with their patients, especially their female patients.

Treating the whole patient. "Some alternative modalities tap into what the British call *remembered wellness*, which I find to be a much more palatable term than *the placebo effect*," Dr. Engler says. "Placebo is a powerful agent. Beneficial results can be seen in 60 to 90 percent of diseases, including asthma. We need to incorporate a balanced view of humans. Each one of us is a physical, mental, and spiritual being, and all these elements are critical to healing in the 21st century."

Improving patient compliance. "I'm always stunned by the patient participation that alternative practitioners enjoy," Dr. Engler says. "We have difficulty getting patients to comply with a twice-a-day regimen. The complexity the alternative community demands of its patients is overwhelming, yet people go do it. What are they doing to get patients to participate in the process that we're not doing as well?"

idea, come to the table, and let's build an integrative medicine."

Putting It All Together

It's truly an exciting time in the world of medicine. At clinics and labs throughout the country, doctors and researchers are now working to determine the best treatments from both conventional *and* alternative medicine. To sort out what works and what doesn't, they're subjecting alternative allergy therapies to the gold standard of conventional medicine: double-blind, placebo-controlled studies.

Although their work is far from complete, they're finding that some alternative therapies—including herbalism, Traditional Chinese Medicine (TCM), and even homeopathy—might have more than a placebo effect.

Further, more of them are embracing the "hygiene hypothesis," which theorizes that allergies are largely a consequence of the oversanitized Western lifestyle. They're finding that lifestyle changes, especially in the areas of diet and exercise, can relieve allergies and reduce patients' dependence on conventional drugs.

Worldwide, some of the most exciting research into complementary and alternative

When Allergies Get Serious, Don't Go It Alone

Until now, people with allergies have had only two real choices: either subscribe to some doctor's dogma—conventional or alternative—or engage in self-experimentation with vitamins, herbs, and other self-help therapies.

Studies show that about half of people with allergies seek medical treatment, whereas the other half chart their own course.

We say that both of these approaches are outdated. Blindly following any doctor's orders can leave you feeling frustrated, powerless, and closed off from other self-help therapies that might help you become allergy-free. On the other hand, being your own guinea pig can be downright dangerous, especially if you have asthma.

A study conducted by the department of medicine at the University of California, San Francisco, found that patients who self-treated their asthma with herbs, coffee, black tea, or over-the-counter medications were up to *3½ times* more likely to end up in a hospital emergency room as were patients receiving conventional asthma treatment.

Clearly, if you have a serious allergic condition, playing with self-treatment is like playing with fire.

medicine for allergies and asthma is being conducted in countries such as Finland, Australia, and Japan. In the United States, promising studies are under way at the federally funded Center for Complementary and Alternative Medicine Research in Asthma at the University of California, Davis.

So far, no one has discovered a magic bullet for the treatment of allergies and asthma. But as researchers have learned more and more about the complex ways that nature and nurture conspire to produce environmental hypersensitivities, there's a growing consensus that conventional treatments can be combined with lifestyle interventions to create an effective allergy-treatment plan.

Proponents of this "blended," or "integrative," medicine believe that it has the potential to be greater than the sum of its parts. They believe that a complementary approach has the greatest potential to stem the burgeoning epidemic of sneezing and wheezing.

Note: To locate the natural remedies at a glance in this book, look for the ✦ icon.

Exploring the Best Alternative Therapies for Allergies

To identify the most promising alternative therapies for allergies and asthma, University of California researchers have read thousands of research papers on the use of complementary and alternative medicine. Since most of the papers did not meet the team's rigorous standards, they surveyed conventional doctors, alternative practitioners, and patients.

The researchers found that allergy patients were most likely to be interested in dietary changes and dietary supplements. So they decided to investigate vitamin C, magnesium, and about a dozen other supplements, including red grape extract, American ginseng, Siberian ginseng, goldenseal root, astragalus root, silymarin, bacopa, elderberries, shilajit, moomiyo, bovine thymus, and bovine colostrum.

In addition, they are investigating the allergy-fighting potential of foods such as yogurt, reishi and maitake mushrooms, wheat grass juice, various anti-inflammatory oils, and—attention, chocolate lovers—cocoa. Before you stock up on chocolate bars, though, consider that it might not be the chocolate itself that's helpful, but one of its many extracts.

The researchers are also evaluating mind-body therapies such as hypnosis, massage, and biofeedback.

So far, there have been some tantalizing preliminary results. For example, one small study showed that subjects who ate a cup of yogurt containing active starter cultures each day had 25 percent fewer colds and one-tenth as many allergy symptoms. This supports the hygiene hypothesis notion that probiotics, or "good" bugs, might help restore balance to our oversanitized gastrointestinal systems.

Unfortunately, there have been no announcements of any major breakthroughs. Setting up, conducting, and evaluating any given therapy in a way that can withstand the withering gaze of scientific scrutiny is a process that takes years.

Still, researchers are hopeful that some initially disappointing therapies will eventually prove to be winners. Among the most promising contenders is wheat grass juice, a pollen-rich concoction made from the tall Western grass that actors commonly chew in cowboy movies. Now a staple item at many juice bars, wheat grass juice is a rich source of antioxidants. Although initial trials have been disappointing, researchers still hope that it will prove to be a potent allergy fighter.

In general, experts believe that people with allergies and asthma shouldn't rely on any single food or supplement. They say it's healthier to adopt a varied diet rich in antioxidant foods and anti-inflammatory oils. Instead of gobbling vitamin C and vitamin

The Risks of Combining Conventional and Alternative Medicine

Just because conventional allergists are warming up to some alternative practices, that doesn't mean they buy into the whole natural-is-better philosophy.

"Natural does not mean free of side effects," cautions Renata Engler, M.D., chief of the allergy and immunology department at the Walter Reed Army Medical Center in Washington, D.C.

Alternative medicine, especially herbal medicine, can occasionally have adverse reactions. That's why Marianne Frieri, M.D., Ph.D., professor of medicine and pathology at State University of New York at Stony Brook and director of the allergy/immunology training program at Nassau University Medical Center/North Shore University Hospital, requires all her allergic patients on herbal medicines to be careful with cross-reactive seasonal pollens and take periodic liver function tests.

If you're going to integrate conventional and alternative medicine, you have to do so intelligently. In most cases, it's best to start with conventional medicine before branching out into complementary therapies. Even then, you should try complementary therapies only under the guidance of your allergist or primary care physician.

A pills, for example, people with allergies and asthma might be better off eating more broccoli because it contains a wide variety of antioxidants and other anti-inflammatory compounds.

Although alternative strategies can work wonders, experts say that the goal should be to complement conventional therapy, not replace it. Allergists are especially reluctant to stop conventional treatments in patients with asthma. It's just too serious a disease. Since uncontrolled asthma can be life-threatening, doctors argue that it must be reined in with con-

ventional treatments before complementary and alternative treatments are introduced.

In the rest of this chapter, we'll introduce you to some specific alternative healing systems and explore the most promising treatment options each offers for people with allergies. Then, in succeeding chapters, you'll see how natural, self-help measures can work synergistically with conventional medicine to make you feel better, reduce your dependence on allergy drugs, and speed you toward your goal of becoming allergy-free.

Here are some reasons to avoid treating your allergies the other way around.

- **Adverse reactions.** Herbs can cross-react with conventional drugs, cause toxic reactions, and even make your allergies worse. "In large doses, ephedra and lobelia have been linked to paralysis of the respiratory system," Dr. Engler says. "There have been reports of homeopathic remedies causing sudden wheezing or cough. And chamomile can worsen symptoms in ragweed-allergic patients."

- **Delay in getting definitive treatment.** If you have asthma, failure to control inflammation can lead to permanent lung damage. "If someone with asthma is not being treated well conventionally, they may seek out the alternative arena and fail to get the quality care that is available in our arena," Dr. Engler says.

- **Financial loss.** Since complementary and alternative treatments aren't usually covered by insurance, they can be a significant expense. And there's no guarantee that they'll work. In recent years, the field has become glutted with practitioners who advocate a wide variety of unproven and, in some cases, disproven therapies. This plethora of procedures makes it difficult for patients to sort out the wheat from the chaff, leaving them vulnerable to a cash-only cottage industry that makes the whole field look bad.

Promising Natural Approaches

Here are some alternative therapies that have undergone scientific study and may appeal even to the most conventional practitioners.

• Herbs and Spices

There are a number of herbal supplements and spices that show promise for relieving the symptoms of allergies and asthma. Here are the top contenders.

Cinnamon. Small doses of this spice can stimulate respiration in people with asthma or allergic rhinitis. Animal studies show that it can prevent a variety of allergic reactions, including some types of anaphylaxis.

Coleus forskholii. In one report, this Ayurvedic herb seemed to have a powerful bronchodilator effect with fewer side effects than conventional drugs.

Garlic. The bodacious bulb has been shown to enhance production of anti-inflammatory chemicals.

Ginkgo biloba. A controlled study of this herb demonstrated decreased asthma triggered by dust mites. It may also protect against exercise-induced asthma.

Licorice root. Not to be confused with "licorice" candy (which contains anise), this herb contains a natural steroid that reduces cough and inflammation. But if taken for longer than 2 weeks, it can cause hypertension (high blood pressure).

Saiboku-to. This Japanese asthma remedy contains 10 herbs. It has been shown to help some people with asthma get off or reduce steroids, but it has lots of side effects, including pneumonia.

Tylophora indica. Human and animal studies show that this Ayurvedic herb—also known as *Tylophora asthmatica*—is as effective as epinephrine for asthma, although it frequently causes side effects such as mouth soreness and nausea.

• Homeopathy

A decade ago, the National Institutes of Health challenged conventional researchers to compare homeopathic medicine to conventional treatments for chronic illnesses such as allergies and asthma. Unfortunately, few studies have been conducted, since most conventional researchers believe that homeopathy is pure piffle. In general, conventional doctors believe that homeopathy doesn't work because it *can't* work.

Homeopathic allergy remedies are prepared by dissolving small amounts of allergenic substances in water. The solution is then diluted until not a single molecule remains of the original allergenic substances. The resulting "remedy" is then used to desensitize patients to the allergens via its effect on the whole body through a local injection.

Although conventional doctors are skeptical of homeopathy, they acknowledge that it is becoming increasingly popular in many nations, including the United States.

Since there's little risk in taking such diluted remedies, some conventionally trained physicians are willing to entertain the notion that it might help. "I don't know why it works, but I've read several texts on the dilution theory, and it's as if you might be giving low-dose oral immunotherapy," says Marianne Frieri, M.D., Ph.D., professor of medicine and pathology at the State Univeristy of New York at Stony Brook and director of the allergy/immunology training program at the Nassau University Medical Center/North Shore University Hospital in East Meadow and Manhasset, New York. "Think about it. You use very small concentrations and alter the immune system, which is what we're doing by giving our initial injections during the buildup phase for allergen immunotherapy."

"I have lots of patients who use homeopathic remedies," says Gailen Marshall Jr., M.D., Ph.D., director of the division of allergy and clinical immunology at the University of Texas–Houston Medical School. "It seldom hurts patients, and it may help them overall. Whether or not there's any biological effect, though, I don't know."

Here are the results of some recent studies on the usefulness of homeopathy in treating allergic rhinitis and asthma.

• In California, researchers conducted a double-blind, placebo-controlled study of 32 patients with allergic rhinitis. Half were treated with a homeopathic nasal gel (Zicam Allergy Relief) containing Luffa operculata, Galphimia glauca, Histaminum hydrochloricum, and Sulfur. The other half were treated with a placebo nasal gel. (A placebo is a fake medication.) Researchers determined that the Zicam-treated group's symptoms improved 52 percent compared with a 19 percent improvement in the group treated with placebos.

• In England, researchers conducted a double-blind, placebo-controlled study of 50 patients with allergic rhinitis. Half were treated with an oral homeopathic remedy containing a dilution of dust mite, tree pollen, and cat dander. The other half were treated with placebo pills. Here's what the researchers concluded: "Compared with placebo, homeopathy provoked a clear, significant, and clinically relevant improvement in nasal inspiratory peak flow, similar to that found with topical steroids." In plain English, that means the homeopathic remedy cleared up the subjects' stuffy schnozzes as effectively as steroid sprays.

• Not all studies have shown improvement with homeopathic remedies, however. For example, researchers in Germany reviewed three double-blind, placebo-controlled trials of a total of 154 asthma patients. Half were treated with three different homeopathic remedies. The other half were treated with placebo pills.

Although two trials showed slight improvements in homeopathy-treated patients, the third trial showed no difference. The researchers concluded that there wasn't enough evidence to reliably assess the role of homeopathy in asthma treatment.

• Mind-Body Therapies

For people with allergies and asthma, stress presents a double whammy. Not only does it place the body in a state of alarm—the so-called fight-or-flight response—it also increases production of the allergy antibody immunoglobulin E (IgE), which means more sneezing and wheezing. In extreme cases, it can even increase a patient's susceptibility to the most lethal form of asthma: status asthmaticus.

As a result, conventional allergists have shown increased interest in mind-body therapies that help patients simmer down. "We've forgotten the mind-body connection," Dr. Marshall says. "Medicine is a ministry as well as a practice, in my opinion. If we don't minister to the minds of our patients as well as their physiologic systems, then we are doomed in terms of any meaningful success."

In alternative practices, the following mind-body therapies play a central role in allergy treatment.

• Acupressure
• Acupuncture
• Breathing exercises
• Chiropractic
• Guided visualization
• Hypnotherapy
• Massage
• Meditation
• Osteopathy
• Reflexology
• Yoga

The results of these therapies vary. Small-scale studies suggest modest benefits from acupuncture, breathing exercises, guided visualization, hypnosis, and massage. Some therapies, such as acupuncture for children with asthma, may produce only short-term improvements, while other therapies, such as a comprehensive yoga program for adolescents with asthma, appear to have more far-reaching effects. Still other therapies, however, such as chiropractic for children with asthma, have been found to be ineffective.

Since stress has been shown to exacerbate allergies and asthma, you'd think that standard stress-management therapies would be helpful. But California researchers were unable to find any group benefits from hypnosis or massage in the treatment of asthma. When they measured airflow, they found no objective difference between the groups that received mind-body therapies and those that didn't.

On an individual level, though, some doctors believe that mind-body therapies can make a measurable difference.

The greatest potential of such therapies

is on a psychological level. Because they feel good, these therapies encourage patients to take better care of themselves in other ways. For some patients, that might mean better compliance with a conventional asthma regimen. For others, it might mean adopting a leaner diet or a meaner exercise program. No matter how they take charge of their allergies, the simple fact that they've chosen to do so is empowering.

The more patients become involved and the more self-care they practice, the better they do, experts say. How much of that is compliance and how much is in the mind is hard to define.

And despite what laboratory instruments might say, nothing can stop the suffering like soothing human touch. A single caress can relax the muscles and mind, not to mention twitchy airways. As proof, Dr. Engler points to a successful program that teaches parents to give massages to children with asthma. The massages are administered at night, since that's when asthma attacks are most likely to strike.

"Massages are wonderful," Dr. Engler says. "What is the harm of sharing them? It reduces fear and increases connectivity—that unmeasurable quality that occurs between the caregiver and the patient."

• Traditional Chinese Medicine

Allergy medicine started in China when ancient healers discovered the wonders of ephedra. Today, ephedra is still a mainstay of TCM treatments for allergies and asthma. Doctors of oriental medicine typically combine ephedra with licorice and ginseng.

Scientists have only recently begun studying such combination remedies, at least in Western countries. The new research suggests that they may be a useful alternative to conventional medicines and cause fewer side effects.

For example, researchers from the University of Sydney in Australia studied 58 patients with allergic rhinitis. Half received a TCM formula while the other half received a placebo. At the end of the trial, the researchers concluded that the TCM formula, known as BIMIN, is effective in treating rhinitis, which makes it the first herbal medication that has been proven to be effective for this condition in a rigorous scientific trial.

Likewise, TCM remedies have shown promise for treating asthma. Researchers from the Mount Sinai School of Medicine of New York University in New York City and Johns Hopkins University School of Hygiene and Public Health in Baltimore studied the effects of two TCM formulas—Ding-Chuan-Tang (DCT) and Jia Wei San Zi Tang (modified Three Seeds Decoction, or MTSD)—on mice with asthma. They found that the formulas significantly reduced IgE antibody production and relieved the wheezy rodents' asthma. "These preliminary findings suggest that antiasthma TCM formulas may have potential for alternative or complementary treatment of allergic asthma," the researchers concluded.

• Vitamins and Minerals

Unlike alternative practitioners, conventional allergists have been slow to recommend supplements that may help treat allergies and asthma or mitigate the side effects of conventional drugs.

For example, some alternative practitioners have recommended taking extra vitamin C to prevent cataracts, a potential side effect from the long-term use of corticosteroids, says Dr. Engler.

But conventional doctors are waking up. The weight of scientific evidence now clearly shows that some supplements are especially useful for people with allergies and asthma. They include:

Calcium. Although this mineral might not have any direct benefits, Dr. Engler says that the recommended daily amount can prevent another side effect associated with long-term use of inhaled corticosteroids: osteoporosis.

Magnesium. Studies show that magnesium levels are low in people who have asthma, so magnesium supplementation has the potential to help open congested airways.

Vitamin C. In addition to preventing cataracts, this antioxidant improves lung function. People who have asthma, especially, may need more of it than those who do not, say researchers at the Center for Complementary and Alternative Medicine Research in Asthma.

PART TWO

The Allergy-Free ENVIRONMENT

Outwit
Allergy Triggers
WHEREVER YOU ARE

AT TIMES, TRYING TO COPE with allergies can feel like a struggle between you and the vast environment around you. And at first glance, the odds would seem to be stacked in the environment's favor.

For starters, the elements that set off an attack of allergic rhinitis (hay fever) or asthma, to name just two allergic ailments, are generally too small to be seen by the naked eye. Under a microscope they're grotesque: the spiderlike dust mite and its excrement, the bristled ball of pollen, the icky glob of a mold spore. But in the everyday world, they're virtually invisible as they waft into our noses and lungs and grind into our eyes and skin.

Add to the mix those wisps and droplets of irritating chemicals that you so often encounter—as well as the traces of nuts, milk, and wheat that can set off food allergies—and you may face a veritable army of hard-to-detect allergy triggers.

In addition, changing times could be encouraging the growth of even more of these allergy triggers. According to recent government research, rising amounts of carbon dioxide in the atmosphere may have doubled the amount of airborne ragweed pollen—a potent allergen—during the last several decades.

Even indoors, the odds don't get much better. The newer homes that many of us live in may put us at greater risk for allergy because they offer less ventilation, which tends to encourage the growth of mold and dust mites.

It's time to turn the odds in your favor.

Though you may not be able to see these harmful particles and tiny critters, you *can* learn to instinctively sense where they lurk—then make their hideouts inhospitable to them. You can also take simple, easy steps to bolster your defenses to protect yourself from allergen and irritant attacks.

In this section, you'll learn how to outwit allergy and asthma triggers no matter where you are.

At home: You'll cut down on your coughing, wheezing, and other symptoms when you turn your bedroom into an allergen-free oasis, learn how to cope with the animal dander from your pets, and choose safe cleaning products.

You will also learn how to choose devices and products such as air filters and dehumidifiers that efficiently make your home more allergy-proof—and avoid others that don't.

In your yard and garden: When you're outdoors, you may be driven to distraction by the countless types of mold spores and pollen as well as some of the products commonly used on lawns and gardens.

You'll breathe easier, though, when you follow advice on how to find out exactly which types of airborne allergens bother you, surround yourself with low-allergy plants and flowers, fight pests the natural way, and shield yourself with a dust mask while you're outdoors.

At work: When you head off to your job, you could be picking up far more than a paycheck. Your workplace may be exposing you to substances that can give you allergies or asthma or aggravate a condition you already have.

By protecting yourself from harmful elements at your workplace and gathering vital information about your surroundings, you can save yourself some misery—and maybe even your life.

While traveling: When you travel, your new surroundings can pose both familiar and novel threats that may be tougher to contend with because you're away from home.

But with planning, you can learn to take a detour around allergy and asthma triggers in airplanes, cruise ships, cars, hotels, the great outdoors, and other vacation surroundings.

The Allergy-Free HOME

ON THE SURFACE, your home might be so neat and tidy that you'd be proud to give your boss—or even the President—a tour of the place if he ever showed up for a surprise visit.

But if your home is anything like the typical American residence, a trained eye with a microscope might find a teeming world of allergy- and asthma-triggering particles buried in the carpet, resting on the couch, and floating through the air. Better get a hankie for Mr. President!

Don't feel bad. This isn't necessarily a reflection on your housekeeping skills. The way many homes are constructed and maintained encourages the buildup of a wide array of allergens.

Some homes are just built too well. In the late 1970s, the energy crisis led to more tightly constructed homes to cut down on air leaking in and out. Though this may have led to smaller utility bills, less ventilation keeps more allergens indoors and increases the humidity in the home. And humidity encourages the growth of two major indoor allergens: dust mites and mold spores.

On the other hand, some older buildings have seen healthier days. When residents live in homes that have had generations of wear, more and more allergens tend to build up, according to Jay Portnoy, M.D., chief of allergy, asthma, and immunology at Children's Mercy Hospitals and Clinics in Kansas City, Missouri.

Adding to this situation are a few items without which many people feel a home isn't complete: carpeting and house pets. Allergy experts frequently regard carpets as vast, persistent reservoirs that can contain billions of dust mites, which are tiny relatives of the spider, along with the allergenic feces they produce.

About 30 percent of U.S. households

have a cat, and slightly more own a dog. Furry pets shed a steady amount of lightweight, allergenic protein onto their skin and hair that then floats throughout the house. The major cat allergen comes from the sebaceous glands, which produce oil on the fur. Allergies to cats are more bothersome than allergies to dogs. Pet birds and rodents are also sources of allergens.

Rounding out the list of common allergens, particularly in densely populated urban areas, is the lowly cockroach. As if their other flaws don't make them an unwelcome enough visitor, roaches leave be-

hind a trail of allergy-triggering secretions, fecal pellets, and body parts. And if you manage to kill them, their bodies slowly decay, which can release more allergens that float through the air. In inner cities, mice occupy second place after cockroaches on the allergen list. A study from the Johns Hopkins Medical Institutions noted that there was detectable mouse allergen in at least one room (usually the kitchen) in 95 percent of the 608 homes tested.

In addition to these offenders, many of us stock our homes with products that release odors and particles—from air fresheners,

Go Duct Hunting Wisely

Cleaning out the heating and cooling ducts in our homes just seems like it would be a good idea. After all, who knows what evil substances are lurking back in the dim recesses of the ductwork, floating out into the very air we breathe?

Most likely, not too much. Though you may feel relieved and somehow safer after paying to have those ducts sucked clean, it's probably not going to do anything to improve your allergy or asthma symptoms, says Jonathan Bernstein, M.D., associate professor of medicine at the University of Cincinnati, who educates other allergists through the Allergen Control Network (ACN). The ACN is an organization of allergists committed to environmental control measures and the education of their patients.

People who watch as their ducts are cleaned see the stuff that's coming out and think "That's what I'm breathing in!"—but in fact it's not what they're breathing in, says Dr. Bernstein. It's what's sitting in their ducts.

Further, according to the Environmental Protection Agency (EPA), this ductwork tidying may set you back $450 to $1,000—money you could spend on other allergy-reduction tactics that could have bigger health benefits.

household cleaners, and perfumes to wood- and gas-burning appliances—that can irritate our airways. These can make us even more sensitive to the effects of dust, dander, and other allergens floating around.

So what's the allergic homeowner or renter to do? One approach is to rip out the carpets, send the pets packing, hose down the home with roach killer and fungicide, and order a credit card's worth of gizmos from an allergy-supply catalog.

But that's the wrong approach. We'll help you embark on the task of reducing the allergens in your home in an informed and organized fashion so that you can save time, hassle, and money.

Haste Makes Waste

During a conversation, one woman revealed to Jonathan Bernstein, M.D., associate professor of medicine at the University of Cincinnati, that she had spent hundreds of dollars on what she thought were appropriate measures to rid her home of allergens—and she didn't even know what she was allergic to.

Worst of all, some cleaners spray sterilizing chemicals into the ducts to kill bacteria and mold. These chemicals may drift through your home and cause health problems, both Dr. Bernstein and the EPA warn.

That said, sometimes you *should* get your ducts cleaned. Consider a cleaning in any of the following situations, according to the EPA.

• Vermin such as rodents or insects are thriving in the ducts.

• The ducts are blocked with debris, or you see dust blowing out of your vents.

• The cleaning company can prove that a sizable amount of mold is growing in sheet-metal ducts or other parts of your heating and cooling system. This is often the case in ducts that are damp. If you have mold growing on fiberglass ducts or fiberglass insulation lining the ducts, you should have any contaminated material removed and replaced, the EPA says.

Before you hire a duct cleaner, be sure that the company is experienced in working with systems like yours and that workers won't use sterilizing chemicals or sealants until they discuss it with you. In addition, make sure they comply with recommendations from the National Air Duct Cleaners Association and, if dealing with fiberglass components, the North American Insulation Manufacturers Association.

She's not the only one falling prey to ideas that sound better than they are. Here are a few examples.

• A major manufacturer of household cleaners recalled a brand of powder and spray designed to kill dust mites in carpets because it was triggering asthma attacks and skin irritation in hundreds of people. Ironically, it seemed to most affect people with pre-existing allergies and asthma—the crowd that has a special reason to kill mites in the first place.

• Some types of air-cleaning devices can generate ozone, which at ground level is a pollutant that can irritate your lungs.

• After hearing convincing sales pitches, homeowners may be lured into having the ductwork in their houses cleaned of dust and debris, which is a potentially expensive yet often unnecessary procedure. According to Dr. Bernstein, duct cleaning may be useful in homes with certain problems in the ducts, such as water damage or airflow restriction, but it's not recommended as a general frontline approach to reducing indoor allergens. Plus, the technicians sometimes spray the ducts with chemicals that can cause breathing problems.

The bottom line? Don't charge off on your own, blindly trying to turn your home into an allergy-free zone. "For people who suspect they have allergies, it's a much better solution to see an allergist to evaluate their allergies so that proper recommendations regarding environmental control can be made," Dr. Bernstein says.

Symptoms of indoor allergies include a stopped-up or runny nose, itchy eyes, and breathing trouble. Symptoms can also include chronic nasal stuffiness and drainage at the back of your throat, and sometimes even skin problems. These problems tend to last year-round as opposed to the seasonal misery of pollen allergies, and they're often worse in the morning.

If you think you might be allergic to something in your house, an allergist can help determine what, if anything, you're allergic to; how serious your allergies are; and what kinds of modifications to your home are likely to be worth the effort.

"Right now, the marketing of environmental-control products has overtaken the actual science," Dr. Bernstein cautions. "Establish the allergist as the environmental-control consultant, not the ads in the newspapers or the heating/ventilation/air-conditioning guy."

Where to Start to Finish Off Indoor Allergens

The reaction of the body to allergens is like its reaction to a wound that is not cleaned. If you don't remove the dirt from the wound, it won't heal. The same with allergens. If you don't remove the allergens, they can spell trouble, causing allergy and asthma symptoms. Your task is to bring the level of allergens down to where it won't trigger these problems.

"It's not a difficult thing to do, and it's not exorbitantly expensive," explains Dr. Bernstein, who founded the Internet site Stopallergy.com, which carries products and provides information, and the Allergen Control Network, which educates doctors on environmental issues.

But reducing allergens in your home *does* require you to make changes in your lifestyle and stick with them. And you'll need patience. It may take several months before you feel allergy or asthma relief, since many allergens fade away slowly once their source is removed.

In addition to any recommendations your doctor might have to help your specific needs, Dr. Bernstein offers these three general suggestions for bringing down the level of allergens in your home. We'll elaborate on all of them in the sections that follow.

Make your bed a safe haven. This is where you spend about a third of your day, burrowed deeply into sheets, blankets, and pillows atop a comfortable mattress—all of which may be saturated with dust mite allergen.

Keep your home dry. Most homes have three of the four requirements that mites need to thrive: nesting sites like carpets and mattresses, human skin cells to eat, and a comfortable temperature. The fourth variable—the humidity that gives them moisture—is often what determines whether they'll multiply in your home or not.

A recent National Institute of Environmental Health Sciences study found that about 43 million homes, or 49 percent of the houses, in America have enough dust mite allergen in the bedding to potentially cause allergies. And about 13 million of these homes have enough allergen in the bedding to trigger an asthma attack.

If you keep the relative humidity in your home between 30 to 50 percent—probably best accomplished by using an air conditioner and possibly a dehumidifier—you can help ensure that your home isn't included in those statistics.

Filter out the bad stuff. According to Dr. Bernstein, it's important to have proper filtering throughout your home to snatch up allergens. This could include a vacuum equipped with filters to keep it from spraying out allergens as fast as it sucks them up, clean and well-working filters on your furnace and air conditioner, and a freestanding air filter in your bedroom that traps airborne allergens. Filters will trap allergens from cats and dogs, although they will miss the heavier dust mites and their allergens, which do not hang about in the air.

These general steps will get you started, but the process doesn't end here. As you deal with allergens, try to remove their source whenever possible. Cleaning up the

Fascinating **fact!**

Just like a stuffy nose and wheezing can make you go batty, bats can trigger a stuffy nose and wheezing. Researchers in Argentina conducted a study examining people with allergies and asthma who lived in tall buildings and old houses in Buenos Aires. The cause of their allergy misery? Bat feces.

problems *after* they're in your environment—such as by dusting, vacuuming, and buying air filters—isn't as effective as rooting out the origin of the allergens.

For example, if you're allergic to your pet, the best option health-wise is to find another home for it. Not surprisingly, though, Dr. Bernstein has found that many people can't bear to part with this beloved member of the family.

If you can't stand the thought of losing your pet, then keeping it outside is another option. Bear in mind, though, that this strategy isn't as effective, since the allergens will still get into your house on clothing. Finally, if you can't keep your pet outside, then at least reduce the threat to your health by keeping it out of your bedroom and, if possible, having a nonallergic family member wash it regularly to minimize the allergens it disperses. (Talk to your veterinarian about how to keep your pet's skin

At a Glance: The Best Ways to Allergen-Proof Your Home

Here's a quick summary from our allergy experts of the simplest, most effective steps you can take to turn your home into an allergy-free zone.

- Each time you take a shower, make sure the bathroom is ventilated to the outside from the overhead fan or an open window.
- Vacuum at least weekly.
- Wash your indoor pets, especially cats, at least weekly, after discussing this with your vet.
- Wash your sheets and pillowcases weekly and your blankets every 3 weeks, all in water heated to at least 130°F. Wipe down or wash protective covers on your mattress and pillows monthly.
- Dust all the flat surfaces in your home, from tabletops to floors, each week with a damp cloth or mop. Wipe down window shades or wash the curtains weekly.
- Clean your kitchen weekly, wiping down the stovetop, countertop, and cupboards.
- Replace your furnace or air-conditioner filter monthly while in use or according to the manufacturer's directions.
- Wash your kids' stuffed animals in 130°F water once a month. If they can't take the stress of washing, put them in a plastic bag in the freezer for a few days each month.
- Have your fireplace and chimney professionally inspected before the heating season each year. Also have your window or wall air conditioners and fuel-burning heaters and water heaters inspected each year.

from getting too dry from the frequent washing.)

Similarly, you'll be much better off if you make your home unattractive to roaches from the start, by sealing up their entry holes and keeping the living areas free of food crumbs and water, than if you try to kill them and clean up their mess *after* they enter.

Finally, as you make your home a healthier environment, you may need to limit the amount of household cleaners and other chemicals you use that send fumes wafting through the air. As you'll read later, these chemicals can work hand in hand to aggravate your allergies and asthma.

You may want to see how effective your efforts are by using a diagnostic or detective kit that analyzes and measures levels of allergens. After you've been tested for allergies by your doctor, you may want to use the kit to see if those allergens are actually in your house. After you've made some of the changes in your home that are suggested here, you can test again to see how much reduction you've accomplished. Allergen detective kits cost about $100, and they are available from Stopallergy.com.

Read on for an overview of simple steps that you can take around the house—broken down by room or area—to reduce allergens or prevent them in the first place.

Outside the Home

As you start to hunt down sources of allergens in your home, pay close attention to the changes you can make *outside* to keep problems from cropping up on the inside.

Slam the door on roaches. Seal any crevices, holes, gaps, and cracks around the outside of your house that would give the allergen-shedding bugs the chance to slip inside your home. That includes openings around drains, in woodwork, and under doors.

Close down the roaches' watering hole. Any source of water can lure roaches into your home, since they require water to thrive. Cut off their drinks, and your home becomes less attractive to them.

Send rain down the drain. To prevent mold, you need to ensure that the rainfall and other precipitation that hits your house winds up away from it—not in it. To do so:
• Keep the gutters free of leaves, obstructions, and standing water.
• Make sure that the gutters don't leak into the eaves of your roof, where they could pour water into your walls.
• Check to see that the downspouts that siphon water from the gutters carry it away from the house, and that the landscaping in your yard is sloped so the water keeps flowing away. If it doesn't, it could wind up in your basement.

Chill out properly. If you have window or wall air conditioners, get them cleaned and serviced by a professional before the warm season begins. Be sure to keep the coils and drain pans clean and drained according to the manufacturer's instructions so that they don't store water.

Walk all over a doormat. To cut down on allergens that you track into your home from the outside, place doormats outside all the doors leading into your home and ask everyone coming inside to use them.

In addition, you can borrow a trick from *Mister Rogers' Neighborhood* and take off your "outside" shoes at the door and put on footwear worn only in the house.

Don't fill your laundry with allergens. If you hang up clothes and bedding to dry outside, they may pick up pollen and

Be Your Own Detective with a Walk-Through Home Inspection

Even though many homeowners can instinctively point to an allergen hot spot in their homes, they tend to wait for an official confirmation before they have the problem fixed, marvels Jay Portnoy, M.D., a Kansas City, Missouri, allergist who has inspected allergy-ridden homes. He is chief of allergy, asthma, and immunology at Children's Mercy Hospitals and Clinics in Kansas City.

Instead, take the initiative and use your eyes and nose to give your home a checkup. You'll want to pay particularly close attention to the following signs that point to possible mold or other allergen and irritant sources.

- Musty odors, moisture, or water stains in your basement, bathrooms, attic, and crawl spaces
- Musty odors, moisture, or water stains around air conditioners, dehumidifiers, refrigerators, carpets, or ductwork
- Carpet on concrete floors, which is especially prone to picking up moisture and allowing allergens to thrive. Also carpeting that's been damaged by heavy traffic, moisture, or pets
- Firewood in or around your home, which is a potential source of mold, bugs, fungi, and moisture
- Gutters and downspouts that are obstructed with leaves, for example, or that don't properly drain water away from your home
- Any building material that is rotting, a possible sign of moisture
- Dirty filters on your furnace or air conditioner
- Neglected humidifiers attached to furnaces or freestanding units
- Any signs of roaches, such as dead bodies, live roaches, or fecal pellets (they look like coffee grounds)

other outdoor allergens that you'll unleash indoors when you bring in the laundry. Use a clothes dryer instead, says Dr. Bernstein.

Inside the Home

The following general tips are ideal to use throughout your house, but some of them may be especially important in certain places. For example, you should keep the humidity low throughout your home, but you also need to monitor traditionally damp areas like the bathroom and basement with extra vigilance.

Keep cool and dry. Warm, damp surroundings are great—if you're a flower in a greenhouse. But if you're a person with allergies, you should keep your home cool and dry to decrease mold and dust mite growth and roach intrusions.

After an 18-month study, Larry Arlian, Ph.D., professor of biological sciences and director of the microbiology and immunology graduate program at Wright State University in Dayton, Ohio, found that levels of mites and other allergens dropped significantly in homes where the relative humidity was kept below 50 percent. To maintain this level, you may need to use your air conditioner along with a dehumidifier.

For treating the air throughout your entire home, Dr. Arlian recommends a high-efficiency dehumidifier, which can remove about 12 gallons of water a day from the air in your home. These cost about $1,000, so check with your doctor first to see whether the dehumidifier will help you enough to be worth the cost. If you need to reduce the humidity only in a damp spot, like the basement, a smaller dehumidifier should suffice.

To track the humidity level in your home, you can buy a gauge with a digital readout, called a hygrometer, for about $30. These are available at hardware stores or from allergy supply companies.

Keep a clean dehumidifier. These machines can become a breeding center for mold if you don't care for them properly. If you use a dehumidifier, be sure to empty out the water daily—or better yet, have the machine run directly into a drain if possible. Also, clean it regularly according to the directions supplied by the manufacturer.

If you must have carpets, think small. Obviously, hardwood, tile, or linoleum floors are ideal for people with allergies, but if you still feel the need for a soft surface in places, lay out a few washable throw rugs. Just be sure to wash them regularly in water heated to at least 130°F. This kills dust mites and washes out the allergens they produce, Dr. Arlian says. Anything cooler won't do the trick. (To find out how to check the temperature of your water, see "What's the Temperature of Your Wash Water?" on page 82.)

Researchers in Australia found that eucalyptus oil added to the laundry will kill mites. The downside is that your clothes will smell like eucalyptus for a few days, says Dr. Arlian. The researchers suggest the following eucalyptus wash once a year: In a small, lidded jar, add one part dishwashing detergent to three to five parts eucalyptus oil. Shake well. If the detergent won't dissolve, you need to try a different detergent. If it does dissolve, add a teaspoon of this mixture to a glass of water; the resulting milky solution should remain opaque for at least 10 minutes. If your detergent passed these tests, mix one part detergent in four parts eucalyptus oil. Place your bedding in the washing machine and fill it with water. Add the eucalyptus oil and detergent mix to the water and allow to soak for 30 minutes to an hour. Then go through the regular washing cycle.

Although there are no studies to show the effectiveness of grapefruit seed extract (GSE), some allergists suggest that 30 drops of GSE added to a load of wash may help kill dust mites. GSE is available in many health food stores.

Say goodbye to stuff that's not dry. If any carpeting in your home gets wet—from a flood or a burst pipe, for example—thoroughly clean and dry it within 24 hours. If you can't do this, you should remove the carpeting, since mold is likely to take hold of the material and stubbornly defy your best efforts to get rid of it.

Also toss out drapes, stuffed toys, ceiling tiles, and upholstered furniture if they get soaked and you can't immediately get them cleaned and dry. If items with hard-to-clean spots like mattresses, straw baskets, or wicker furniture get soaked, get rid of them as well.

Vacuum, vacuum, vacuum. All carpets trap dust, and your wall-to-wall carpet will slowly increase in weight as time goes by

What's the Temperature of Your Wash Water?

Dust mites on washable fabrics will die if the material is washed in water that is at least 130°F. If you're not sure if your washing machine is mustering up 130°F water, run a load of clothes on the hot-water cycle and use a meat thermometer to check the temperature of the water. To do this, interrupt your wash cycle by lifting the lid after your washer has filled. Be sure the agitator has stopped moving. Keeping your hand out of the water, place the meat thermometer's probe in the water until the temperature indicator stops rising.

If you have children in the house and have set your hot-water temperature below 130°F to keep them from getting scalded, take your bedding, throw rugs, or other items to a laundry facility with sufficiently hot water.

and it collects more material. Deep inside the lush jungle of the carpet, hordes of dust mites can congregate, causing you big allergy problems.

The mite population and the allergens they produce are so entrenched in the depths of the carpet that you're not going to put much of a dent in their numbers even with extended vacuuming. A vacuum cleaner just removes those on the surface or very near the surface. But when you combine regular vacuuming with low humidity in your home and other precautions, the allergy levels in your household will decline— possibly low enough so that they won't trigger your symptoms, Dr. Arlian says.

If parting with your carpet isn't an option, vacuum it at least once a week, suggests Dr. Bernstein, or let a family member or friend who doesn't have allergies do it. A vacuum that has a special double-lined bag, a HEPA (high-efficiency particulate air) filter, or a combination of both will trap more of the allergens that it lifts out of the carpet. Finally, you should wear a dust mask while vacuuming, or leave the room while someone else is doing the chore.

Go easy on the mite killers. In the laboratory, some chemicals show promise in reducing the number of dust mites and related allergens in carpets. Benzyl benzoate, for instance, kills the critters, and tannic acid breaks down the proteins they leave behind.

But because the conditions in your home might be much different from those in the laboratory, these products may not be very effective on your carpet, warns Dr. Arlian and other allergen researchers. For example, the ingredients might not be able to reach down into the carpet where they're needed the most, or the length of time you have to leave the chemicals in the carpet can be inconvenient.

Make your home a no-smoking zone. "The smoking issue, I think, is relatively easy," says Anthony Rooklin, M.D., an allergist and clinical associate professor of pediatrics at Thomas Jefferson University in Philadelphia. "Smoke is a significant irritant. The less smoke that one is exposed to, the less irritant."

Secondhand smoke can trigger an asthma attack and aggravate symptoms in people with allergies. In addition, tobacco smoke has been shown to make asthma worse in preschool children—and may even cause it.

Ventilate your house . . . maybe. If humidity isn't a problem in your area, you may want to open your windows and doors and flip on window or attic fans to air out your house and help blow away pollution and allergens. Just make sure when you open the windows that you don't violate the ever-important guideline of keeping your home's humidity below 50 percent.

If you're allergic to pollen that might come in through the open window, you can buy a pollen-proof screen to keep the stuff out of your home. These are available through allergy supply companies such as Allergy Control Products, National Allergy

Supply, Stopallergy.com, Allergy Solutions, and others.

Don't operate a chemical storehouse. Many products around the household, like paints, varnishes, waxes, fuels, cleaners, disinfectants, and hobby supplies, contain organic chemicals. Even if the containers are closed, they can release some pollution into your home that can irritate your lungs and throat.

Don't keep old, unnecessary chemicals around the house. If you no longer need them, dispose of them according to the laws in your area. If you need a product only occasionally, just buy as much as you'll need right away.

Run a low-odor household. Even if they smell good, use caution with products in your home that give off smelly fumes—or avoid them outright. These include aerosols, paints, perfumes, cleaners, candles, and air fresheners. They may irritate your airways and make your allergies and asthma worse. If a product bothers you, stop using it and replace it with an unscented alternative.

Dust you must. Clean the hard surfaces and shiny floors in your home weekly with treated dust rags, damp mops, or rags. Don't use a dry cloth or a feather duster, since you'll just fling the allergens in the dust back into the air.

Decorate sparingly. Ceramic figurines, stuffed animals, wicker baskets, and dried flowers may help you express your personality, but they also collect dust. Use them as sparsely as possible.

Keep your filters clean. Regularly clean or replace the filters on your furnace and air conditioners according to the manufacturers' instructions. Generally, when they're in use, you'll need to replace them (or clean them if they are the reusable type) monthly.

Don't drown your plants. Some researchers and doctors recommend houseplants as a way to clean pollutants out of your indoor air, though just how much practical value they have on a home-by-home basis is still unknown. If you do keep plants in the house, be sure not to overwater them, as the damp soil may encourage allergens. A layer of pea gravel will help reduce evaporation from the soil. Less evaporation means that less mold and bacteria from the soil can become airborne, says Gabriella Kusko, an environmental health specialist in the allergy, asthma, and immunology section at Children's Mercy Hospital in Kansas City, Missouri. Pea gravel is available at plant nurseries and garden centers.

Borrow a nose. "People are the best air-quality monitors of them all," Dr. Portnoy says. "If you walk into a house and smell mold, there's a problem."

Unfortunately, we often become used to a musty scent in our own homes and can't smell it, he says. After you've been away from your home for a while, give it a critical smell for a musty odor when you return—or ask someone else to walk through and give you an opinion.

The Bedrooms

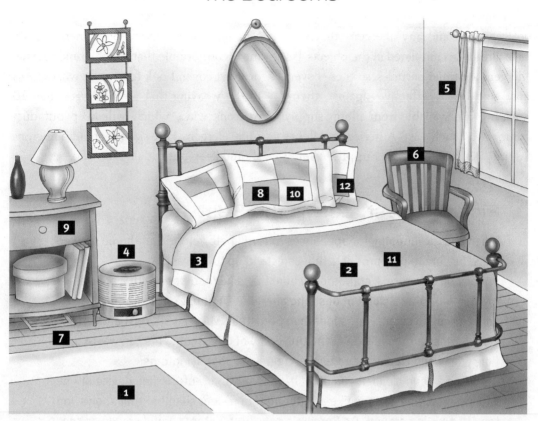

You and your family probably spend about one-third of the day in your bedrooms, bundled up in sheets, pillows, and other bedding that can hold a rich stew of allergens. That's why many experts recommend that when you're allergy-proofing your home, you make your earliest and most extensive efforts in the bedrooms.

1. Keep your pets out. If you're allergic to your pet but can't bear to part with it or keep it outside, at least keep it out of your bedroom and other areas of the house where you spend a lot of time.

Don't expect this to solve your problems, though. Even if you restrict your pets to certain rooms, the allergens they produce will float throughout your house.

2. Encase your sleeping place. Your mattress is a dust mite's dream home. It is soft and warm, retains moisture, and is full of your cast-off skin flakes for mites to munch on. Other allergens, like those from pets, also tend to accumulate in your mattress.

To reduce your exposure to allergens, slip allergen-proof encasings over your mattress, box spring, and pillows, Dr. Arlian suggests.

These keep new dust mites and their output from entering your bed and form a barrier between you and any allergens that may have already accumulated in the objects. Pet allergens are tinier particles, so these covers may not be as effective against them. Encasings are available from allergy supply companies such as American Allergy Supply, National Allergy Supply, Allergy Control Products, and Stopallergy.com.

You can find effective fabriclike encasings that allow air to flow through them and are more comfortable than a hot, crinkly plastic or vinyl cover. Look for a style with spaces in the weaving that are no larger than 10 microns wide, which will keep out dust mite allergens. Pore sizes of about 6 microns should keep out cat allergen, too.

Pick the Best, Leave the Rest

When you go shopping for appliances that will help you rid your home of allergens, be sure to pick products that can stand up to the task.

Vacuum cleaners. A standard vacuum that's not equipped with a special bag or filter will spray a cloud of dust and allergens right back out into the area you're trying to clean, warns Jonathan Bernstein, M.D., an allergist and associate professor of medicine at the University of Cincinnati. This can waste the time you spend cleaning and further aggravate your symptoms.

To find a good cleaner, you don't have to buy a top-of-the-line device or one with eye-catching options like a water filter or a clear chamber that shows you the dirt whirling around, Dr. Bernstein says. But neither should you go as cheap as you can—these might not have enough suction or be built for durability.

When *Consumer Reports* tested vacuums in May 2000, seven of the nine upright vacuums that won the highest marks from the magazine were in the $190 to $300 range, and all of them were dubbed very good to excellent in terms of the minimal amount of dust they blew out. Uprights tend to do better on carpets, while canister vacuums perform better on bare floors.

Try vacuums with HEPA (high-efficiency particulate air) filters or electrostatic filters that screen allergens out of the air before they blow back out of the vacuum, recommends Dr. Bernstein. And instead of using a regular bag in the device, buy a double-lined bag to cut down on the dust that even gets to the filter.

Air cleaners. If you decide to buy a freestanding air cleaner to put in a room, go for one with a HEPA filter or an electrostatic filter, Dr. Bernstein recommends. These are known as mechanical filters. The material in the HEPA filter is so small

3. Clean your sheets with lots of heat. Wash your bedding in water heated to at least 130°F; this kills dust mites and washes out the allergens they produce, Dr. Arlian says. Wash your sheets and pillowcases weekly, wash your blankets every 3 weeks, and wipe down or wash protective covers monthly.

If you have children in the house and have set your hot-water temperature below 130°F to keep them from getting scalded, take your bedding to a laundry facility with sufficiently hot water.

4. Run your air through a filter. A freestanding air filter in your bedroom may help you breathe easier, depending on a few key variables. Cat and dog allergens are relatively light and are able to stay aloft for sev-

that it traps particles. The electrostatic filter creates static electric charges as the air passes through it, and the charges attract and trap the particles. These filters trap ions but do not emit ions.

Don't confuse these with an electronic filter or ion generator, which may emit ozone, a gas that can irritate your lungs and cause other lung problems, says Dr. Bernstein. These are electronic devices, not mechanical, and they emit ions. Ion generators can also make particles in the air cling to walls and furniture, soiling them. Ion generators produce ozone. The ozone chemically changes gases that have an odor so that they no longer smell, but the gases are still present and can cause harm.

The Environmental Protection Agency says that at levels that don't exceed public health standards, ozone is not effective at controlling indoor air pollution. There are no published studies to show that ion generators are effective in reducing allergen levels or killing mites, says Larry Arlian, Ph.D., professor of biological sciences and director of the microbiology and immunology graduate program at Wright State University in Dayton, Ohio.

When you're choosing a specific brand and type, keep these factors in mind.

- The product's speed in processing the air. Be sure to match the capacity of the unit to the size of the room where you'll be using it. The more frequently it can process all the air in the room, the better.
- Its efficiency at removing particles from the air.
- The sound level it makes. Some can be distractingly noisy.
- The cost of replacement filters, and how often you should change them.

eral hours, so an air filter can be useful if you're allergic to these troublemakers. (Remember, though, that the filter will be most effective if the source of the allergens is completely removed from the house.)

On the other hand, if you're allergic to dust mites only, air filters probably won't help you much. Dust mite allergens are heavy, so they hang in the air only a few minutes after they're jostled from their hiding places. Thus, they're not floating around for the filter to draw them in.

HEPA filters are the most efficient. They grab more than 99 percent of particles as small as 0.3 micron, which is about one-third the size of a particle of tobacco smoke.

When you use an air filter in your room, remember to always close doors that lead to other rooms so the machine won't be over-burdened with too much air to clean.

5. Banish the blinds. Avoid venetian blinds, which can harbor hard-to-reach dust. Instead, hang curtains that you can wash weekly in 130°F water or vinyl window shades that you can wipe down each week.

6. Steer clear of soft seats. Don't keep upholstered furniture in your bedroom. Instead, use wooden or metal chairs that can be wiped down to remove dust.

7. Filter your vent. To filter dust out of the air, place a vent filter under the plate that covers the heating and cooling vent in your bedroom. Be sure to change it regularly.

Just what effect these filters will have on reducing allergens or improving symptoms is unknown, Dr. Bernstein says, but they're inexpensive and don't significantly hamper the airflow from the vent. Vent filters are available from allergy-care catalogs such as Allergy Solutions, Walter Drake, Practica, WEB Products, or Comfortliving.

8. Pick your pillows and comforters wisely. Doctors traditionally have told people with asthma not to use feather pillows, as bird feathers can provide a home for dust mites. That advice, however, may be wrong. Studies found that dust mite levels were higher on pillows with synthetic stuffing than on feather pillows, maybe because feather pillows have more tightly woven coverings to keep the feathers in, which also keeps mites out. This issue needs further study. For now, experts say that a synthetic pillow with an allergy encasing is just as effective as a feather pillow.

Most sources still recommend that you use pillows and comforters stuffed with synthetic fiber, like Dacron. Whether you choose feathers or synthetic stuffing, if you're allergic to mites, put your pillows and comforters in special allergen-proof pillowcases and duvets. Allergy-proof encasings for mattresses or pillows are sold by Allergy Solutions, Stopallergy.com, Allergy Store, Tools for Living, and Janice's.

9. Stow your gewgaws away. Books, CDs, stuffed animals, and other knickknacks may give a bedroom charm, but they also gather dust and the allergens hidden in it. Keep all these items in drawers or closed cabinets. This will make it easier to keep the bedroom free of dust.

10. Wash away the pollen. During the time of year when plants are unleashing pollen, wash your hands whenever you come inside to keep from spreading pollen indoors. If you're allergic, wash your hair before you go to bed to keep pollen off your pillow.

11. Debunk the mites. If your kids sleep on bunk beds, the child on the bottom bed might be breathing in a double dose of allergens from both beds. Consider either trading in the bunk for two regular beds or encasing both beds in allergen-proof covers and following the previously men-

Clean Your Home Naturally

If the odors from household cleaners and other products irritate your airways, you can experiment with unscented versions or clean up with the following natural alternatives, says Gabriella Kusko, an environmental health specialist in the allergy, asthma, and immunology section at Children's Mercy Hospital in Kansas City, Missouri. Ridding homes of chemicals also reduces the chances of accidental poisonings. Ten percent of poisonings are attributed to cleaning substances.

Some people may find that they are sensitive to a few of these products, so use them cautiously at first.

Instead of . . .	Try . . .
Disinfectant	A solution of 1½ cups of borax in a gallon of hot water, or 10 drops of grapefruit seed extract in a gallon of warm water
Drain cleaner	½ cup of baking soda poured down the drain, followed by ¼ cup of vinegar and ½ cup of salt. Let it bubble for 15 minutes, then carefully pour hot (not boiling) water down the drain. Be sure to cover your face and hands.
Fabric softener	¼ cup of vinegar added to the rinse water
Furniture polish	2 tablespoons of olive oil mixed with 1 tablespoon of vinegar and poured into a quart of warm water. Keep it in a spray bottle. When you use it, heat the bottle in a bucket of warm water to help the solution work better, then spray it onto a polishing cloth and use it on the furniture. Apply to a small test area first.
Glass cleaner	½ cup of vinegar mixed with 1 gallon of warm water. Fill a pump spray bottle and use on the windows and other glass surfaces.
Laundry whitener	Borax
Scouring powder	Baking soda on a sponge
Stain remover	Hydrogen peroxide, sea salt, or lemon juice (test a hidden area first for colorfastness)
Toilet bowl cleaner	1 cup of borax and ¼ cup of vinegar or lemon juice poured into the bowl. Let it sit for 2 hours and scrub with a brush.

tioned guidelines on regularly washing the bedding.

12. Give Teddy a bath. If stuffed animals are going to remain residents of your kids' bedrooms, wash them in water heated to at least 130°F once a month (the stuffed animals, of course, not the kids). You can find specially made critters that withstand the wear and tear of frequent washing in allergy-care catalogs.

An alternative is to put the stuffed animals in plastic bags and place them in the freezer for a few days each month, Dr. Arlian says. This won't clean off the existing allergens, but it will kill off the current crop of dust mites.

The Kitchen and Dining Room

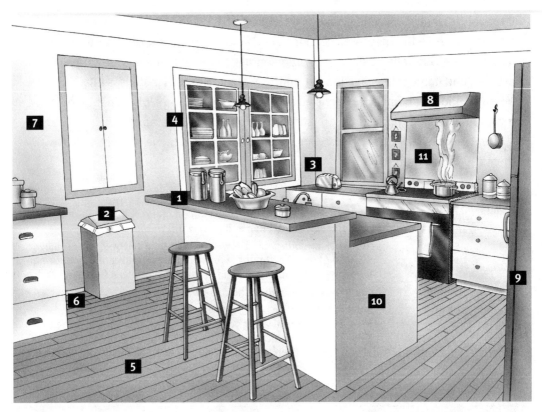

Of all the rooms in your house, the kitchen is where cockroach allergens—that unappetizing mixture of debris, like roach saliva, excrement, and body parts—are most commonly found. This isn't the nicest thing to think about as you prepare a meal, but it does show you the importance of taking steps to keep from attracting the bugs.

Also, as you make your kitchen healthier,

keep an eye out for mold sources and irritating chemicals.

1. Roach-proof your food. When you're feeling hunger pangs, you'll likely head for your kitchen—and so will any roaches residing in your home. Make sure that you store your food in sealed, airtight containers so it won't attract roaches, and don't leave leftovers lying out in the open. This goes for your pets' food, too: Put away their food dishes when they're finished eating.

It's much better to keep roaches out of your home in the first place than to kill them off once they've arrived, Dr. Bernstein says. As those dead roaches decompose into dust, they'll add more allergens to your home.

2. Put a lid on your trash. Where you see trash, roaches see a feast. Be sure you use a garbage can with a lid, and dispose of trash regularly. The same goes for your recycling bin.

3. Get crumbs where they hide. Your crumbs are a roach's dinner. Regularly clean under stoves, refrigerators, toasters, and other places where crumbs can gather.

4. Don't let dishes get crusty. Wash your dishes in hot, soapy water soon after you use them.

5. Scrub those floors and cupboards. Mop the kitchen floor and wipe down the countertops, stove top, cupboards, and other surfaces at least once a week. Also, don't forget about your dining room floor. If someone around your table has a habit of dispersing bits of food onto the floor—that lima bean casserole you tried to feed your 3-year-old, for example—be sure to sweep or vacuum these away after the meal. Roaches have no qualms about eating off the floor.

6. Battle roaches with smarts. Before you or an exterminator starts spraying pesticides to kill roaches, try boric acid and poison baits. Boric acid is a white powder that's odorless and not very toxic to people and pets. But it's extremely fatal to roaches when they crawl over it and then clean it off their legs and antennae. Pick up boric acid in a squeeze bottle with a narrow applicator tip, shake it, and puff out a very light dusting—roaches won't walk through a big pile of it—under sinks, the refrigerator and dishwasher, and other roach hangouts. The thin layer should be barely visible. Just be sure to keep it off the countertops or any spot where food is prepared. Avoid breathing the dust, wash thoroughly after handling, and read all label cautions.

Poison bait trays are also a good choice for roach control, since they're essentially odorless and the poison is in a child-resistant plastic container so you and your family aren't exposed to it. The roach will eat the poison and carry it back to the nest, where it will kill more roaches. Place the bait in spots where the floor meets the wall under sinks, dishwashers, stoves, and refrigerators. Bait traps said to work well are Max Force bait traps, Raid, Raidmax, Roach Motel, and Biopath.

7. Call in the pros. If you've done all of the above and still can't rid your home of roaches, it may necessary to call in an exterminator. To minimize your exposure to chemicals, ask the exterminator to spray only in infested areas, and gather up your pets and family and get out of the house during the spraying. Make sure to air out your home afterward.

8. Be a fan of your fan. Moisture from bubbling pots on your stove and steamy exhalations from your dishwasher encourage mold growth, dust mites, and roaches. Be sure to use the exhaust fan in your kitchen to suck away humidity when moisture starts rising in your kitchen. Ideally, this exhaust fan—and the one in your bathroom—will blow outside, not into the attic.

9. Avoid the cold mold. Nasty mold, which may look like a black goo, can grow on the rubber seal around refrigerator and freezer doors. Be sure to clean it off if you spot it. And if your refrigerator has drip pans, clean them regularly, too.

10. Choose your cleaners wisely. Your kitchen gives you another opportunity to choose unscented or nontoxic household cleaners. Stop using any product that causes tightness in your chest, coughing, a burning or runny nose, or other allergy symptoms, cautions Susanna Von Essen, M.P.H., M.D., associate professor of pulmonary and critical care medicine at the University of Nebraska Medical Center in Omaha. Take special care with spray-on oven cleaner, which often can cause these kinds of problems, she says.

Baking soda, an abrasive pad, and some good ol' elbow grease is the safest cleaner for ovens, says Kusko.

11. Cook your food, don't gas it. Gas stoves and ranges can release into your home carbon monoxide, nitrogen dioxide, and other pollutants that can irritate your respiratory system. If you have a gas appliance, use the exhaust fan while cooking. If the flames in the burners start burning with yellow tips instead of blue—signaling inefficient combustion—have a technician from your gas company adjust them. Also, never use the gas stove to heat your home.

The Living Room

Your living room should be a place where you can relax and breathe easily—not where you have to worry about irritating allergens in the air. Here's how to make sure your family room is family-friendly.

Keep your fireplace in place. In addition to generating carbon monoxide, an odorless gas that can be fatal in high levels, fireplaces and woodstoves can also produce nitrogen dioxide and airborne particles. Nitrogen dioxide can irritate your eyes, nose, and throat and cause shortness of breath, and the tiny particles can further irritate your lungs.

If you have a woodstove, make sure that the doors are tight-fitting. Burn only aged or dried wood, and never set fire to chemically treated wood. Open your fireplace's flue when you're using it, and have the flue and chimney inspected annually for obstructions, cracks, excess creosote, damage, or signs that smoke is blowing back into your home. Finally, make sure that you have properly working smoke and carbon monoxide detectors in your home.

The Bathroom, Laundry Room, and Closets

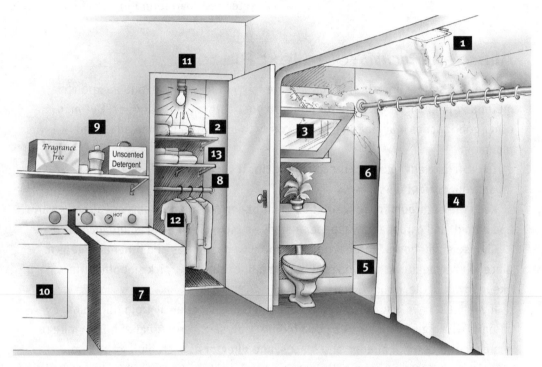

The main allergen-reducing tactics in the bathroom are avoiding dampness and minimizing mold growth.

1. Turn on the fan. Taking a shower or bath puts moisture into the air and condensation on surfaces, encouraging a range of allergens. To help prevent this, flip on the exhaust fan before you turn on the water.

2. Harvest piles of damp stuff. Don't let damp clothing and towels accumulate. Launder them to discourage mold growth.

3. Pick a natural freshener. If you need to rid the room of odors, open a window or turn on the exhaust fan instead of spraying chemical air fresheners. These can release harmful gases into the air.

4. Bring down the curtain on mold. Shower curtains can make an excellent hangout for mold. If you notice growth on your shower curtain, replace the curtain, clean it in the washing machine on a hot-water cycle with a cup of bleach, or scrub it with an irritant-free household cleaner and rinse well.

5. Bleach the mold away. If you find mold on a hard surface, and the odor of bleach doesn't irritate your airways, scrub the mold away with a solution of 1 part bleach to 10 parts water.

6. Be the squeegee man. Use a small squeegee to remove water from shower walls and the floor of the shower or tub after every use.

You would think that with all of the hot water and soap found in a laundry room, it

Allergen-Proof Your Next Place

Most of the suggestions in this chapter are fairly quick, simple, and inexpensive methods of making your home friendlier to your asthma and allergies. But many other good tactics may be too large or costly to use without some advanced planning.

You can take advantage of the following tips if you ever build a new home or remodel your current one.

Keep the bathroom free of carpet and wallpaper. Most bathrooms are already warm and humid, and carpet and wallpaper just give mold a hiding spot where it can thrive.

Choose shiny floors. Carpets trap dirt and give dust mites and other allergens a place to accumulate. When you're choosing a floor covering, pick smooth surfaces, like hardwood, tile, or linoleum.

If you must have wall-to-wall carpeting in a room, steer away from thick, shaggy carpets, which give dust mites a good hiding spot, says Larry Arlian, Ph.D., a mite researcher, professor of biological sciences, and director of microbiology and immunology graduate program at Wright State University in Dayton, Ohio. Instead, pick a low-pile, less-dense carpet—like the kind you might see in the lobby of a hotel. You'll be able to vacuum it more effectively. And avoid laying carpet on a concrete floor. These are especially prone to growing damp easily, letting mold take hold.

Choose low-gas ingredients. Pick types of wallpaper, paints, and other building materials that put off fewer gases into your indoor air.

Knock on wood. Pressed-wood products, like those you might find in cabinets, furniture, or mobile-home furniture, may contain formaldehyde, which can waft out of the wood as an irritating gas. Before you buy any of these items, ask about the formaldehyde content. And if you can, choose types that are sealed with a polyurethane or other waterproof sealant since this will cut down on the gas released.

would be the last place that you'd need to worry about allergens. But you had better tread carefully: The chemicals found in fabric softeners and permanent-press clothes can act as irritants if you have a sensitivity to them. Fortunately, a washing machine full of hot water is one of your best defenses against allergens throughout your home.

7. Take your washer's temperature. If you're not sure if your washing machine is mustering up 130°F water (necessary for killing dust mites), run a load of clothes on the hot-water cycle and use a meat thermometer to check the temperature. (See "What's the Temperature of Your Wash Water?" on page 82.)

8. Wash permanent-press clothes before you wear them. Permanent-press clothes are treated with formaldehyde at the factory to help keep them wrinkle-free, and some of the chemical can float out of the clothes as an irritating gas. A single article of clothing is unlikely to cause you trouble, Dr. Rooklin says, but if it does, wash clothing when you bring it home so that it will release fewer chemicals for you to breathe.

For the same reason, you may want to avoid ironing permanent-press clothes. Have someone who is not sensitive to formaldehyde press them for you.

9. Opt for smell-free products. If chemical odors bother you, be sure to choose unscented detergents and fabric softeners.

10. Be sure the clothes dryer blows outside. This one's pretty straightforward: Your dryer should be vented to blow the mois-

ture from your wet clothes outside your home and not anywhere inside it.

Even though they are a relatively small part of your house, you shouldn't forget the closets when you're embarking on your quest to ferret out allergens.

11. Leave the light on. Because mold thrives in damp, dark places, you should try to leave the lights on in your closets, when practical. This helps to remove air moisture and keep the spores at bay. Also, periodically leave closet doors open to let fresh air circulate.

12. Air out dry-cleaned clothes. Since the chemicals used to dry-clean your clothes may release gases after they leave the cleaner's, let clothes air out before you bring them inside and hang them in your closet. If you repeatedly notice a strong chemical odor in your clothes when you pick them up, alert your dry cleaner. If the smell persists, try taking your clothes to a different cleaner. Finally, if another way to clean your clothes is acceptable, like washing by hand, use it.

13. Use wire shelves. Wire shelves in your closet will allow better ventilation and collect less dust than wood shelves.

The Basement

As with the bathroom, your main concern in the basement should be keeping it dry so it doesn't encourage mold growth.

Ventilate. Make sure that plenty of warm,

dry air circulates through your basement to make it less mold-friendly.

Dehumidify. Your basement may be the spot in your home that most needs a dehumidifier. If so, keep the appliance well-cleaned and remove the water every day.

Stop the drips and leaks. If you notice water leaking from pipes or seeping into your home from outside, get the problem fixed right away.

Don't run a mold farm. People often store items in their basements and forget about them, leaving a rich spot for mold to grow and spread, says Dr. Portnoy. Avoid storing your clothes, books, papers, and other stuff in damp areas. Periodically check the items you do have tucked away to make sure they're not growing moldy. If porous items like wicker or upholstered furniture start sprouting mold, throw them out. Keep in mind that it's very hard to root out the problem once it has started.

Be the Allergy-Free Detective

How many potential allergy-provoking problems can you spot in this garage and workshop?

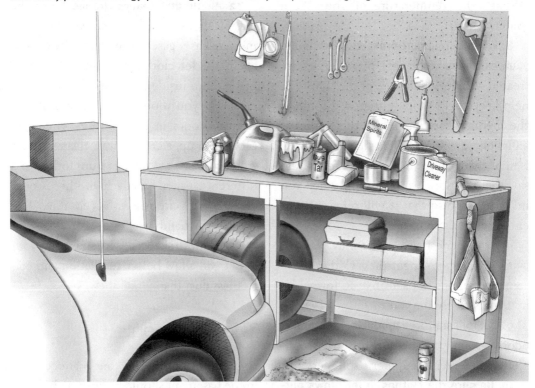

1. moldy rags on floor; 2. old chemicals stored on table; 3. paint can not closed tightly; 4. car engine shouldn't be left running in garage; 5. room should have a window or exhaust fan; 6. tools should be cleaned outside or in an area with good ventilation

The Crawl Space

Don't forget to check the crawl space of your home; it can be a source of mold.

Laminate it. If you have a crawl space under your home, cover the dirt with plastic sheeting to keep moisture out of the house. Make sure that plenty of fresh air is flowing through the area, and use your nose to check for a musty odor.

The Garage

If you live in a house with an attached garage, be aware that about 30 percent of the fresh air in your home enters through it, Dr. Portnoy says. So keep it as clean of allergens and irritants as you can.

Start your engines—outside. A running vehicle in your garage can send deadly carbon monoxide wafting through your home, which can be fatal to anyone inside if the level of the gas gets high enough, Dr. Von Essen says. So don't leave any gas-burning motor running in the garage. Carbon monoxide poisoning can happen even if you leave the garage door open when the car is running.

Ditch your damp possessions. If you store household items in your garage, be sure they stay dry and mold-free. If porous or hard-to-clean items get damp and moldy, pitch them.

Store chemicals safely. Instead of leaving unneeded chemical products in your garage, buy only what you'll use quickly, and get rid of old, unwanted products in a legal, responsible manner. Check with your municipality to find out the date of the next household hazardous waste collection.

The Hobby Room or Workshop

Your hobby should be fun—not irritating to your respiratory tract. Check out the following safety tips for your workshop or hobby room.

Be cautious with chemicals. Chemicals in solvents, paint, glue, and epoxy can release irritating and cell-damaging gases. Open a window or turn on an exhaust fan when you use these products, and reseal the containers tightly when you're finished. In addition, clean your messy tools outside.

Be extra cautious with methylene chloride. Aside from causing cancer in animals and being a suspected human carcinogen, this ingredient, which is found in paint strippers, adhesive removers, and spray paints, turns into carbon monoxide in your body. Be sure to get as much ventilation as possible when using this chemical, and don't get it on your bare skin, Dr. Von Essen warns.

The
Allergy-Free **YARD**

IF THE PLANTS filling the yards, neighborhoods, and open spaces across the countryside could uproot themselves during breeding season and go searching for a mate, people with allergies would be spared a major source of misery.

But these trees, weeds, flowers, and grasses are stuck firmly in one place, and when they feel the urge to procreate, they're unable to personally meet to share their genetic material. So seed-bearing plants use a method they *can* perform magnificently, from the lowly weed to the proud oak: Male plants make a contribution in the form of pollen and let it sail out into the world, hopefully to land on a female plant of the same species.

Since this is such a hit-or-miss manner of reproducing, some plants tilt the odds in their favor by producing copious amounts of pollen, which can float away on the wind for miles. But all too often, one of us hapless

humans gets in the way. On a warm, sunny day, we might inhale the lush aroma of spring just as a hodgepodge of invisible pollen drifts by. Our breath catches it. And instead of landing on an awaiting plant, the pollen vanishes into the dark recesses of our noses.

If you aren't allergic to a particular type of pollen, you probably won't ever know when you've inhaled it. But if you are, you may soon burst into a blossoming bouquet of sneezes, wheezes, and coughs.

Don't grab a hoe and take revenge on the nearest flower just yet, though, since not all plants are harmful to the allergy-prone. Nor are they the only source of outdoor allergy triggers. Mold spores, which grow readily and abundantly outside from coast to coast, are also a common cause of allergic reactions.

Considering the sheer magnitude of all the pollen-making plants in the world and the hiding spots for mold, we have no chance of completely keeping these allergens out of our lives. After all, there is always the neighbor's lawn, with its unmowed areas of overgrown weeds, or the grove of trees a mile away.

You can—and should—however, take steps to minimize the sources of pollen and mold in your yard. Since these can attack you repeatedly at close range, their allergy-triggering effects tend to be more powerful than the ones caused by faraway sources.

"If you're in close proximity to an allergen, you're going to get more of it. The less you're exposed, however, the better off you are," says Warren V. Filley, M.D., of Oklahoma City, a board-certified allergist, clinical professor of internal medicine at the University of Oklahoma Health Sciences Center, and former president of the Oklahoma Horticultural Society.

While you're reducing allergens in your surroundings, you should also bolster your own defenses to protect yourself from any remaining problems that could cause a sneezing or wheezing attack.

First, though, we need to understand how these tiny allergy triggers travel and how they interact with your body.

The Birds and the Bees of the Flowers and the Trees

Each time a pair of humans brings a baby into the world, the journey from the couple's first introduction to creating a child follows a completely unique version of "boy meets girl."

Similarly, most of the plants surrounding us connect and reproduce in ways that are a rich variation on a similar theme, according to David Bradshaw, Ph.D., professor of horticulture at Clemson University in South Carolina. (Some plants, such as moss, reproduce on their own, or *asexually*, which does not concern us here. We'll be talking only about types that share pollen to reproduce.) How exactly these plants go about making their offspring helps determine how likely they are to trigger your allergies.

In some types of plants, one individual may be male, bearing pollen-making structures called anthers, while another individual is female, bearing pollen collectors called stigmas, along with ovaries containing eggs that must interact with the pollen to form seeds.

When pollen lands on a female flower's stigma, it will release some proteins and enzymes that identify what type of pollen it is. If the recipient is the right species, a little pollen tube will grow down to the ovary.

An example of a species with male or fe-

Fascinating fact!

Looking for a pollen-free area of the planet to call home? Good luck. The stuff has been found floating in the air 400 miles out at sea and 2 miles up in the sky. And even if you go to the ends of the earth, you'll still find it. In fact, scientists who study weather patterns in the Antarctic dig ice cores out of the landscape to examine pollen embedded in the samples and estimate when the winds blew the pollen there.

male plants is the ginkgo tree. The male trees make a lot of pollen, while female trees make an extremely foul-smelling fruit. Most people who plant ginkgoes choose the male plant to avoid the smell—only to add more pollen to their environment. Go figure.

Other species have both male and female organs on the same plant. Some of these plants can pollinate themselves, but others still require pollen from another plant to ensure diversity, Dr. Bradshaw says. Corn is an example of a species that bears female and male flowers on the same plant. When you shuck a fresh cob of corn,

the silks are the tubes that carried pollen to the ovary, and each kernel of corn is a fertilized egg.

While the goal of pollination is fairly straightforward—to make sure that pollen from the male flowers gets to the female flowers—plants use a variety of methods to get this done. For example, some may depend on the wind to carry their pollen all over the surrounding area. Others create their pollen with the intent of letting bees, other insects, and birds carry it from flower to flower. This makes a big difference in whether or not a plant will cause you allergy grief.

A Pest-Free Lawn, Naturally

Each time you squirt chemicals like herbicides and pesticides in your yard, you may be putting yourself one step closer to an allergy attack.

When chemicals irritate your system, they can leave your body less able to fend off allergens, warns Warren V. Filley, M.D., of Oklahoma City, a board-certified allergist, clinical professor of internal medicine at the University of Oklahoma Health Sciences Center, and former president of the Oklahoma Horticultural Society. The allergen and the irritant combine to have a more powerful effect. "Both of them together could make a person miserable, when one or the other alone would just give the person some mild symptoms," he says.

When you need to knock out a pack of bugs or a cluster of weeds that's threatening your treasured lawn or garden, keep these hints in mind.

Fight nature with nature. You can handle some insect pests, like aphids and spider mites, with a blast of water. Adjust the nozzle on your garden hose and squirt the plants vigorously enough to shake off the bugs, but not so hard that you damage the plant. It's best to wash the plants early in the day so both plants and ground dry out before mold can grow. Doing this in the evening can harm plants and promote mold growth.

Plants that rely on bees and other creatures create a sticky pollen that will cling to the visitor as it makes the rounds of flowers to eat nectar. To attract them, the plants tend to have bright, sweet-smelling flowers—nature's little billboards that shout, "Free food here!" As a result, this pollen follows a confined path and usually stays out of your nose. That's why plants with colorful flowers generally don't cause allergic reactions.

The drab, inconspicuous plants, on the other hand, are more troublesome. They know that bugs aren't likely to visit, so they compensate by churning out huge amounts of light, airy pollen—the better to hitch a ride on wind currents.

Around the country, those people who are allergy-afflicted curse different plants. For example, aggravating many Texans is the juniper tree, says Mary Jelks, M.D., a retired allergist in Florida and author of *Allergy Plants That Cause Sneezing and Wheezing*. The juniper grows in abundance there, and males can put off so much lightweight pollen that the tree appears to be billowing smoke.

In Michigan, trees like maple, elm, oak, walnut, hickory, birch, and sycamore cause a good deal of the allergy misery, says Lawrence Sweet, M.D., head of adult clin-

You can also buy friendly bugs, such as lady beetles, in bulk from garden supply catalogs and stores and unleash them in your yard to eat harmful insects. (Be aware, though, that for some people, even the seemingly innocent lady beetle can cause allergic reactions. For more on this, see "Lady Beetles: Cute but Not Harmless" on page 270.)

Use care with pyrethrins. While this bug spray is regarded as a semiorganic alternative to chemicals, it's derived from a plant that's related to ragweed. Often people with ragweed allergies will have a serious allergic reaction to pyrethrins, Dr. Filley warns.

Sacrifice an individual to save the group. If you find that one plant is becoming a chewed-up haven for bugs, you might as well pull it up and toss it away to save the rest, suggests Dr. Filley.

Use mulch. If you know that you're not allergic to mold spores, which grow heavily in mulch, go ahead and use the material. Spread a 4-inch-deep layer of mulch in your flowerbeds and around trees to keep weeds down. As long as you don't dig in it and disturb it, you won't release many mold spores into the air, Dr. Filley says.

ical allergy at William Beaumont Hospital in, of all places, Royal Oak, Michigan.

And the malcontents that make up the ragweed family spread trouble all around our nation, except for the Pacific Northwest.

Most plants will produce pollen for about 4 weeks, according to Dr. Jelks. Unfortunately, they don't all do it in one 4-week burst of activity. Instead, they spread it out across the warm months.

Trees pollinate from January to June in the southern states and from March to June farther north. Grass starts getting busy across the country between March and May and pollinates until late summer or fall. As for weeds, their pollen season doesn't de-

Playing the Numbers

If you eagerly scan through your morning newspaper for the pollen counts like a lottery player looking for the winning numbers, you might be setting yourself up for a sneezing fit later. Because unlike lottery numbers—either you're a winner or you're not—pollen counts have a hazy effect on your life.

For starters, those numbers may be telling you what the pollen levels were 1 or even 2 days ago, says Warren V. Filley, M.D., an allergist in Oklahoma City who helped establish the National Allergy Bureau, a nationwide network of counting stations, under the American Academy of Allergy, Asthma, and Immunology.

Some of these stations count and report only pollen, while others sample pollen and mold spores. Here's how the system generally works.

At a certified counting station, a device such as a Burkhard spore trap or a Rotorod Sampler will be used to suction pollen and mold particles from the air.

Next, a technician will use a microscope to examine the number and types of particles that the testing equipment picked up in the previous 24 hours. Mathematical equations are used to determine how many particles per cubic millimeter were sampled. That number, or its rating level (absent, low, medium, high, or very high), is then given to the media, who fit the report into their schedule, Dr. Filley says. While a radio or television station may broadcast it that day, the newspapers will probably print it in the next morning's issue.

The media, however, don't always report that the number is already dated and instead promote it as that day's count, Dr. Filley says. But if the weather changes after the count is taken, it could completely alter the amount of pollen in the air.

Further complicating the way the pollen count affects you is how far you are from the counting station. If you live miles away near a cluster of pollen-producing trees,

pend so much on latitude, but it tends to begin from spring to early summer and runs until the fall.

Even when a plant has stopped pollinating locally, the trouble may not be finished. Sometimes Dr. Jelks, who measures pollen counts, will notice that a specific type of pollen has dwindled in her area, but then, several weeks later, a weather front will blow the same kind of pollen in again from plants hundreds of miles north.

In short, pollen-producing plants are virtually everywhere, and they can bother people in other towns, counties, or even states. We're talking about *a lot* of pollen. Just how much is a lot?

the number of allergens surrounding you could be hundreds of times higher than the official report.

The good news is that if you use the pollen counts correctly, they can be helpful in managing your allergies. Here are some tips for making the most out of the pollen count.

Get pollen counts from the freshest source possible. This will probably be television or radio instead of the newspaper, Dr. Filley says. Be sure you know where the pollen was counted and how old the results are. If you're in doubt, call the newspaper office or broadcast office.

Use the counts as a guideline to plan your activities, not a clear-cut rule. If you know you're allergic to elm, for example, and the elm pollen counts have started to rise in recent reports, then start taking practical steps to avoid the pollen. But don't let a single count keep you huddled in the basement for the next few days.

Look outside. If the weather has changed markedly, the pollen may have, too: If it has been raining since the pollen was counted, the actual number has probably dropped. If it has grown sunny and windy, the true count is probably higher.

Use another number as well. If your local media carry the ozone levels for your area, pay attention to them, too, suggests Mary Jelks, M.D., a retired allergist in Florida and author of *Allergy Plants That Cause Sneezing and Wheezing*. Ozone can inflame the mucous lining in your nasal passages and create tiny openings that give pollen more chances to enter your body.

In addition, ozone and other pollutants can change the proteins in pollen to make it more likely to trigger an allergic reaction. Thus, if the ozone level and the pollen levels are both high, limit your time outdoors, she suggests.

Think you see a lot of stars when you look up into the nighttime sky? You're seeing only about 3,000. In comparison, a single ragweed plant can produce a *million* grains of pollen. Multiply that one stalk by a nation full of weedy lots, grass-stuffed lawns, and tree-swollen forests, and you get a sense of just how much pollen can be floating through the air during the growing season.

But pollen isn't the only pesky outdoor allergen. Add mold spores to the list, too. These make their home in nearly every climate, and you can find them floating outdoors year-round in the South and on the West Coast. They hit their peak in July in warm states and October in cooler states.

At the risk of bringing more tears to any itchy, watering eyes out there, Dr. Jelks says that in many climates you can find 1,000 mold spores for each grain of pollen in the air.

Now we know that this stuff is out there. But how does it do what it does to us?

The Inner Voyage

The hickory tree—notorious in the South for its allergenic effects—produces grains of pollen that Dr. Bradshaw describes as tiny balls covered with bristly Velcro. And ragweed pollen looks sinister, too—sort of like a microscopic version of a spiny sea urchin that would give you a sore foot if you stepped on it at the beach.

When these little bundles dig into the moist, delicate membranes inside your nose, they release materials as a way of inquiring what type of flower you are. But your body, which most definitely is *not* a flower, will react violently if it is overly sensitive to the material.

"We put forth this allergic reaction, which is sort of our body saying, 'I have to fight you away. You're invading me,'" Dr. Jelks says. If your body regards the pollen—or mold spore—as a threat, special cells found in great quantities in your nose, lungs,

Medicate Wisely

If you take medications to minimize your allergy problems, be sure to follow your doctor's advice on the best way to use them. Generally, though, when you know you're going to be exposed to an allergy trigger like pollen, the sooner you take your medications, the better off you'll be, says Warren V. Filley, M.D., of Oklahoma City, a board-certified allergist, clinical professor of internal medicine at the University of Oklahoma Health Sciences Center, and former president of the Oklahoma Horticultural Society. If you take them early, you may stop or prevent the symptoms with a smaller amount of medication. If you wait until later, you'll be so miserable that a whole lot of medication will do little to make you feel better, he says.

and eyes will unleash a flood of inflammatory chemicals in response.

This process can leave you with allergic rhinitis, also known as hay fever or seasonal allergies. Its symptoms, like sneezing, wheezing, a stuffy nose, and itchy, watery eyes, are synonymous with misery. This disorder can also lead to asthma, a serious condition in which the airways in your lungs grow inflamed when you breathe in pollen, mold, or other allergens and irritants, leaving you short of breath.

About 40 million Americans have allergic rhinitis, and more than 15 million have asthma. Most people with asthma have both conditions. Fortunately, when you reduce the sources of allergens in your surroundings and take some other simple precautions to protect yourself, you help decrease the opportunity for these disorders to give you grief.

Fix Your Yard—And Yourself—To Bring Down Allergies

Now that you know how outdoor allergy triggers operate, you can follow some basic guidelines to cut down on potential attacks.

Get tested. Talk to your family doctor or allergist about finding out exactly which plant or mold causes you problems, says Dr. Filley. "Rather than saying, 'I need to avoid all these trees and all these shrubs,' you may need to avoid only certain ones, or you may not need to avoid any at all," he notes.

If, for example, you find out that you're allergic to elm pollen, you can learn which weeks out of the year elms in your area pollinate, so you can limit your time outdoors then and be ready to take allergy medication. Or, by knowing what you're allergic to, you and your doctor can decide if you should get shots that desensitize you to that allergen, Dr. Filley says.

In a skin test, the doctor or staff member will place a drop of a diluted allergen sample onto you—like grass or tree pollen—then gently prick or scratch your skin beneath it and watch to see if an itchy red bump rises up on your skin. If it does, you're sensitive to that allergen.

Educate yourself. Pick up a plant identification book and use it to familiarize yourself with the trees, weeds, and other plants around your yard. When you do so, you might be a step ahead of your physician in recognizing troublesome plants. Ironically, Dr. Jelks has visited other allergists' offices and noticed ragweed growing around the parking lots.

Go for plants that feel at home. Dr. Jelks is a steadfast supporter of a landscaping philosophy that can save you not only from allergy misery but also from some hard labor in the yard.

When you plant foliage, stick with low-allergenic varieties that are native to your region. Native plant lists can be obtained from your local Native Plant Society. For starters, they tend to require less care, which means you won't be outside nurturing them

(continued on page 108)

Know Your Pollen Enemies

Since each of our immune systems has its own way of reacting to intruders like pollen, experts can't list every plant that will give people the sniffles and sneezes—or tout others as always safe.

"In medicine, you never say never, and you never say always," explains Warren V. Filley, M.D., of Oklahoma City, a board-certified allergist, clinical professor of internal medicine at the University of Oklahoma Health Sciences Center, and former president of the Oklahoma Horticultural Society. "Although there are certain kinds of plants that traditionally produce allergy, an individual with allergic tendencies can become allergic to basically anything."

For example, even though colorful flowers typically don't cause allergies, florists who work with them frequently may begin to sneeze and wheeze every time they're near. And if strong-smelling flowers like honeysuckle or lilac simply irritate your sinuses, you'll want to avoid them even though they're not producing a true allergic reaction.

Many plants, though, are a common enough source of misery to compile them into a warning list, and other plants are generally regarded as safe enough to recommend to the public. Here's a list of some generally trouble-free or generally troublesome plant choices, as given the thumbs-up or thumbs-down by Dr. Filley.

Note: Before you plant any of the trouble-free choices, ensure that they're well-suited for your climate.

Trouble-Free Trees

Carolina cherry laurel
  (*Prunus caroliniana*)
Cherry, plum, and peach
  (*Prunus* spp.)
Crab apple (*Malus* spp.)
Crape myrtle
  (*Lagerstroemia indica*)
Dogwood (*Cornus* spp.)
Flowering pear (*Pyrus* spp.)

Golden-rain tree
  (*Koelreuteria paniculata*)
Holly (*Ilex* spp.)
Magnolia (*Magnolia* spp.)
Persimmon (*Diospyros virginiana*)
Redbud (*Cercis* spp.)
Spruce (*Picea* spp.)
Tulip poplar (*Liriodendron tulipifera*)
Washington hawthorn (*Crataegus phaenopyrum*)

Troublesome Trees

Acacia (*Acacia* spp.)
Ash (*Fraxinus* spp.)
Australian pine (*Casuarina* spp.)
Birch (*Betula* spp.)
Cedar, cypress (*Cupressus* spp.)

Elm (*Ulmus* spp.)
Hackberry (*Celtis* spp.)
Hickory (*Carya* spp.)
Juniper (*Juniperus* spp.)
Maple (*Acer* spp.)

Mesquite (*Prosopis* spp.)
Mulberry (*Morus* spp.)
Oak (*Quercus* spp.)
Olive (*Olea europaea*)
Palms: Canary Island date palm
   (*Phoenix canariensis*), queen palm
   (*Arecastrum romanzoffianum*), and
   Everglades palm (*Acoelorrhaphe
   wrightii*)

Pecan, hickory (*Carya* spp.)
Poplar, cottonwood (*Populus* spp.)
Sweet gum (*Liquidambar* spp.)
Sycamore (*Platanus* spp.)
Walnut (*Juglans* spp.)
Willow (*Salix* spp.)

Trouble-Free Ground Cover

Ajuga (*Ajuga* spp.)
Bishop's weed
   (*Aegopodium* spp.)
Cotoneaster (*Cotoneaster* spp.)
English ivy (*Hedera helix*)
Honeysuckle (*Lonicera* spp.)

Hosta (*Hosta* spp.)
Lamb's-ears (*Stachys byzantina*)
Moneywort (*Lysimachia nummularia*)
Monkey grass (*Liriope* spp.)
Pachysandra (*Pachysandra* spp.)
Vinca (*Vinca* spp.)

Troublesome Ground Cover

Bermudagrass
   (*Cynodon dactylon*)
Fescue (*Festuca* spp.)
Johnsongrass
   (*Sorghum halepense*)
June or bluegrass
   (*Poa pratensis*)

Orchard grass (*Dactylis glomerata*)
Perennial ryegrass (*Lolium perenne*)
Redtop (*Agrostis ternis*)
Sweet vernal grass (*Anthoxanthum
   odoratum*)
Timothy grass (*Phleum pratense*)

Trouble-Free Shrubs

Azalea, rhododendron
   (*Rhododendron* spp.)
Barberry (*Berberis* spp.)
Blue spirea (*Caryopteris* spp.)
Boxwood (*Buxus* spp.)
Butterfly bush (*Buddleia* spp.)
Camellia (*Camellia japonica*)
Flowering quince
   (*Chaenomeles* spp.)

Glossy abelia (*Abelia* × *grandiflora*)
Holly (*Ilex* spp.)
Hydrangea (*Hydrangea* spp.)
Japanese aucuba (*Aucuba japonica*)
Spirea (*Spiraea* spp.)
Viburnum (*Viburnum* spp.)
Weigela (*Weigela florida*)
Yucca (*Yucca* spp.)

Troublesome Shrubs

Bayberry (*Myrica* spp.)
California lilac
   (*Ceanothus cuneatus*)
European or purple elder
   (*Sambucus nigra*)

Japanese maple (*Acer japonicum*)
Privet (*Ligustrum* spp.)
Sweet fern (*Comptonia* spp.)

as often and breathing in as many outdoor allergens, Dr. Jelks says. Plus, you generally won't have to water native plants as much, which will help you keep down mold growth in your yard.

As a cautionary note, just look to parts of the Southwest desert region. "People there often try to bring in things that aren't native to the area, because the plants reminded them of home. Others had the problematic attitude of 'Anybody can grow that cactus in Tucson. I want to grow something nobody else can grow,'" says Dr. Filley. Long ago, allergy sufferers flocked to Arizona to find relief. But many newcomers brought in high-allergenic grasses and plants like mulberry and olive trees, and now some cities there are filled with allergy sufferers.

Plant ground cover. Many people with outdoor allergies stir up trouble when they

Protect Yourself against Pollen

An ideal way for a person with pollen and mold allergies to handle lawn-mowing, leaf-raking, and other grubby yard chores is to watch from indoors as a family member or neighbor does them.

But if you can't rouse anyone in the house to work outdoors—or the neighbor kid has hiked his rates—you can do it yourself with less risk of an allergy attack when you follow some simple precautions.

Be the masked man (or woman). Wear a disposable mask—similar to what surgeons wear—to keep pollen, mold spores, and other debris out of your mouth and nose, says Warren V. Filley, M.D., of Oklahoma City, a board-certified allergist, clinical professor of internal medicine at the University of Oklahoma Health Sciences Center, and former president of the Oklahoma Horticultural Society. A simple paper mask will work, but make sure that the mask you use fits snugly against your face, with no open spaces around the edges to let the offending substances enter.

In addition, wear a set of goggles to keep airborne grit out of your eyes, Dr. Filley suggests. They, too, should form a snug barrier against your face.

If you wear contact lenses, consider using eyeglasses instead when working in the yard, since just a few grains of pollen under your contacts may give you a terrible case of itchy, watery eyes. Some goggles will slip on over a pair of eyeglasses.

Cover yourself. Wear a long-sleeved shirt, long pants, and gloves while working in the yard. As soon as you're done, take them off and immediately wash them.

fire up the lawn mower, Dr. Filley says. The whirring blades turn grass into an airborne spray and send dust, debris, and mold spores aloft. Obviously, if you can decrease the size of the area you need to mow, you'll churn fewer allergens into the air.

Try covering a portion of your yard with a low-allergenic ground cover that you won't need to mow, like ivy, pachysandra, sedum, vinca, or ajuga. You can then embed stepping-stones or concrete tiles into the foliage to create a walkway through it.

Minimize the mold. If you're allergic to mold spores, be careful to keep your lawn clear of anything that will trap moisture and give the mold an ideal spot to run rampant, warns Arlene Schneider, M.D., chairperson of the department of allergy and immunology at the Long Island College Hospital in Brooklyn. Troublesome areas in-

Wash your problems away. Once you've shed your clothes, hop into the shower and thoroughly wash off any allergens that may be clinging to your skin and hair, Dr. Filley suggests.

You can also get rid of intruders that have gotten *inside* you by rinsing out your nose with salt water. "I tell patients it's like hosing out the garage," says Dr. Filley.

To be prepared for your next allergy attack, create a hypertonic saline nasal solution by combining 1 liter of distilled water, 1 tablespoon of canning salt, and 1 tablespoon of baking soda. Mix well and store in a sealed container. (You can also create an alternative nasal rinse solution with $\frac{1}{3}$ teaspoon of salt and 8 ounces of tepid water.) Be sure the water is lukewarm before using; test the water with a clean finger to make sure it's not too hot or cold.

Then, use a bulb syringe, nasal rinse bottle, or nasal adapter for a Waterpik to wash out your nose up to four times a day using several full bulbs (or 2 to 4 ounces per nostril). These products are available online or at your local drugstore. Lean forward and let the water run back out. Continue until the water runs out clear or your sinuses feel cleaned out. Be sure to keep the throat closed while doing this and gently blow your nose between rinses. Do not swallow the water, and allow excess water to drain by bending your head below your waist if needed. Don't forget to clean your syringe, rinse bottle, or Waterpik between each use with hot water and detergent. Make a fresh solution at least once a day.

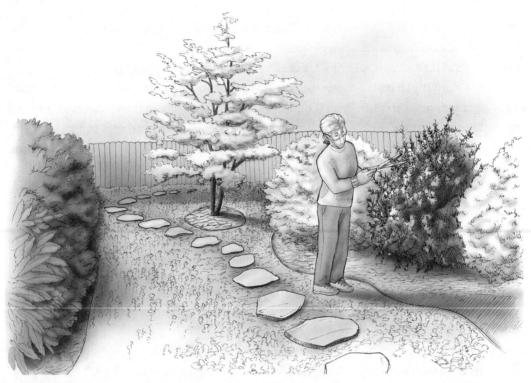

In this yard, allergens are kept to a minimum by using a ground cover of ajuga instead of grass and by planting relatively trouble-free trees and shrubs such as dogwood, boxwood, bayberry bushes, and glossy abelia shrubs. In addition, mulch is spread in 4-inch layers to deter weed growth.

clude piles of cut grass, mounds of fallen leaves, and layers of mulch.

When you rake leaves or cut your grass, be sure that the refuse is bagged and disposed of according to your local ordinances; don't let it accumulate in your yard. Also, if mold sets off your symptoms, don't maintain a compost pile, since it provides prime real estate for mold to grow, Dr. Schneider says.

Be vigilant. Keep an eye out for any new weeds or grasses that appear in your yard. For example, ragweed commonly pops up where the dirt has been disturbed, like around roadways and construction sites, Dr. Jelks says. If you dig in your yard, watch to make sure this highly allergenic plant doesn't make a home there.

Be a creature of the evening. If you're going to work in your yard, concentrate your chores in the late afternoon or early evening hours, when you'll encounter fewer allergens in the air, Dr. Sweet says.

Keep problems outdoors. If the pollen and mold spores outside bother you, don't invite them inside. For example, run your air conditioner during the warm months instead of opening your windows. And don't hang bedding and clothing outside to dry, since they'll collect allergens that you'll then set loose in your home, Dr. Jelks says.

The
Allergy-Free
WORKPLACE

THE CURIOUS PHYSICIAN watched the laborer clean out his sewage system with great haste and asked what seems like a painfully obvious question: Why are you working so fast? Because, answered the cleaner, spending too much time in such a harsh environment irritates the eyes and can cause blindness.

Thus marked a key moment in the birth of occupational health, way back in the late 1600s. The Italian physician, Bernardino Ramazzini, went on to investigate illnesses commonly found in a wide variety of professions, including painting, farming, fishing, nursing, and food processing.

More than 300 years later, these same occupations still figure prominently in lists of workplaces that can cause or worsen allergic conditions such as skin rashes, runny nose and itchy eyes, asthma, and anaphylaxis.

Many job sites use substances that can irritate the lungs, nose, skin, or eyes or that can find their way into the body and cause the immune system to react. At least 250 substances are known to cause occupational asthma, and the list of usual suspects is growing longer each year as more products are found to be troublesome.

Some occupations are known for particular ingredients that sicken hordes of workers. Chemicals called diisocyanates, which are used in spray painting and the production of plastic and polyurethane items, are the leading cause of occupational asthma in industrialized countries. Latex products are causing many nurses, doctors, and other health care workers to develop reactions—from skin irritation to life-threatening shock. And an enzyme used in detergent was the culprit behind an epidemic of asthma in workers who handled the stuff in the 1960s and 1970s.

If an allergen or irritant punches your clock when you start work for the day, the solution may or may not be simple. In certain cases, you may be able to shield yourself with masks, gloves, and other protection. If your exposure to this allergen or irritant is more considerable, you may be able to persuade your employer to change your workspace or move you elsewhere in the company.

But for many people who are miserable, sick, and at risk, the stakes are simply too high to stay exposed to an allergen or irritant. The single best solution for your health is to just get away from the substance. That could mean that if your employer can't or won't make accommodations that would prevent your symptoms, you may need to find a new job or career.

These may be tough solutions, but it's a difficult problem. Fortunately, a doctor with good detective skills can help identify what's making you sick, and government benefits may provide money while you're out of work and help train you for a new field of employment.

And you can do a lot to protect your health by taking notes, collecting vital information about your workplace, and maintaining a good relationship with your employer.

The Major Players

A look at how your job can contribute to major allergic conditions—asthma, skin problems, and allergic rhinitis—will show just how complicated workplace allergies can be. For more detailed information on these diseases, see the chapters devoted to them.

• Asthma

As the sawmill operator slices the tree trunk into boards amid a shower of sawdust, he feels the familiar chest tightness of an approaching asthma attack.

If your workplace gives you breathing problems along with your paycheck, it's a problem you should take very seriously.

"There are now several known reported cases of people who died from occupational asthma after it was diagnosed," says William Beckett, M.D., professor of environmental medicine at the University of Rochester in New York.

Around the world, at least 10 percent of the asthma cases that affect adults may be linked to the workplace. This includes both previously healthy people who come down with asthma that's directly related to their jobs and people who have a preexisting asthma condition that worsens from substances at work. Both are health risks and should be treated the same medically.

Sometimes, the asthma is due to an allergen. This usually requires months or years of exposure to the offending substance before you get sick, because your body's immune system requires time to work up the allergic response to it. This is the type of situation found in veterinarians who become allergic to cat dander and sawmill workers who develop asthma from wood dust.

Your asthma symptoms may pop up an hour after you're exposed to the trigger and vanish within 1 to 3 hours after you're away from it, or it may take several hours more for your symptoms to show up and go away. Making this even more troublesome, your symptoms may return 12 hours after you recover from the first bout.

The Troublesome Coworkers List

Given the virtually limitless number of occupations and substances used in them, a comprehensive list of potential allergens and irritants is impossible to assemble here. But here's a sample of some of the chemicals and other substances famous for giving skin, nose, and lung grief to workers in particular fields.

Potential Allergen or Irritant	Occupation
Acrylate	Adhesive handlers
Amines	Shellac and lacquer handlers
Anhydrides	Users of plastics, epoxy resins
Animal allergens	Veterinarians, animal breeders, lab workers, seafood processors
Antibiotics	Health care workers, pharmaceutical workers
Cereal grains	Bakers, millers
Chloramine-T	Janitors, cleaners
Dyes	Textile workers
Enzymes	Detergent handlers, pharmaceutical workers, bakers
Ethylenediamine	Beauticians, plastics and rubber workers
Fluxes	Electronic workers, solderers
Formaldehyde and glutaraldehyde	Hospital workers
Gums	Carpet makers, pharmaceutical workers
Insects	Grain workers, dock workers, and farmers
Isocyanates	Spray painters, insulation installers, and plastics, foam, and rubber workers
Latex	Health care workers, glove makers
Metals	Solderers
Persulfate	Hairdressers
Platinum salts	Platinum refiners
Psyllium	Pharmaceutical workers
Tobacco leaf	Tobacco farmers and processors
Wood dust	Forest workers, carpenters

But asthma in the workplace isn't always caused by allergens. Irritants like hydrochloric acid and sulfur dioxide can cause you to start wheezing immediately after you encounter them. A reaction that occurs after you inhale a large amount of an irritant, such as toxic fumes or gas during a chemical spill, is called RADS, or reactive airways dysfunction syndrome. This can have long-term, disabling consequences.

Another cause of asthma is breathing in certain airborne chemicals, like some insecticides used in farming, which cause the natural substances histamine and acetylcholine to build up in your body and constrict your airways.

Certain factors will increase your chances of getting work-related asthma. Being atopic, or predisposed to having allergic diseases, puts you at greater risk.

Smoking also makes you more likely to get occupational asthma, makes it worse once you have it, and gives you a harder time proving that it's work-related.

If you have asthma linked to the workplace, you'll probably notice your symptoms worsening through the week and improving through the weekend. But the problems can drag on through the weekend, making them appear to be continuous (and making the diagnosis trickier).

• Skin Problems

After the hairdresser gives yet another permanent to a customer, her itchy, burning hands start to give her fits.

Occupational skin diseases account for up to 20 percent of all reported work-related diseases. Of these skin problems, by far the most common is contact dermatitis caused by irritants and allergens. When we look more closely at contact dermatitis, we find that three-quarters of the time it's caused by an irritant, and the rest of the time it's from allergens.

Most often, when Vincent S. Beltrani, M.D., sees patients with occupational skin problems, they work as hairdressers, who by the nature of their job frequently have their hands wet with water and chemicals. Dr. Beltrani, an allergist and dermatologist in New York, also sees plenty of bartenders and food handlers who often have their hands immersed in soapy water.

Water and soaps are sources of irritant contact dermatitis, as are solvents, resins, greases, fiberglass, acids, and alkalis. Allergic contact dermatitis may be triggered by ingredients in rubber and epoxy, cosmetics, and poison ivy and oak. Some substances can affect you as both an irritant or an allergen.

Irritant contact dermatitis tends to show up from minutes to a couple of days after you come into contact with the harmful substance. The borders of the resulting rash are often sharply defined, and it generally fades away within 4 days.

Allergic contact dermatitis, however, will strike only people already sensitized to a substance. It feels extremely itchy and may leave red, fluid-filled blisters. The rash, which isn't as sharply defined as those caused by irritants, may take 1 to 6 days to show up after you touch the substance, and it may take weeks to go away.

Another skin condition that can result from your work surroundings is urticaria, or hives. These show up within minutes to an hour after you touch the offending substance, and they disappear within a few hours. Latex and foods like seafood, fruits, and cheese can trigger this.

The people most at risk for these skin problems are people with atopic dermatitis, a condition in which the skin is extremely sensitive and overreacts to substances it encounters, Dr. Beltrani says.

If you've ever had atopic dermatitis, even as a baby, think twice about taking a job like hairdressing or cooking, where you'll frequently have your hands wet or encounter irritants and allergens, Dr. Beltrani recommends.

• Allergic Rhinitis

The graduate student sneezes as she looks through itchy eyes at the laboratory rats in the cages surrounding her.

All those lab rats used for experiments often get their revenge on the white-coated workers who push them around: Lab workers are one of the groups most commonly hit with work-related rhinitis, and the rats are most often the culprit.

Better known as hay fever, allergic rhinitis strikes with symptoms like runny nose and congestion, sneezing, itching in the roof of the mouth, and itchy, watery eyes. It can be triggered by allergens, annoying scents like perfumes, irritating fumes and particles like cigarette smoke and coal dust, and blasts of concentrated, damaging chemicals like chlorine.

It's certainly not just a problem of lab workers either. Psyllium, an ingredient in laxatives, can cause rhinitis in workers who manufacture the stuff and nurses who give it to patients. Guar gum, used to thicken foods and make dye stick to carpet fibers, can induce rhinitis in workers.

As far as work-related conditions go, however, rhinitis is generally not given as much attention as asthma, perhaps because it's not as dramatic and potentially serious an illness. Because it does cause unpleasant symptoms—and may show up before or alongside asthma—you should definitely take action if it strikes.

If you have rhinitis that's linked to your workplace, you'll probably notice the symptoms at work, but they may appear later in the evening, since your body may take a while to react to the allergens and irritants. And while you'll typically feel better on your days off and vacations, lingering symptoms may take several days to disappear.

Now that we know what these work-related conditions look like, it's time to learn what to do about them.

This is the hard part.

Show Occupational Allergies Who's Boss

As you've already read in this book and will see again, leading an allergy-free life requires a certain amount of detective work. And if you're trying to cope with workplace allergies, your investigative, observational, and interpersonal skills may play a crucial role in how well you succeed.

In this section, experts will give you the lowdown on how to work with your doctor, your employer, and the workers' compensation system to get what you need.

• Your Doctor

Bernardino Ramazzini, the founder of occupational medicine whom we discussed earlier, was famous for visiting his patients' workplaces, no matter how unpleasant. And modern-day experts stress the importance of the doctor making an on-site visit to make observations.

In the real world, though, persuading a busy doctor to come to your workplace is about as likely as getting a company-sponsored foot rub at the end of the day.

In fact, because of the time it takes a doctor to diagnose your problem, verify that it's work-related, and come up with a solution—and possibly speak for you in a legal proceeding—you may have a hard time getting the help you need even at a doctor's office, says Dr. Beltrani, who is also associate clinical professor of dermatology at Columbia-Presbyterian Medical Center in New York City.

"The sad thing is, fewer doctors are willing to handle this type of stuff," he says. As far as occupational skin conditions go, most doctors don't want to deal with it because they make twice as much money treating a cosmetic problem.

Larry Martin, M.D., a pulmonary specialist and workers' compensation examiner in Cleveland, agrees that not all doctors are overjoyed at taking on an occupational-illness case. So if you have a choice, make sure early on that your doctor has the knowledge and time required to do a thorough job, he suggests. Your primary care doctor might not be the best person for this kind of task.

While an allergist is a good choice for any of these conditions, a dermatologist may be the best choice for skin problems, a pulmonologist for lung problems, and an ear-nose-and-throat doctor for rhinitis. You might also bring in an occupational-medicine specialist for additional expertise in how to handle your situation.

Since time is short, the more information you bring to the doctor's office, the better. Here's what you should collect.

• Your history. "The more documentation patients bring, the better the doctor can make an assessment," Dr. Martin says.

Provide your doctor with detailed information on previous illnesses, any personal or family history of allergy, the medications you're taking or have used, and your habits such as smoking. Also include meticulous descriptions of your present and previous job duties and workplace surroundings.

• A diary. Keep very careful notes about your work schedule and when you develop symptoms, whether at work or on your own time. This will help establish when your symptoms arise, Dr. Beltrani says. And it may even show that you're allergic to something that's not work-related.

• MSDS. This is the acronym for "material safety data sheets." Companies that use certain chemicals are legally obligated to keep these sheets, which describe the substance and offer safety information, available.

Not only should you use these to educate yourself on how to handle any chemicals around you at work, you should show them to your doctor, says Emil J. Bardana Jr., M.D., head of the division of allergy and clinical immunology at Oregon Health Sciences University in Portland and an expert on occupational allergies. Dr. Bardana says that these sheets are essential for educating yourself on the nature of the chemicals you are handling at work, their potential adverse health effects, and the recommended protection.

"If you suspect a health problem, bring the MSDS to your physician so he can become familiar with the chemical agents and their properties. Many high-tech industries use a myriad of agents that would be impossible to suspect unless the MSDS was available," he says.

Depending on your special circumstances, your doctor will use the information you provide, a physical examination, and possibly a number of tests to help pinpoint the problem.

Asthma. Your doctor may give you skin-prick tests to see if you're allergic to proteins like animal dander or soybeans. With a nonspecific bronchial challenge, a test to show that you truly have asthma, you will have to inhale histamine or methacholine to see if your lungs overreact.

The doctor may also ask you to use a peak-flow meter—an inexpensive, simple device that measures how well you can breathe—at home and at work, recording the results.

The gold standard for proving occupational asthma, though, is to expose you to specific suspect substances and observe your reaction. This, however, takes special equipment and medical professionals who can help you if you react badly to the substance.

Skin problems. Your doctor may choose to test you with an array of possible allergens by placing them on your skin and covering them with a patch, Dr. Beltrani says. Since the standard available arrays of test allergens can't possibly cover every substance you may encounter, you may need to bring in samples of suspected products from work for the test, he says.

If you have contact urticaria, the doctor may choose to test you by pricking a bit of the suspected substance into your skin.

Rhinitis. Again, the doctor may skin-test you to see if you're allergic to particular proteins.

In a simple test called a nasal challenge, your doctor exposes your nose to a suspected substance, then takes a look inside to note any changes and possibly measures how well you can blow air through your nose.

Whether your condition hurts your lungs, skin, or nose, the single best solution

Troubles May Await You at Work

If you're having symptoms like stuffy nose, tightness of the chest, sore throat, fatigue, headache, nausea, skin irritation, and burning eyes, your workplace may be suffering from the so-called sick building syndrome, according to the American Lung Association.

This often-mysterious problem can be caused by a number of factors, including mold, which can grow in the air ducts; carbon monoxide from garages and loading docks; secondhand tobacco smoke; and gaseous volatile organic compounds released from carpets, photocopying machines, cleaning fluids, and many other sources.

Some of the things that you can do if you suspect that your building's air quality is poor or the building is making you sick are the following:

- Avoid blocking the air supply and return vents in your office.
- Clean up water spills immediately or report them to the proper authority. Water gives mold a place to grow.
- Store food properly, and empty your garbage daily.
- Talk with your coworkers, supervisor, or union official to find out if other people are complaining about the same problems, and if so, make sure your supervisor or company health administrator knows.
- Talk to your doctor about your symptoms.
- Report the problem to your state or local health department.

Your office manager or facility manager may take such steps as evaluating the air-supply system in your building and fixing any problems, ensuring that office equipment and products that give off fumes are properly ventilated or low-pollution options are chosen, and establishing smoking rules so that secondhand smoke stays away from workers.

They may also need to bring in specialists to examine the building and question the occupants to determine possible problems.

to nip a workplace allergy in the bud is to get away from the troublesome substance, says Dr. Beckett. Simply treating your symptoms with medications is just masking a bad situation. And if you have asthma, exposing yourself to more triggers could have fatal results.

Given your individual circumstances, however, you might not have to quit your job and find another. Instead, you may be able to modify your job with your current employer to make it suitable.

Since many of us have a limited say over our work environment during our shift, it's crucial to work with supervisors to come up with a solution.

• Your Employer

If your doctor can prove that a substance at work is harming your health, ask him to report this to your employer, along with a recommendation of what kind of changes you require, says Gary Rischitelli, M.D., J.D., assistant health professor at Oregon Health Sciences University and adjunct professor of law at Lewis and Clark College in Portland.

Your employer has to do something to help you make necessary changes, but it doesn't have to be exactly what you'd prefer. That means if an employer can think of a cheaper or in any way less burdensome way to meet the requirements, he can do that, Dr. Rischitelli says.

Certain laws may give you a hand here. OSHA (Occupational Safety and Health Administration) requires companies to keep a safe environment, and that includes maintaining certain chemicals in the air below a particular level, Dr. Beckett says.

But not all potentially harmful substances are regulated. The chemicals known as isocyanates are, but the wheat flour that gives some bakers asthma isn't, Dr. Beckett says. Plus, Dr. Rischitelli points out, OSHA is designed more to protect workers in general than to protect an isolated worker with a special need.

You may find more help from the Americans with Disabilities Act (ADA), which puts a pretty substantial burden on the employer to try to accommodate the individual, Dr. Rischitelli says. If, however, you have a garden-variety case of allergic rhinitis or dermatitis, your condition may not be serious enough to invoke the ADA. You'll be more likely to benefit if you have significant asthma, he says. And the bigger and more well-off your company is, the more responsibility it has to accommodate your needs.

Whether or not these legal benefits support you, your requests may fall on more sympathetic ears if you start off with a cooperative attitude toward your supervisors instead of considering them adversaries. Save your lawyer for later, since having a lawyer involved early on can create an adversarial posture that might not be conducive to getting what you want, Dr. Rischitelli recommends. Only when negotiations are at an impasse, or there's employer retaliation for any of your actions, is it advisable for a lawyer to get involved.

Occupational-medicine doctors take three levels of approaches to protect workers, Dr. Rischitelli says. The most favored is to use engineering controls, in which changes are made to the workplace itself. This could entail, for example, enclosing a dust-making machine in a box, adding a vacuum system that sucks up the dust, or improving ventilation to the area.

Earlier in this chapter we mentioned a wave of asthma cases in the detergent industry. These problems were dramatically improved, in part, with these kinds of changes.

The next-best solution is administrative controls, he says, in which the ailing person is transferred to a different work environment. This could mean doing the same job for a shorter amount of time each day, taking a different job, or working in a different building.

For example, lab workers who are sensitive to mice typically react to the protein in the urine and might be able to just dissect the animals, as long as the workers are kept away from urine-soaked cages.

The choice that doctors like least, but one that employees often have to accept because it's the easiest for the employer, is to wear protective equipment. That includes wearing a mask or respirator to keep out dust or wearing gloves to keep hands dry.

If you must wear a protective device, talk to your company's industrial hygienist, if it employs one, about what kind of mask to use and how to use it properly. It's up to the employer to decide if he wants to allow voluntary use of a mask. New OSHA regulations permit a single worker to use a mask, if necessary, in the absence of a comprehensive respirator program, but the employer must meet the OSHA standard, which includes providing information on proper use and limitations of the mask. Sometimes these are complicated masks that require filters or cartridges that must be changed regularly, Dr. Beckett says.

Whatever option he chooses, your employer will have plenty of potential reasons to try to accommodate you. The cost of compromise may be less than the cost of finding and training a new worker. Plus, if your employer realizes that you'll have a good case, he may not want to risk the time and money involved in the workers' compensation and other benefits needed to get you healthy and working again, Dr. Rischitelli says.

• Workers' Compensation

If your condition forces you out of your job, you may be entitled to workers' compensation benefits. This is a form of insurance, varying from state to state, that your employer takes out on you. If your workplace causes you an illness or injury, workers' comp is intended to provide you with some of your wages if you can't work (temporarily or permanently) and to pay for your medical care, Dr. Beckett says.

The amount of money you may receive will depend on your *medical loss*, which is how your condition hampers a bodily function like breathing, or by your *wage loss*, which is how your condition impairs your future employment possibilities. Some states will base the decision on a combination of the two.

Since the laws governing these benefits vary from state to state and case to case, this section can offer only general advice.

Odds are, when you decide to take the plunge into workers' comp, you'll want to take a lawyer with you and keep your doctor's number handy. Your company or its insurance carrier probably isn't going to just hand you a bag of money, and they and their hotshot attorney likely will argue against your diagnosis.

Getting compensation for an occupational allergy can be difficult. It's not an obvious injury like a broken arm, and it's further complicated by whether the workplace caused you to have a brand-new condition like asthma or if it just triggers a condition you already had. Your exposures to allergens and irritants outside work further muddy the issue, and so do habits like smoking. And allergy fakers who have gone through the system before you can make defending your legitimate claim even tougher.

A slam-dunk, easy-to-prove case would go like this: You've never been around green coffee beans in your life, and you've never had asthma. You go to work for a company where you shovel green coffee beans all day, and you develop asthma. Tests prove that you're sensitive to green coffee beans. Thus, you can easily prove that you're entitled to some benefits, Dr. Rischitelli says.

But if you're a smoker who's had asthma all your life, and you take a new job in an office and your asthma gets worse, but with no particular triggers, you'll have a much tougher time showing that you're deserving of financial compensation. Not all states' laws will help you out if you have a preexisting condition that's merely aggravated by your workplace.

This is why it's so important to keep careful notes of your symptoms and work schedule, as well as safety sheets and labels of substances you work around. These can help your doctor and lawyer make a convincing claim that your workplace caused you damage and you need help recovering from it.

In addition to workers' compensation, your state may offer job-retraining benefits. If the only task you know how to do is shovel coffee beans and you become allergic to the stuff—or if emergency surgery is your whole life and you become allergic to latex—you may qualify for assistance in learning how to do a new job.

Allergy-Free
TRAVEL

TO PREPARE TOURISTS for unplanned excitement ranging from hurricanes to revolutionary uprisings, the U.S. State Department offers safety recommendations for travel to dozens of countries.

For people with allergies and asthma, though, travel doesn't have to be to an exotic locale to bring threats of discomfort or even danger. A cross-country airline flight, a weekend at a hotel across the state, or even holiday dinner at Grandma's can all expose travelers to a trunkload of allergens and irritants.

Fortunately, with thorough preparation—and a willingness to speak up when you aren't pleased with your accommodations—you can help ensure a vacation free of sniffling, sneezing, and wheezing, says Stanley Goldstein, M.D., a Long Island allergist who has been giving his patients travel advice for 20 years.

"If people do their homework, then they really can go anywhere and avoid all of the potential problems that they could have," Dr. Goldstein says. "The most important thing is pre-travel planning."

General Guidelines for Your Journey

When you're traveling, the changes in your daily routine and lifestyle can make you vulnerable to allergy problems. Overeating, drinking too much, and becoming caught up in the novelty of being away from home can make you lower your guard against food and environmental allergens, says Dr. Goldstein. So enjoy yourself, but don't neglect the measures that you normally use to protect yourself from allergy symptoms while you're at home. Along with those measures, check out these additional tips, which will help you take a vacation while leaving your allergies at home.

Police for pollen. Something more than fun could be in the air at your vacation spot—mold and pollen could be lurking there as well. Pollen levels surge at different times around the country, and warm, moist areas like vacation hot spots in Florida, Hawaii, and California may be a haven for mold spores.

If you're allergic to these outdoor allergens, check the maps below to see if grasses, ragweed, trees, or weeds are pollinating where you're going. You can also get current pollen and spore counts by contacting the National Allergy Bureau of the American Academy of Allergy, Asthma, and Immunology at (800) 9-POLLEN or (877) 9-ACHOOO.

Learn the lingo. If you're heading for for-

WEED POLLEN SEASON

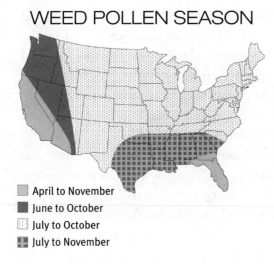

- April to November
- June to October
- July to October
- July to November

RAGWEED POLLEN SEASON

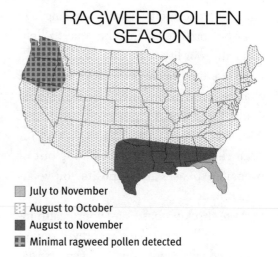

- July to November
- August to October
- August to November
- Minimal ragweed pollen detected

TREE POLLEN SEASON

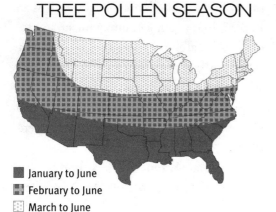

- January to June
- February to June
- March to June

GRASS POLLEN SEASON

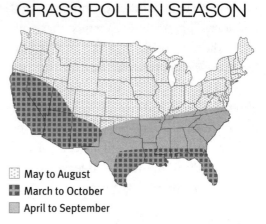

- May to August
- March to October
- April to September

eign shores, you may want to write down a list of phrases in that country's language to help describe your allergies, recommends Andrew Trofa, M.D., an infectious disease and travel medicine physician in Somers Point, New Jersey. For example, you may want to include such comments as "I am allergic to peanuts" or "Breathing smoke makes me very sick" to read to a chef or hotel manager.

A foreign-language dictionary or phrase-book, Internet resources, or a local language professor or teacher may be able to help you with your list.

Ensure that you're insured. If there's a chance that your allergies or asthma could force you to postpone or cancel your trip, consider purchasing travel insurance to take the financial sting out of prepaid expenses and deposits you've already made.

Also, check to make sure your health insurance will follow you wherever you're going and will handle any emergencies that arise. If it won't cover asthma or allergy medical costs in another country, strongly consider supplemental insurance that will. Read the fine print to make sure it will cover pre-existing conditions.

Get checked out. If you have questions about traveling and health that only your doctor can answer—or your allergy or asthma symptoms are out of control and your medication needs tweaking—Dr. Goldstein recommends a pre-trip checkup with your doctor or allergist to help prevent problems.

Bring your medicine cabinet with you. Obviously, if you're taking regular medications and other remedies, be sure to bring along enough to last for your trip.

Make sure the medications are in their original containers—the ones that have your name on them. This is especially important when you're traveling internationally and are taking a controlled substance, like cough medicine with codeine; in this case, the name on your medications should be the same as the name on your passport to avoid questions from authorities. In addition, you may want to carry an extra set of prescriptions in case you lose your medication and need to refill it.

Finally, if you're in another country and need your physician to phone in a prescription, make sure she requests the generic form. The trade name for the drug might be different from what it is in the United States.

Stick with the sticker. If your doctor has prescribed a shot of epinephrine, such as an EpiPen, that you inject into yourself in case of life-threatening food or insect stings, asthma attacks, or other emergencies, be sure to bring it with you and have it available at all times. The pen-size device can keep you alive until you get medical attention.

Bring a mask, too. The last time he was visiting India, Rajiv Narula, M.D., medical director of International Travel Health Consultants in Poughkeepsie, New York, saw plenty of locals wearing masks to help protect themselves from air pollution.

If you're going to a city or region blanketed by pollution, a disposable dust mask or a surgical-style mask can help filter out some of the airborne particles. These can be particularly helpful if you're out during rush hour, Dr. Narula says.

Wear useful jewelry. If you have a severe allergy—especially to medications—consider wearing a MedicAlert bracelet or necklace to give crucial information to any health care providers who might treat you. These are usually recognized internationally.

In a Car

As you cruise down the highway with the radio blaring your favorite tunes, your car may feel like your home away from home. But as with your home, you need to take some steps to make your car as allergy-proof as possible.

Step out of the car, please. If you live in a damp environment that encourages mold growth, or you're bothered by dust that could blow out of your car's vents, open your car windows and turn the air conditioner or heater on full blast for 10 minutes before you get in and drive away, Dr. Goldstein says.

This is especially important at the beginning of the heating or cooling season to blow dust out of vents that haven't been used in a while.

Put a lid on it. If you're allergic to dust mites and have upholstered seats in your car, you may want to put vinyl seat covers over them to seal in the mites and the allergens they produce. Be sure to keep the covers wiped clean of dust.

Drive protected. If you have allergies to pollen and mold, be sure to travel with your windows rolled up to avoid picking up any sneeze-making hitchhikers. Use your air conditioner if you need a breeze.

Drive in the off-hours. If you can be choosy about when you drive, take to the road in the early morning or late evening, especially if you're going through densely populated areas, Dr. Goldstein says. Fume-spewing traffic is lighter at these times, and the air quality is better, providing less threat to your asthma or allergies.

Remember that the car isn't for wet storage. Mold thrives in damp areas, so don't stash any wet towels, clothing, swimsuits, or shoes for long periods of time in your car or trunk, Dr. Goldstein says.

Rent from nonsmokers. If you're going to rent some wheels for your trip, ask if the agency offers smoke-free cars so you can breathe clear air as you hit the road.

Protect yourself from pets. If you've found ways at home to keep your pets from troubling your allergies—like keeping them outdoors—you may have trouble traveling with them in the car, since you'll essentially be stuck in a sealed metal box with the allergens, Dr. Goldstein says.

If you can't avoid this scenario, be sure to roll down the windows to ensure you'll get some fresh air (if you're not allergic to outdoor allergens, of course), and pretreat yourself with the necessary antihistamines, inhalers, or other preventive treatments you usually use to minimize your symptoms.

Bring your own nebulizer. If you use a nebulizer to treat your asthma, consider getting a portable type that plugs into the cigarette lighter of your car or uses a battery pack.

In a Plane

Contrary to what you might believe, your allergy symptoms are *not* at the mercy of the airline when you're on a plane. There are a number of simple things that you can do—both prior to and during your flight—to ensure that your trip through the clouds is a pleasant one.

Keep your supplies with you. When you get on the plane, make sure that any medications and other supplies you need to treat your allergies and asthma are packed into a kit in your carry-on bag and not checked in your luggage, Dr. Narula suggests. Otherwise, if you're flying to Sweden and your luggage is Oklahoma-bound, you'll be out of luck if your allergies kick in somewhere over the Atlantic Ocean.

Wash out your nose. Because the air in planes tends to be extremely dry, carry a squirt bottle of saline nasal spray to use every hour you're on board to keep your nasal passages moist and comfortable.

Wash out the rest of you, too. Guzzle plenty of water and juice while you're on the plane. If you don't take in plenty of fluids, you run the risk of starting your vacation dehydrated and not as strong and healthy as you could have been. Being dehydrated can really set you off on the wrong foot if you're visiting a hot, tropical area, Dr. Trofa says.

Make sure that the drinks you're tossing back don't contain alcohol or caffeine, since these work as diuretics, further draining you of fluid.

Watch for surprise smokers. Flights on all U.S. airlines are smoke-free, as are flights on all foreign carriers to or from America.

If, however, you manage to get on an international flight that still allows smoking, ask well in advance for a seat that's as far away from the smoking section as possible. "It seems almost ridiculous to get a seat one row behind a smoking section, because that doesn't lend any avoidance of cigarette smoke," Dr. Goldstein says.

Think before you fly. If you're having asthma flare-ups, you're better off waiting until you get them back under control before you fly, Dr. Goldstein says. When an airplane is flying at 35,000 feet, the amount of oxygen in the cabin is as thin as if you were at 5,000 to 8,000 feet above sea level.

One of Dr. Goldstein's young patients who was having asthma symptoms the day before going on a plane trip with his mother developed breathing problems during the flight. When his mother discovered with a measuring device that the oxygen in the boy's blood was too low, the plane's staff had to give him oxygen to prevent an emergency landing.

Let them know you need O₂. If you have severe asthma that requires you to use oxygen regularly and you must fly, make sure you work this out in advance with the airline. They can't refuse to let you travel, but you do need to let them know beforehand so they can make the proper arrangements.

Pack your own food. If you have food allergies, it's very difficult to be sure that any snacks or meals the airlines serve are safe. The airlines get their food from vendors, so no one on the plane will be able to be sure what may be tucked away in the ingredients. Instead of taking a chance, stick a safe snack in your carry-on bag to enjoy during the flight, says Dr. Goldstein.

In a Hotel

You may be a "guest" at a hotel, but remember that you're also a customer. As such, don't hesitate to make sure you get a room that meets your health needs.

Choose a room you won't rue. Call to reserve a room ahead of time, and ask the hotel for a designated smoke-free and pet-free room. While this won't guarantee that your room has nothing to set off your allergies, it can tilt the odds in your favor.

While you're at it, ask for a room well away from the indoor pool, since rooms near the pool tend to be more damp and mold-friendly, Dr. Goldstein says.

Check before you sign. Take a look around the room before you agree to sign for it. If you detect a problem that's going to trigger your symptoms, go back to the front desk and request another room, Dr. Goldstein suggests.

If you feel nervous about doing this, remember: You're the customer paying for the room—and if it aggravates your allergies, you'll be the one paying that price, too.

Bring your own protection. If you use special coverings on your pillow and mattress at home to keep you away from allergens in the bedding, consider using them at the hotel. It might be too cumbersome a chore to put the mattress cover on if you're going to be in the room only a day or two, but slipping on an allergen-proof pillowcase is easy in any situation.

While you're at it, you may reduce your risk further by bringing your own pillow and sheets from home, too.

In the Great Outdoors

A retreat in the great outdoors provides you with plenty of fresh air and a chance to commune with nature. But before you put on your backpack and hiking boots, take a moment to read the tips below.

Be a happy camper. If you're pulling your damp tent and sleeping bags out of a musty basement before you head into the woods, some of the wildlife you'll encounter might be mold spores. To increase your odds of having a pleasant stay, set up your tent in the sunlight and let it air out and dry before you head off to camp, Dr. Goldstein suggests. If your sleeping bag is washable, take the time to launder it. But whether you wash it or not, air your sleeping bag out so it's dry. When you come home, air everything out well again before you pack it away.

Stay safe up high. Like on a jet, the oxygen in the air gets thinner as you go into the mountains. If your asthma isn't controlled, consider holding off on a trip to the mountains until you're breathing easy again, Dr. Goldstein says.

Arrive alive on your dive. If you have asthma and want to scuba dive, make sure that your breathing has been under good control for at least a week beforehand, Dr. Goldstein says. And that doesn't just mean that you're feeling well; your peak-flow meter results and blood-oxygen levels should be good, too. (For more information on using a peak-flow meter, see Asthma on page 222.)

If you have any concerns about your ability to dive safely, visit your doctor a week before your trip.

Stay safe in the sun. If you have atopic dermatitis, be sure to protect your skin from the outdoor elements. This includes not staying out in the sun long enough to burn (you're at the greatest risk between 10:00 A.M. and 4:00 P.M., when the sun's rays are most intense) and wearing sunscreen with an SPF of 15 or higher for extra protection. In addition, be sure to keep your skin properly lubricated so it doesn't dry out. (For more tips on atopic dermatitis, see Symptom Solver: Skin Problems on page 411.)

On a Cruise

Water, sun, great food—what's not to like? To enjoy your adventure on the high seas, first check out the following tips.

Stick to your routine. Cruises offer several benefits to people with allergies and asthma, Dr. Goldstein points out. You have plenty of food and drink choices; a medical staff is nearby; you can keep your medications handy and easy to find; and the pollen level in the air tends to be slight when you're away from shore.

On the other hand, as you're enjoying the high life on the high seas, don't forget to keep your guard up against the foods, drinks, and environmental conditions that could set off your allergies or asthma, he warns.

Check out the docs before you leave the

dock. Contact the medical department of the cruise line well in advance to ensure that your ship will have a doctor and staff who will be able to treat any potential allergic problems that arise.

Talk to the food staff. Make sure when you hit the buffet table that the food you're selecting won't trigger any allergies. Talk to the chef if necessary. And as always, if you can't be sure the food won't give you problems, don't eat it.

Be safe in sun and surf. The sun and salty air out at sea can dry out and irritate your skin if you have atopic dermatitis. So be sure to keep your skin properly lubricated and safe from the sun. Use moisturizing creams and sun-blocking agents.

On a Bus or Train

Whether you're going to be speeding through the countryside or a city, travel on a bus or train requires you to take some precautions prior to your journey.

Remember that planning's a must on the train or bus. If you're taking a trip on a bus or train, your options are limited for avoiding the chemical irritants they carry, such as the smell from cleaning products, Dr. Goldstein says.

Be sure to take any preventive treatments you normally use, such as antihistamines and inhalers, when you can't avoid asthma and allergy triggers. And if outside allergens

don't bother you and you are able to open the windows, go ahead and do it.

At the Table

Whether your food has been prepared by Aunt Sal or a chef trained at Le Cordon Bleu in Paris, unless you ask about the ingredients, you won't know whether or not the food is safe for you to eat. So speak up—your health depends on it.

Stay focused at the family table. Even when you're eating at a family gathering, don't assume that your loved ones doing the cooking have followed any stringent food-allergy guidelines that you might have. Check to ensure that the meal you're eating doesn't have nuts (which frequently pop up in holiday foods), milk, wheat, or other ingredients that trigger your allergies.

Act like a private investigator at restaurants. Ask every question needed to satisfy your curiosity about whether your food will be free of allergy-provoking ingredients. Talk to the food server, the chef, the manager, or whoever will be able to assure you that your food will be safe.

You may want to do this in a phone call ahead of time during a nonhectic hour of the day at the restaurant. That way, the staff will have time to acknowledge your needs and prepare for your arrival.

Stick with simple choices. If you're severely allergic to a food, steer away from extravagantly prepared dishes that offer more hiding spots in which a drop or crumble of a disastrous ingredient could lurk.

In Another Person's Home

Being a courteous guest—and one who gets invited back—usually means not asking about your host's housekeeping routines. But if you have allergies, a few politely worded inquiries could mean the difference between a pleasant stay and one interrupted by allergy or asthma attacks.

Feel free to ask for good housekeeping. When you and your allergies are going to spend the night at a friend's or relative's home, it can be tough to broach the subject of your allergies without the risk of of-

fending your hosts. "How can you tell your grandma to clean her house?" Dr. Goldstein asks. "People are just reluctant to say anything."

As you learned earlier in this book, a tidy house and a low-allergen house are two different things. But if you arrive pointing out problems with the arrangements, you could soon have an awkward visit on your hands.

Be sure to discuss your needs ahead of time. That way, your friends or relatives will have plenty of time to prepare their home so it won't trigger your allergies or asthma. Remind them that these requirements are medically necessary and you're not just being picky. If they need more convincing, photocopy relevant pages from this book and mail them to your hosts.

PART THREE

The
Allergy-Free
LIFESTYLE

Learn How to Lower Your
ALLERGIC RESPONSE

IN THE PREVIOUS PART, we taught you how to allergy-proof your environment. You learned natural and effective ways to delete the dust mites in your bedroom, clobber the cockroaches in your kitchen, and murder the mold spores in your basement. You also learned how to transform your lawn and garden from an allergy horror into an allergy oasis and how to stay allergy-free while traveling.

Hopefully, you've already started putting some of that advice into practice. Unfortunately, not even the most scrupulous environmental control can protect you from all allergens all of the time. So now comes a more difficult task: allergy-proofing yourself.

You may have been told that there's nothing you can do to make yourself less allergy-prone. Some conventional doctors will tell you that eating a better diet, exercising regularly, and reducing stress might improve your overall health. A few of them may be-

lieve that even the most beneficial lifestyle changes can't change your hypersensitive immune system.

While it's true that you can't buy a new immune system off the rack like you'd buy a new air cleaner, a growing body of evidence shows that how you eat, exercise, and unwind has a profound effect on your allergic response.

Think of it as rain accumulating in a barrel. By adopting a healthier lifestyle, you automatically reduce the level of physical and psychological stress (the rain) that accumulates in your body (the barrel). As a result, you're better able to tolerate exposure to pollen, mold, and other allergy triggers before they overflow, sending you into fits of sneezing and wheezing.

In the following chapters, we'll show you how the typical Western lifestyle contributes to your allergies. And we'll show you how a few simple lifestyle changes can tame even the twitchiest immune system. Since children are especially hard hit by allergies and asthma, we've also included a chapter for parents of allergic infants, children, and teens.

Here's a preview of what you'll find in this part.

The Allergy-Free Diet. Whether you know it or not, you're probably eating a nutritionally "at-risk" diet that aids and abets the allergic response. When you eat the wrong foods, you flood your system with inflammatory chemicals. Since your immune system is already working overtime to produce its own inflammatory chemicals, a poor diet can only double your allergic displeasure. In this chapter, you'll learn about the foods that make your allergies worse, the foods that make your allergies better, and ways to create a nutritionally sound, low-fat, anti-inflammatory diet that's right for you.

The Allergy-Free Supplementation Schedule. Although it's best to get essential nutrients with a knife and fork, we recognize that this isn't always possible. So in this chapter we discuss many of the dietary supplements that are used to treat allergies. Here you'll find an overview of allergy-fighting vitamins, minerals, bioflavonoids, herbs, and other supplements—along with recommended daily dosages.

The Allergy-Free Exercise Plan. Although exercise can cause problems for people with allergies, especially those with asthma, experts say it's an allergy trigger that you should not avoid. By improving your cardiovascular fitness, you increase your lung capacity, decrease your need for medications, and control your weight. Study after study show that a leaner frame is associated with fewer allergy symptoms. In this chapter, you'll learn which exercises are best (and worst) for people with allergies and asthma. For good measure, we've included an all-purpose 30-minute total-body workout.

Allergy-Free Stress Busters. Although stress doesn't cause allergies, it's often a fellow traveler. Just knowing you're allergic to natural substances that cause most people no harm can make you feel like a second-class citizen. When you add in the stress caused by actual allergy symptoms—and the stressful side effects caused by some allergy drugs—it can make you want to raise a white flag. But there's no need to surrender. In this chapter, you'll find the 10 best mind-body therapies for people with allergies, from biofeedback to yoga.

The Allergy-Free Child. If you have allergies, the last thing you want to do is pass this affliction on to your children. New research shows there are steps you can take to delay or reduce the odds. In this chapter, you'll see what you can do during pregnancy and infancy to reduce your child's risk of developing allergies and asthma. If your child already has well-established allergies or asthma, you'll learn the best ways to manage the disease at home, in school, and during those rebellious teenage years.

The
Allergy-Free
DIET

SUPPOSE YOU'RE ALLERGIC to pollen, mold, and dust mites. Sure, it's no fun being allergic to these phantom menaces. But you probably consider yourself luckier than the poor souls who can't eat a plate of shrimp without swelling up like the Michelin Man.

At least you're not allergic to *food*. Even so, you need to be careful. Just because you can eat shellfish with impunity (and lots of extra cocktail sauce), it doesn't mean your diet has no effect on your allergies or asthma.

"Even if you don't have food allergies, diet still plays an important role in your health," says Robert Rountree, M.D., a holistic physician in Boulder, Colorado, and coauthor of *Immunotics*. "Sixty percent of the immune system resides along the lining of the intestines, so it's doubly important to keep the gut healthy."

Eating the wrong kinds of food riles up your immune system. You might as well be dining on pollen pâté, mold meringue, and dust-mite dessert.

Conversely, eating the right kinds of food can actually calm down your immune system. Your allergies and asthma might improve so much that you can reduce or even eliminate some of your medications.

How Diet Can Make Your Allergies Worse

Allergies and asthma are diseases of inflammation. You become sensitized to one or more substances in your environment, and your immune system reacts to them by sending out a flood of inflammatory chemicals. The process is not unlike the "friendly fire" that claims many casualties in war.

In a sense, the histamines, prostaglandins,

135

and other inflammatory chemicals released by your immune system are misguided missiles. Although their target is allegedly a "foreign" invader, they do the most damage to you. The result: itchy eyes, a runny nose, congested lungs, skin problems, digestive problems, and a host of other unpleasant symptoms.

"Underlying these symptoms is an inflammatory disorder—a problem that results from excessive inflammation in the body," Dr. Rountree says. "It's as if the eyes, nose, and lungs are on fire."

If this "friendly fire" isn't halted, the inflammation becomes chronic. "The immune system becomes an agent of destruction," says Dr. Rountree. "The fire gets out of control, and normal tissue gets damaged."

A poor diet can make this inflammation worse.

If you don't eat enough fresh fruits and vegetables, foods rich in magnesium, or oily fish, your allergies and asthma will probably get worse. Further, eating too many of the wrong things, such as too much saturated fat or processed foods filled with salt and other additives, will also probably aggravate your allergies and asthma.

• The Problem with Saturated Fat

Suppose you eat a chocolate doughnut during a morning coffee break. Before you get back to your desk, your stomach acids are already starting to break down the doughnut's whopping amount of saturated fat. You might not think that this will have any effect on your allergic rhinitis (hay fever), asthma, or eczema. If anything, you're probably more worried about the effect it might have on your weight, cholesterol, and coronary arteries.

But doughnuts—and other fatty foods—have other, less obvious ways of biting you back.

After fat by-products are digested, they undergo further processing in the liver before moving on to the rest of your body. Then they run amok like a gang of saboteurs, forcing your body's chemical plants to produce harmful substances.

The end result of this subversion: inflammation.

If you have allergies and asthma, you already have enough inflammatory chemicals floating around in your system. The last thing you need is a diet that triggers the release of even more of them.

If you subsist on a diet of hamburgers, fries, and other fatty foods—in short, the typical Western diet—it's like putting out a fire with gasoline. In general, animal fats are more likely than plant fats to feed the fire, but there are exceptions. Some plant oils—sunflower oil, for example—contain large amounts of saturated fat.

So the next time you eat a bacon double cheeseburger, don't just think about the effect it'll have on your waistline. Consider the effect it'll have on your lungs.

The Traditional Healthy Asian Diet Pyramid

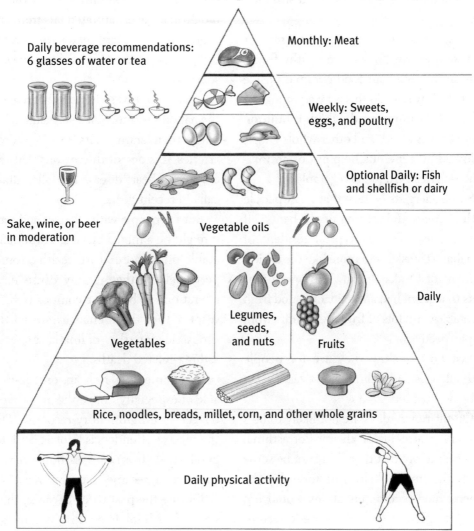

Daily beverage recommendations:
6 glasses of water or tea

Monthly: Meat

Weekly: Sweets, eggs, and poultry

Optional Daily: Fish and shellfish or dairy

Sake, wine, or beer in moderation

Vegetable oils

Daily

Vegetables

Legumes, seeds, and nuts

Fruits

Rice, noodles, breads, millet, corn, and other whole grains

Daily physical activity

Better Choices: The Asian Pyramid

Like most doctors, allergists have seen the serious consequences of eating what they call a nutritionally at-risk diet.

Just a generation ago, Americans considered fast food a luxury. Today, many people are so squeezed for time that they consider fast food a necessity.

Allergists are especially concerned about the dietary habits of their most vulnerable patients: children. African-American children, in particular, have a disproportionate risk of not only developing asthma but also dying from it.

A poor diet only makes a bad situation worse.

If you're eating Homeric (i.e., Homer Simpson) proportions of unhealthy foods, consider turning your food pyramid upside down. One way to do this is by adopting the so-called Asian pyramid, which is built on daily servings of rice and other whole grains, followed by generous helpings of antioxidant-rich fresh fruit and vegetables.

Some allergists believe that most people with allergies and asthma might benefit if they ate less like the typical resident of Omaha, Nebraska, and more like the typical resident of Osaka, Japan. They note that diets that are rich in antioxidants, good fresh vegetables, and lots of fruit are healthy from all perspectives.

Just how healthy they are for people with allergies and asthma, however, has yet to be determined.

On their own, diets are not likely to be a primary treatment for allergies or asthma. This isn't to say that there may not be some foods that might help. But for now, the generic food recommendations would not be a lot different from the generic recommendations for good, healthy nutrition. So it's probably best to think of diet as part of a global strategy to put an end to your sneezing and wheezing.

Omega-6: A Mixed Blessing

Thanks in part to the medical community's recommendations for a healthy diet, Americans are eating less saturated fat than they did 30 years ago. Saturated fats from animal sources have to a large extent been replaced by polyunsaturated fats from vegetable sources.

In general, this switch has been good for the nation's health. Since vegetable oil is less likely than animal fats to clog coronary arteries, it is one of the reasons that the incidence of heart disease has fallen dramatically in recent years.

But for people with allergies and asthma, it might be a mixed blessing. Although vegetable oil is more heart-healthy, some experts believe that it may cause harmful alterations in body-fat composition. They suspect that these changes are partly responsible for the dramatic increase in asthma-related deaths.

Vegetable oils rich in omega-6 fatty acids, especially, have been proven to trigger an inflammatory response. One of the biggest offenders is linoleic acid, found in oils made from corn, safflower, soybean, cottonseed, sesame, and sunflower.

During the past three decades, the proportion of linoleic acid in human fat has risen from 8 percent to 15 percent. That's a direct consequence of using vegetable oil in manufactured foods, fast-food frying, and home food preparation—not to mention the widespread use of vegetable oils in margarine, mayonnaise, salad dressings, and ready-to-eat frozen foods. The increasing amount of linoleic acid in our bodies might be one of the reasons that allergists are seeing an increasing incidence of serious and fatal asthma.

People with allergies and asthma need to be especially vigilant when they go out to eat, because restaurant food is often a hidden source of fat, especially rancid fat. According to Dr. Rountree, fat becomes rancid, or toxic, when the bonds in polyunsaturated fats, which are already relatively unstable, come into contact with oxygen. This creates lipid peroxides, a kind of free radical. High heat used in cooking accelerates the process. Like any other business, some restaurants like to save money. One way to do that is to conserve their cooking oil by using it over and over again. By the end of a busy evening, the oil in a restaurant's deep-fat fryer can become terribly oxidized.

As bad as fresh oil is for your body, rancid oil is even worse. Even if you're cooking with an oil that's low in saturated and unsaturated fat, such as extra-virgin olive oil, you should cook with it only once since all oil becomes rancid after repeated use. Such oil is so pro-inflammatory, experts say, that it can punch holes in your cells.

How Much Water Should You Drink?

Dehydration is bad for everyone, but it's especially harmful for people with allergies and asthma.

When researchers at the University of Buffalo studied the effects of dehydration on people with asthma, they found that it increases the risk of asthma attacks even in humid weather.

"No matter what, always drink plenty of water—at least 8 to 10 glasses a day—to keep secretions in your respiratory tract fluid," recommends Andrew Weil, M.D., director of the program in integrative medicine and clinical professor of medicine at the University of Arizona College of Medicine in Tucson. "Drinking plenty of water also speeds up the process of eliminating irritants and toxins from the body."

Individual needs vary, however. In fact, the more you weigh, the more water you lose. To determine how much water is optimal for you, follow these steps.

1. Write down your weight in pounds.
2. Multiply your weight by .04, which equals pounds of water lost.
3. Multiply the result of step 2 by 2 to determine the number of cups you need per day.

You'll need to drink extra water when weather conditions are hot or dry and when you exercise. In addition, remember that caffeine and alcohol sap as much water out of you as they put in. To keep yourself from getting parched, drink an extra ½ cup of water for every cup you drink of caffeinated or alcoholic beverages.

Think about that the next time you dine out fashionably late.

"Milk Mustaches" and Other Things to Avoid

Milk and other dairy products are two big culprits when it comes to irritating your immune system.

"Try eliminating these substances from your diet for a couple months and see what happens," suggests Andrew Weil, M.D., director of the program in integrative medicine and clinical professor of medicine at the University of Arizona College of Medicine in Tucson. "The protein in cows' milk, specifically, is a frequent offender, and in those with overresponsive immune systems, it may be an overlooked cause of problems."

Also consider cutting back on the so-called white foods—that is, foods made with white sugar, white flour, white potatoes, and so on. "All those things sap your immune system," Dr. Rountree says. "Eliminating refined carbohydrates is the first step in keeping the intestines healthy."

Of course, that's easier said than done. Hiding the sugar bowl might be psycholog-

Clear Your Pantry of These Allergy-Provoking Items

Just as some things in your diet can help to alleviate your allergy or asthma symptoms, others might be linked to worsened symptoms. Since many alternative and environmental doctors believe that the following items can promote inflammation of the gastrointestinal tract, try to decrease your consumption of them.

Milk and cheese. Milk protein is a common irritant of the immune system.

Omega-6 fatty acids. Although you need some of these acids for good health, they can intensify inflammation and other immune responses. Foods that are high in omega-6's include cottonseed, corn, and sunflower oils and processed foods such as mayonnaise and salad dressings.

Protein. Regardless of whether it comes from animals or plants, it should account for no more than 10 percent of your daily caloric intake. Observe the recommended daily allowance of no more than 50 grams.

Saturated fats. Whether they come from plant or animal sources, they trigger the release of inflammatory chemicals.

Trans fats. Rates of asthma and allergies in teens are highest in countries where people eat the most trans fats. Avoid products—including some that are supposedly fat-free—if the ingredients list includes partially hydrogenated oil.

ically satisfying, but it probably will put only a small dent in your annual sugar intake. The problem is the large amount of sugar found in processed foods.

"A hundred years ago, or even 75 years ago, we ate around 5 pounds of sugar a year. Now we eat at least 150 pounds of sugar a year, and more often than not it comes from corn instead of cane," notes Allan Lieberman, M.D., an environmental-medicine doctor in North Charleston, South Carolina. "I dare you to go to a supermarket shelf and look at any processed food label and not find corn-syrup solids," he says.

Finally, some food additives can be as nettlesome as the foods themselves. Because of this, people with allergies and asthma should take special care to read *all* the fine print on food labels. Although sulfites and food coloring such as tartrazine (also known as yellow dye no. 5) have been linked to allergies and asthma, such sensitivities aren't common in all allergy- or asthma-prone individuals.

Many allergy patients have learned to avoid foods and beverages containing sulfur dioxide because it can trigger an asthma attack. That's why manufacturers place

Foods that are rich in trans fats include peanut butter, bread, muffin mix, cookies, and corn chips.

In addition to the foods listed above, you might be wise to avoid the following items. Though more research still needs to be done, some health practitioners believe that these foods can increase your risk of developing such controversial conditions as candidiasis hypersensitivity, leaky-gut syndrome, and multiple chemical sensitivity.

Alcoholic beverages. Some health care practitioners believe that overconsumption of distilled spirits can lead to leaky-gut syndrome. Wine drinkers probably needn't worry, however, as long as they stick to no more than one glass per day.

Caffeinated beverages. Some health practitioners believe that drinking more than one cup of coffee a day increases your risk of developing leaky-gut syndrome.

Meat and poultry. These foods often carry residues of antibiotics and hormones that can affect immunity.

Sugar. In the view of some health care workers, a sweet tooth can cause leaky-gut syndrome.

warning labels that read "contains sulfur dioxide" or "contains sulfites" on wine and other products.

The Price of a Poor Diet

Repeated insults to your gastrointestinal tract might lead to a condition that environmental-medicine doctors and alternative practitioners call leaky-gut syndrome. According to proponents of this controversial diagnosis, the lining of your gut is supposed to be thick with mucus. Eating the wrong foods thins out the mucus, allowing partially digested food particles to pass into your bloodstream, which can cause allergic reactions anywhere in your body. "Leaky-gut plays a major role in the development of allergy," Dr. Rountree says.

A poor diet also disturbs the delicate balance of "good" and "bad" bugs in your gut, increasing the risk of yeast overgrowth.

Stock Up on These Allergy-Fighting Superfoods

You probably already know that foods like broccoli, spinach, and strawberries are good for you—but did you know that they can also help to relieve your asthma and allergies? The following is a list of allergy "superfoods." For better health, try to increase your consumption of them.

Apples. A British study of 2,512 middle-aged men showed that those who ate five apples a week had significantly higher lung function than those who ate no apples. Experts believe apples contain healthy compounds, including antioxidants that improve lung health.

Borage oil, black currant seed oil, and evening primrose oil. These three oils are all rich sources of gamma-linolenic acid (GLA), which has anti-inflammatory properties. In fact, borage oil is the subject of ongoing research at the Center for Complementary and Alternative Medicine Research in Asthma at the University of California, Davis.

Canola oil. Canola oil is a great source of allergy-fighting omega-3 fatty acids. Other plant sources include soybean oil, flaxseed oil, walnuts, and wheat germ.

Cold-water fish. In addition to plant sources, the following fish are rich sources of omega-3 fatty acids: mackerel, anchovies, herring, salmon, sardines, lake trout, Atlantic sturgeon, and tuna. To get the most benefit, either bake or poach the fish. Eat two or three servings per week.

Once the yeast becomes dominant, it can lead to another controversial diagnosis—candidiasis hypersensitivity. According to environmental-medicine doctors, alternative practitioners, and some conventional doctors, symptoms of candidiasis hypersensitivity include chronic fatigue, depression, mood swings, and weak muscles. (For more information, see Candidiasis on page 450.)

Proponents of both diagnoses say that drinking hard liquor is like adding fuel to the fire. "If you're already prone to yeast infections and you drink a lot of alcohol, you're going to get yeast overgrowth," Dr. Rountree says. "Alcohol is pretty much guaranteed to give you leaky-gut."

The risk is highest if you drink distilled spirits. If you prefer wine, you're much less likely to develop leaky-gut if you don't consume more than one glass of wine a day.

In some cases, an unhealthy diet might actually trigger the onset of allergies in

Fruits and vegetables. Any richly colored fruit or vegetable is loaded with antioxidants, vitamins, and bioflavonoids. Eat more blueberries, raspberries, strawberries, cranberries, sweet potatoes, bell peppers, and tomatoes.

Magnesium-rich foods. Some studies have demonstrated that people with asthma are magnesium-deficient. Magnesium-rich foods include spinach, navy beans, pinto beans, sunflower seeds, tofu, halibut, cashews, artichokes, and black-eyed peas.

Olive oil. Since it's monounsaturated, consider using extra-virgin olive oil as your main source of fat.

Spices. Eat ginger and turmeric regularly for their anti-inflammatory effects.

Spirulina. Sure, it's algae, but it's bioflavonoid-rich algae. It's available in tablet and powder form.

Caution: To avoid possible heavy-metal contamination, buy spirulina only from reputable sources. Check the label for a toll-free number for consumer questions or for an indication that it's been analyzed for heavy-metal content.

Yogurt. A study at the University of California, Davis, showed that people who ate 1 cup a day of yogurt with active cultures had one-tenth as many allergies.

Zinc-rich foods. Some studies have demonstrated that people with asthma are zinc-deficient. Zinc-rich foods include plain yogurt, tofu, lean ground beef, lean ham, oysters, crab, the dark meat of turkey and chicken, lentils, legumes, and ricotta cheese.

people who've never had them before. Usually, such people have an inherited tendency to develop allergies, but for one reason or another, they've managed to stay symptom-free. Over the years, however, a diet low in micronutrients and high in refined carbohydrates and rancid fats inexorably takes its toll, causing a buildup of toxins that gradually poison the immune system.

Meanwhile, yeasts and other bad bugs take over the gastrointestinal system, which produces even more toxins. Eventually, the immune system becomes so stressed-out that it can no longer tell the difference between friend and foe. Without warning, it begins attacking harmless specks of pollen, mold, and animal dander as if they posed a mortal danger.

This might explain why some people suddenly start sneezing and wheezing late in life.

The Right Foods to Fight Allergies

People with allergies and asthma often go to extravagant lengths to control their environment. They rip up their carpeting, encase their pillows and mattresses, and install expensive air-filtration systems. Some even pull up stakes and move to a different climate in a desperate and often futile attempt to "run away" from their allergies.

They can become so obsessed with controlling their environment that they forget about living their lives.

A simpler strategy may be to make some less drastic dietary changes. "Diet is easier to work with," Dr. Weil notes, "and it can influence immune reactiveness profoundly."

Holistic health-care practitioners suggest that a nutritious diet can alleviate or prevent allergies and asthma in four ways.

1. It can help control underlying inflammation of air passages.

2. It can dilate air passages.

3. It can thin down mucus in the lungs.

4. It can prevent food-allergy reactions that trigger asthma attacks.

We've already seen how the wrong kinds of fat can make your allergies and asthma worse. Now let's consider how the right kinds of fat can make your allergies and asthma better.

• The Right Fats

Omega-3 essential fatty acids are natural anti-inflammatory agents. They contain eicosapentaenoic acid (EPA), which counters the formation of inflammatory chemicals. Good natural sources include flaxseed oil, salmon, haddock, and cod.

Another beneficial essential fatty acid, gamma-linolenic acid (GLA), also has anti-inflammatory properties. Good natural sources include evening primrose oil, borage oil, and black currant seed oil.

If possible, you should include more of both of these fatty acids in your diet. Dr. Rountree says that you can add a tablespoon of flaxseed oil or walnut oil, for example, to your cereal in the morning or take a supplement of fish oil to get your omega-3's. He recommends a dose of 500 to 1,500 milligrams daily of EPA. As for GLA, he suggests taking 300 to 600 milligrams daily. "Many nutritionists and herbalists find that the combination of omega-3 essential fatty acids along with GLA creates a more potent effect for decreasing inflammation," he says.

• Colorful Fruits and Veggies

People with allergies and asthma also should load up on more fruits and vegetables, especially the Technicolor variety.

The rich blue, green, yellow, orange, and red pigments found in fruits and vegetables such as blueberries, spinach, and tomatoes indicate that they contain antioxidants. One group of these pigments makes up the carotenoid family, including beta-carotene, lutein, and lycopene. The other group consists of flavonoids, such as quercetin (found in the skin of apples and red onions) and proanthocyanidins (the source of the blue in blueberries and red in cranberries).

"Flavonoids have a number of beneficial effects in treating and preventing allergies," Dr. Rountree says. "In addition to their antioxidant properties, they act as anti-inflammatory agents that help balance and restore normal immune function."

Other rich sources of antioxidants are sweet potatoes, bell peppers, broccoli, cauliflower, cabbage, and strawberries.

• Juices

Fruit juice also can be a rich source of antioxidants, but no one juice is better than another.

Even if the label reads "Grape Juice" in big letters, the product may contain pre-

The Best Choices for an Allergy-Fighting Diet

Confused about what you should and shouldn't eat if you have allergies or asthma? Just check out this handy chart.

Instead of . . .	Try this . . .
Animal protein	Plant protein
Caffeinated coffee	Green tea
Chemically treated fruits, vegetables, and cereal grains	Organically grown fruits, vegetables, and cereal grains
Cow's milk	Soy milk and other calcium-rich foods, such as leafy greens and fortified orange juice
Double martini	Glass of wine
Fruit juice with corn syrup, fructose, other sweeteners	Fruit juice that's 100 percent fruit

cious little grape. If you look at the fine print, you might find wording such as "Contains a mixture of juice." On closer inspection, you might discover that the product contains 10 percent corn syrup.

Buy juice in glass containers if you're concerned about possible chemical contamination. Other kinds of containers, especially plastic, can turn an otherwise healthful juice into a toxic brew that can cause a variety of side effects like headaches and dizziness, says George Miller, M.D., an obstetrician in Lewisburg, Pennsylvania, and president-elect of the American Academy of Environmental Medicine.

• Colon-Friendly Foods

If you have allergies or asthma, good fats and antioxidant foods are only part of the dietary equation. To prevent leaky-gut syndrome, you also need to consume colon-friendly substances.

First and foremost, ensure that your diet contains plenty of fiber, especially the unrefined variety. Fiber is as stimulating to the colon as a crossword puzzle is to the brain. Not only does it energize and wake up your gastrointestinal system, experts say, it also makes your bowel "think."

Since so much of the immune system resides in the gastrointestinal tract, a cognizant colon is important to your overall health. High-fiber foods produce contractions called peristalsis. And an active colon is a healthy colon. On the other hand, low-fiber foods produce a lazy

colon that's more susceptible to cancer and other diseases.

The best sources of fiber are whole grains, nuts, and seeds. The outer bran layer of whole grains and seeds offers a unique benefit to your gastrointestinal system: It's rich in fibers that encourage the growth of healthy bacteria such as *Lactobacillus acidophilus* and bifidobacteria. Brown rice and flax meal are especially likely to foster the growth of these "good" bugs.

When you have the right balance of good bugs, your gut stays healthy and digests food properly. By creating an acidic environment, good bugs drive out such "bad" bugs as salmonella, shigella, and *Escherichia coli*.

Too often, though, good bugs are in short supply. As a consequence of the Western lifestyle, we've shifted the balance toward bad bugs that inflame the gastrointestinal tract, increasing our susceptibility to everything from diarrhea to colon cancer.

Today, our systems are more likely to be populated with pro-inflammatory bacteria than were our ancestors' systems. The likely cause, experts say, is increasing exposure to pollution and increasing use of antibiotics. The end result: an explosion of chronic diseases, including allergies and asthma.

• Yogurt: A Natural Way to Restore the Balance

Assuming that you don't have a milk allergy, the best way to restore the balance between good and bad bacteria in your gastrointestinal tract is to load up on yogurt.

When University of California researchers fed patients 18 to 24 ounces of yogurt a day, their allergic symptoms declined by 90 percent.

Granted, that's a lot of yogurt. A typical serving contains only 8 ounces. But researchers concluded that the more yogurt you eat, the better. Since the good bacteria in your gut need to be constantly renewed, you need to eat yogurt regularly in order to get the beneficial effect.

Yogurt—or at least the active cultures it contains—is not only good for your gut, it can also help skin allergies, according to a Finnish study.

When Finnish researchers gave probiotic supplements of those cultures to children with severe eczema, they helped clear up their skin.

Not all so-called yogurt products are beneficial, however. Unlike the yogurts found in the dairy case, frozen yogurt and canned yo-

A Meal-by-Meal Plan for Fighting Allergies

We wish we could provide you with a step-by-step diet that would eliminate your allergies and asthma. Unfortunately, no single diet is right for everyone. Your nutritional needs are unique to you, because no one else has the same combination of genetic and acquired traits of metabolism, nutrition, and immune status.

That said, here's some general, doctor-approved, meal-by-meal advice that can relieve your sneezing and wheezing. Obviously, if you're allergic to any of the foods here, you will want to find a substitute that's safe and just as nutritious.

Breakfast. Build your breakfast around fresh fruits and whole grains. Avoid sugary products and so-called instant foods. Instant breakfast bars, for example, are loaded with corn syrup and preservatives. If you like to drink milk for breakfast, restrict yourself to fat-free.

Lunch. Unless you're a growing child or a pregnant woman, build this meal around fruits, vegetables, and grains. If you must have meat, eat the leanest meat possible. Remember that in most fast-food burgers, the percentage of calories from fat can be as high as 35 percent.

Dinner. Build your dinner around grains, cooked or raw vegetables, and protein from meat, fish, or soy. Trim off the fat or skin from meat and chicken. Avoid oils and fats in sauces and salad dressings. If you customarily have a drink with dinner, have a glass of wine instead of a beer or a mixed drink.

Snacks. If possible, don't indulge in snacking at all. But if you must have a snack, munch on an apple or some raisins.

gurt have no beneficial effect on allergies and asthma; in fact, your allergies could get worse, thanks to the large amount of sugar these two varieties contain. In Europe, these products can't even be called yogurt since they contain no active cultures. Check the container for the words "live active cultures" to be assured of a bacterial boost. Want to go the extra mile for intestinal health? Take acidophilus (also known as *Lactobacillus acidophilus*) capsules, which are excellent for colonizing the gut with good bugs, says Dr. Rountree. In order to get the maximum benefit, he recommends a brand that contains between 2.5 and 10 billion organisms per capsule.

Eating Strategies for Allergy Relief

In addition to consumption of foods like salmon, strawberries, whole grains, and yogurt, alternative practitioners and environmental-minded doctors believe that the following dietary strategies might also help to ease your allergy and asthma symptoms.

Eat regular meals. French researchers have found that adolescents who either skip meals or eat them on the sly are more likely to have asthma. They concluded that irregular eating has a harmful effect on respiratory function. While more research needs to be done to confirm their ideas, eating regular meals is beneficial in so many ways that it's worth giving it a shot.

Consume natural decongestants. Chile peppers, hot mustard, and horseradish are great symptom relievers because they contain chemicals that help thin nasal secretions.

Go vegan. It can be a drastic step, we know. But consider what happened when researchers placed 25 people with asthma on a diet that prohibited meat, fish, eggs, dairy products, coffee, ordinary tea, chocolate, sugar, salt, tap water, apples, citrus fruits, soybeans, and peas. Unrestricted foods included lettuce, carrots, beets, onions, celery, cabbage, cauliflower, broccoli, cucumbers, radishes, artichokes, beans, blueberries, strawberries, raspberries, cloudberries, black currants, gooseberries, plums, and pears. After 4 months, 71 percent of the participants reported significant improvement. After a year, the figure was 92 percent. Most were able to reduce or stop taking asthma medications.

One last note: Although dietary modifications can obviously benefit people with allergies and asthma, they take time to kick in. "People with allergies respond very well to dietary changes. In my experience, these dietary measures can make a dramatic difference," Dr. Weil says. "But don't expect to see a change before 1 month."

The
Allergy-Free
Supplementation
SCHEDULE

IF YOU ARE LOOKING for supplements to treat allergies, your first thought may be to find alternatives to prescription drugs. Some herbs and supplements may help you, but when you are having a bad bout of allergies, they will probably not be as effective at controlling your symptoms as conventional medicine.

A better reason to consider supplements is to accomplish what allergy drugs cannot: addressing the underlying problem of allergies and strengthening your immune system. Here are some supplements that alternative experts say may do just that. As usual, be sure to tell your doctor about any supplements you're taking.

Take a Multivitamin

It seems so simple, but the easiest supplement to take to help alleviate your allergy symptoms is a multivitamin.

"I believe that taking nutritional supplements every day, including a multiple vitamin, a bioflavonoid such as quercetin, and essential fatty acids, helps keep my allergy symptoms at bay," says Robert Rountree, M.D., a holistic physician in Boulder, Colorado, and coauthor of *Immunotics*, which provides natural remedies for balancing and strengthening the immune system.

Look for a multi with about 100 percent of the Daily Value for most nutrients. Take it with a meal so that your body can absorb most of the nutrients. Look for a multivitamin brand, even a generic, that has "USP" (United States Pharmacopeia) on the label. Makers of those vitamins can be prosecuted by the FDA if their products don't contain the amounts promised on the label or fail to dissolve properly.

Here's where it gets more complicated. Other supplements can help mainly respiratory allergy symptoms like sneezing, wheezing, and a runny nose. A second group of supplements can help digestive health and improve allergy symptoms. A third group can strengthen your adrenal glands, which can improve your immune system and relieve allergy symptoms.

Supplements for Respiratory Allergy Symptoms

• Quercetin

Perhaps the most intriguing allergy supplement is quercetin, a type of bioflavonoid, which is chemically similar to cromolyn sodium (Gastrocrom), a drug used to treat allergic rhinitis (hay fever) and asthma.

Mark Stengler, N.D., a naturopathic and homeopathic physician in La Jolla, California, says that quercetin prevents histamine release, much like loratadine (Claritin), a nonsedating prescription antihistamine—when it works. "A lot of people don't take a high enough dosage and wonder why it doesn't work. And when you stop taking it, the symptoms come back," Dr. Stengler says.

The catch? Quercetin works great in a test tube but is poorly absorbed by the body. And it's expensive, costing typically $25 to $30 a month. But even that's not too bad when compared with Claritin, which costs $85 a month.

If you want to try it, take a supplement containing 1,000 milligrams of quercetin, plus 500 to 1,000 milligrams of bromelain, three times a day at the first sign of allergies. Take them as long as needed. Bromelain is an enzyme derived from pineapple that works as an anti-inflammatory. Combining bromelain with quercetin provides a one-two punch against inflammation. Don't take bromelain if you're allergic to pineapple.

Quercetin chalcone may be the most effective form because it's better absorbed by the body than other forms. You probably won't see "chalcone" on the label, however. Ask your pharmacist to recommend a brand containing quercetin chalcone. Dr. Stengler says that if quercetin is going to work for you, you should see results within 1 to 2 weeks. Continue taking it until after your allergy season ends.

• Nettle

Nettle, which is also known as stinging nettle, is Dr. Stengler's favorite allergy supplement: "I use it a lot with hay fever. It's the most effective, hands down." In one study, conducted at the National College of Naturopathic Medicine in Portland, Oregon, researchers gave nettle to some people with hay fever and a placebo (a fake pill) to others. After 1 week, those taking the nettle reported more improvement in their symptoms than those taking the placebo.

Start taking nettle a few weeks before your allergy season begins and continue taking it straight through the season. Dr.

Stengler recommends taking 300 milligrams of nettle leaf each day. If it is going to work for you, you will see an improvement in your symptoms within 2 to 3 days.

• Bee Pollen

Bee pollen is another option for upper respiratory allergy symptoms, says Dr. Stengler.

The effectiveness of bee pollen is more controversial, even in alternative circles, and Dr. Stengler doesn't know just how it works. But he does know it worked for him.

"When I moved to California, the first spring I had really bad hay fever. I tried bee pollen, and within a few days I did get some pretty dramatic relief—no sneezing, no

Supplement Schedule

Choose among the following supplements to ease your allergy symptoms, improve your digestive health, and strengthen your adrenal glands. Those taken by Robert Rountree, M.D., a holistic physician in Boulder, Colorado, and coauthor of *Immunotics*, are marked with an asterisk (*).

- Multivitamin*: daily
- Quercetin*: 1,000 milligrams, plus 500 to 1,000 milligrams of bromelain, three times a day
- Nettle: 300 milligrams daily
- Vitamin C: 500 milligrams daily
- Vitamin E: 400 IU daily
- Methylsulfonylmethane (MSM): 1,000 milligrams three times a day
- Acidophilus: 1 billion to 10 billion viable organisms a day
- Gamma oryzanol: 100 milligrams three times a day
- Omega-3 fatty acids*: 3,000 milligrams of fish oil daily or 1 to 2 teaspoons of flaxseed oil daily
- Borage oil: 300 milligrams each day
- Pantothenic acid: 500 milligrams three times a day with meals
- Zinc: 30 to 40 milligrams daily
- Korean ginseng: 100 milligrams, standardized to include 4 to 7 percent ginsenosides, two or three times a day
- Siberian ginseng: 8 to 10 milliliters of tincture two or three times a day or 300 milligrams in capsule form, standardized to 0.4 percent eleutherosides, two or three times a day
- American ginseng: 1 to 2 milliliters of tincture two or three times a day

runny nose. I stayed on it another month, and the symptoms didn't come back," says Dr. Stengler.

Your best bet is to use local pollen, although Dr. Stengler's was from Canada and seemed to be quite effective. If you have asthma or a history of anaphylactic reactions or are allergic to bee stings, talk to your doctor first. Dr. Stengler recommends 500 to 1,000 milligrams twice daily, starting when your symptoms are bothering you and continuing for at least 2 weeks.

• Ephedra

A traditional Chinese herb long treasured for easing allergy, asthma, and inflammatory conditions, ephedra can be risky in excessive doses, says Dr. Stengler. Its active ingredient, ephedrine, is chemically similar to the body's own epinephrine, which is also known as adrenaline.

Ephedra's effects are similar to pseudoephedrine, a common decongestant and bronchodilator in over-the-counter cold and allergy remedies.

"Ephedra is a reasonable alternative for people who choose a natural route," says Dr. Stengler, who mainly recommends it for acute sinusitis or asthma but not for long-term treatment of allergies. "For the average, healthy person, it's safe. But not if you have heart disease, high blood pressure, irregular heartbeat, diabetes, glaucoma, hyperthyroidism, or a swollen prostate gland," he adds.

If you want to try this herb, get it in an herbal formula that includes licorice root to offset ephedra's toxicity. "In Chinese medicine, it was always used in combination with 8 to 10 other herbs and only in very low dosage," says Dr. Stengler. Long-term use can not only trigger a rebound effect of increased congestion but also overstimulate your adrenal glands, which can lead to a deficiency of stress hormones, he warns.

Because of these dangers, use ephedra only under the guidance of a qualified practitioner.

• Vitamin C

A natural antihistamine, vitamin C blocks the release of histamine, a biochemical that, among other actions, causes constriction of the bronchial tubes, making it difficult to breathe. Take 500 milligrams daily.

• Vitamin E

This nutrient is essential for normal functioning of the immune system, so supplementing with vitamin E could lessen your allergy symptoms. That's because immune cells are highly susceptible to the harmful effects of free-radical reactions. Take 400 IU of vitamin E each day.

• Ginkgo

The herb ginkgo has been used for thousands of years to treat asthma, allergies, and coughs. The flavonoids in ginkgo seem to be responsible for its helpfulness in preventing membrane damage associated with asthma and stimulating relaxation of contracted blood vessels, which are common in asthma attacks. Take 40 milligrams of ginkgo three times per day. Choose a standardized extract containing 24 percent ginkgo flavone glycosides.

• Methylsulfonylmethane

The sulfur-containing compound methylsulfonylmethane (MSM) can help some people with allergies. Dr. Stengler suspects it increases cortisol levels, but its exact mechanism is not known.

Try 1,000 milligrams three times a day. Start taking MSM a few weeks before your allergy season begins and continue taking it straight through the season.

The Digestive Health/Allergy Connection

Improving the health of your digestive tract can reduce strain on your immune system and sometimes reduce your sensitivity to allergies, according to some alternative-minded doctors.

Problems with gut flora are probably one reason that allergies are so common in modern societies, says Michael Lyon, M.D., director of research at Oceanside Functional Medicine Research Institute in Nanaimo, British Columbia, Canada.

One easy way to improve your gut flora is to eat more yogurt. The idea that eating yogurt is good for your health is not new. Ilya Metchnikoff, a Russian researcher, theorized in the early 1900s that eating yogurt promotes health and longevity. Almost a century later, some American doctors studying the effect of yogurt on the immune system found that it can also reduce allergy symptoms.

Researchers from the University of California, Davis, divided 60 people into three groups. One group ate 200 grams of yogurt containing active cultures each day for a year. The second group ate 200 grams of yogurt in which the culture was heat-killed. The third group didn't eat any yogurt at all. Weekly health questionnaires revealed that the group eating the live-culture yogurt had fewer allergy symptoms than the other groups. The group eating live-culture yogurt also had less gastrointestinal distress than the other two groups. Both groups eating yogurt had fewer upper respiratory problems, such as colds, flu, coughing, and wheezing, than the group eating no yogurt.

The key could be yogurt's benefits for your digestive system. Metchnikoff had theorized that the *Lactobacillus* microbes, which turn milk into yogurt, also help make the intestines more acidic, preventing the breeding of harmful microbes.

But why would this affect your allergies?

Leo Galland, M.D., director of the Foundation for Integrated Medicine in New York City, attributes it to the "rain barrel effect": When the immune system is stressed to its maximum capacity, like a rain barrel filled to the rim, just a small amount of new stress, like a few drops of rain, can cause an overflow, or problem in the system, that under other conditions might not be a problem at all. And difficulties in the intestines can help stress the immune system to capacity.

It's not just harmful microbes that can cause problems either. According to some alternative doctors, excessive permeability of the intestinal lining, called leaky-gut syndrome, and parasites can also tax the immune system.

Surprised to read "parasites" there?

"Contrary to popular belief, parasitic infection is not unusual in the United States," Dr. Galland notes. He says that he has seen a lot of people whose allergies vanish once their gastrointestinal problems are treated.

Supplements to Support Digestive Health

• Probiotics

Friendly bacteria, such as the *Lactobacillus* in yogurt with active cultures, are sometimes called probiotics. Besides yogurt, probiotics are also found in a variety of foods, including litchi nuts and fresh sauerkraut.

Perhaps the easiest way to supplement your diet with good bacteria, however, is to take an acidophilus supplement (also known as *Lactobacillus acidophilus*), containing 1 billion to 10 billion viable organisms a day, Dr. Galland says. Because heat, moisture, and sunlight destroy the organisms, buy supplements that have been re-

frigerated and store them in your refrigerator.

• Prebiotics

For best results, you want the probiotics to actually grow in your body. To help this process along, you also need "prebiotics," foods and supplements that promote the growth of the probiotics in your body, says Dr. Lyon. Fiber is the best prebiotic. Oatmeal and other fiber-rich foods are some of the most beneficial prebiotics there are.

Not only does oat fiber promote the growth of friendly bacteria, it also helps heal the gut mucosa, reducing permeability of the intestinal lining.

Fiber comes in two forms: soluble and insoluble. Soluble fiber, such as fruit pectin, is a good prebiotic because it feeds friendly intestinal bacteria. Insoluble fiber, such as wheat bran, does not feed bacteria, but it does help reduce permeability by inhibiting parasites from attaching to the intestinal wall.

Don't overdo it. If you take large amounts of highly soluble fiber supplements, particularly fruit pectin or guar gum, some alternative doctors say that it can actually increase intestinal permeability, perhaps by producing an overgrowth of bacteria. To reduce this risk, you should balance insoluble fiber with soluble fiber.

The best sources of both soluble and insoluble fibers are foods such as unrefined grains, including oats, brown rice, and whole wheat, as well as peas, beans, and squash.

The USDA recommends that adults get about 25 grams of fiber a day. As you increase your fiber intake, start with a small amount and gradually add more over several days to avoid bloating and gas, says Dr. Lyon.

• Gamma Oryzanol

A potent antioxidant, gamma oryzanol is found naturally in rice bran oil. Its antioxidant properties can help tame your allergy symptoms, and it has healing effects on your stomach and intestines. Take 100 milligrams three times a day. It's safe to take this indefinitely, says Dr. Galland.

• Essential Fatty Acids

Essential fatty acids (EFAs) can help control your allergies by reducing inflammation elsewhere in your body. Two major types of essential fatty acids are omega-3 fatty acids—which are found in flaxseed and deep-sea fish such as salmon, haddock, and cod—and omega-6 fatty acids—which are found in vegetable oils like corn and sunflower and evening primrose and borage oils. But you need to find the balance of omega-3 and omega-6 EFAs that is right for you.

Dr. Galland estimates that about one-third of people with allergies have some form of EFA deficiency and can benefit from supplements. When he suspects an EFA deficiency in patients, he generally starts them out with an omega-3 supplement such as flaxseed or fish oil.

"Then I look to see what happens to them, what happens to their skin, their nails, their hair—and also their energy. And depending on their response, I may add an omega-6, such as primrose oil. And then I adjust the levels up or down to fit the individual," says Dr. Galland.

You can safely try this yourself, he says, if you suspect you need EFA supplements. Take the "Do You Need EFA Supplements?" quiz on page 156 to see.

Start with about 3,000 milligrams of fish oil or 1 to 2 teaspoons of flaxseed oil daily. If after 2 to 4 weeks you are still having problems, try adding about 3,000 milligrams of evening primrose oil a day.

Then experiment with increasing or decreasing these levels to find your optimum dosages. Because heat, light, and air turn EFAs rancid, buy oils that are cold- or expeller-pressed and store them in a refrigerator or freezer. Discard 6 weeks after opening. It's safe to take EFAs for life.

Another essential fatty acid, called gamma-linolenic acid (GLA), can help protect and repair your intestinal lining. GLA is one of the beneficial omega-6 fatty acids. It promotes the production of the prostaglandins that protect your digestive tract. Take 300 milligrams each day in the form of borage oil. It's safe to take this indefinitely.

As you are increasing the beneficial essential fatty acids, like omega-3's and GLAs, you can balance your levels more by reducing some of the less-healthy omega-6's, especially from sources of animal fats, which most Americans get too much of. This may reduce inflammation from allergies—at least in theory.

There is evidence that this strategy helps reduce inflammation from Crohn's disease and rheumatoid arthritis. But there are no scientific studies to show that this approach works for true allergies. It might help reduce inflammation from allergies in some people, however, says Dr. Galland.

This approach involves taking fish oil and flaxseed oil supplements, as described, to increase beneficial fatty acids, while sharply reducing your intake of animal fat, especially from beef. You should stick with it for at least 3 months to see results.

Supplements to Strengthen the Adrenals

Another way to reduce inflammation from allergies is to strengthen your adrenal glands' ability to handle stress, says Dr. Stengler.

"When you have allergies like hay fever, in addition to producing histamine, your body uses up a lot of stress hormones, such as cortisol, DHEA, and pregnenolone.

Do You Need EFA Supplements?

Take this questionnaire, developed Leo Galland, M.D., director of the Foundation for Integrated Medicine in New York City, and adapted from his book *Power Healing*.

Answer each question as follows:

Never = 0; Rarely = 1; Sometimes = 2; Often = 3

I experience:

Soft, fraying, or brittle nails __

Dry, scaly, or flaky skin __

Chicken skin (tiny bumps on my arms) __

Dandruff __

Pain or stiffness in my joints __

Dry, lackluster, or unruly hair __

Excessive thirst __

Menstrual cramps __

Premenstrual breast pain __

If you score 5 or more, you may be lacking essential fatty acids.

These have a natural anti-inflammatory effect on the body," says Dr. Stengler. "But when you have a prolonged allergy, that's when you start to deplete these adrenal hormones." By providing your adrenal glands with plenty of raw materials to make hormones like cortisol, you can help them handle the stress and continue fighting inflammation.

• Pantothenic Acid

The most important "stress" vitamin is pantothenic acid, one of the key nutrients used to form hormones like cortisone, cortisol, and adrenaline. Pantothenic acid is a water-soluble B vitamin.

Dr. Stengler recommends 500 milligrams three times a day with meals.

Producing stress hormones also uses up extra vitamin C and zinc. So Dr. Stengler recommends taking 500 to 800 milligrams of vitamin C, 30 to 40 milligrams of zinc, and a multivitamin each day.

• Ginseng

The herb ginseng can relax your nerves, reduce inflammation, and relieve fatigue, says Dr. Stengler. It can even increase your energy and endurance, apparently by increasing adrenal hormone production.

It is important, however, that you pick the right ginseng. It comes in three types: Korean, Siberian, and American. Chinese, panax, and red ginseng are essentially the same as Korean. The Siberian type is not true ginseng, but it contains similar active compounds and has similar effects.

According to Chinese medical theory, these types vary in their "temperature." American is the most cooling, Korean is the most warming, and Siberian is neutral.

"If you get warm real easily, you shouldn't use Korean ginseng. If you get cold easily, it's excellent," says Dr. Stengler. "Korean is also the most stimulating. If you are very hyper to begin with or have insomnia or high blood pressure, it can aggravate those conditions. But if you're low in energy, Korean could be for you."

Siberian is the safest, especially for women. Some experts recommend that women not take other types of ginseng because it can wreak havoc with their hormone levels.

American and Korean ginseng roots develop potency as they grow, and supplements should be from roots at least 4 years old—sometimes called imperial ginseng.

Dr. Stengler recommends taking one of the following: 100 milligrams of Korean ginseng in capsule or tablet form, standardized to include 4 to 7 percent ginsenosides, two or three times a day; 8 to 10 milliliters of Siberian ginseng tincture two or three times a day or 300 milligrams in capsule form, standardized to 0.4 percent eleutherosides, two or three times a day; or 1 to 2 milliliters of American ginseng tincture two or three times a day.

• DHEA

People with chronic allergies may benefit from DHEA supplements, says Dr. Stengler. That's because, as mentioned before, when you have allergies in addition to producing histamine, your body uses up a lot of stress hormones, such as DHEA. To find out if your DHEA levels are low, test first—a saliva lab test works best. These tests are available on the Internet or through your health care provider.

Take DHEA only under the supervision of a knowledgeable naturopathic or medical professional.

"For some people the improvement can be dramatic, especially seniors or people with fatigue," says Dr. Stengler.

After 1 to 2 months, your doctor will retest DHEA levels to see if the dose is appropriate. Men 40 and older should also get a prostate-specific antigen (PSA) test for prostate cancer before starting DHEA and another 3 to 4 months later because DHEA can increase testosterone levels, which may increase prostate cancer risk.

The Allergy-Free
EXERCISE PLAN

IF PEOPLE WITH allergies exercised more, they'd experience an amazing sensation: open sinuses.

"Aerobic exercise is a natural decongestant," says Gary Gross, M.D., an allergist and clinical professor of medicine at Southwestern Medical School in Dallas. "As you exercise, the blood vessels in your nose constrict, so there is more room for air to move through your nose."

That's not all. Exercise may boost your resistance to allergens.

The problem is that people with allergies probably exercise even less than the general population, experts say. "They can't go outside as often," points out Christopher Randolph, M.D., director of allergy and immunology at St. Mary's Hospital in Waterbury, Connecticut. And even indoors, they are besieged by pollen, mold, and other microscopic menaces.

It's easy to see why many people with al-

lergies are averse to exercise. After all, exercise can aggravate a host of allergic conditions, including asthma, allergic rhinitis (hay fever), and hives.

Almost everyone with asthma and as many as 40 percent of those with allergic rhinitis experience some degree of exercise-induced asthma. Symptoms include wheezing, coughing, shortness of breath, and difficulty in taking a breath. Breathing difficulties typically begin 5 to 10 minutes after starting exercise, peak 5 to 10 minutes after stopping exercise, and subside over the next 20 to 30 minutes.

"During exercise, the lung capacity of a person with asthma can drop as much as 50 percent," says James Sublett, M.D., national medical director of the Vivra Asthma and Allergy group practice in Louisville.

In rare cases, exercise can even cause anaphylaxis. Such life-threatening reactions usually occur when a person exercises after eating certain foods. These syndromes go by names such as "wheat-dependent exercise-induced anaphylaxis."

"With the impact that allergies have on quality of life, there's a tendency for people to back off from exercise," Dr. Sublett says. This process often begins in childhood, when children discover to their dismay that they can't keep up with their nonallergic peers on a track or soccer field. "They're the ones who can't do the mile run or who are standing on the sidelines," he notes.

Often, these children get no sympathy from physical education instructors and coaches. "Although there's more awareness now, a lot of people still think these kids are dogging it," Dr. Sublett says.

Repeated humiliations on the playing field can make people so exercise-shy that they swear off any activity that reminds them of gym class. "They don't enjoy the exercise, so they withdraw and become couch potatoes," notes Dr. Sublett. "That leads to the potential for obesity."

The Obesity-Allergy Connection

Studies show a strong link between obesity and allergy, especially asthma. For example, when researchers from the Channing

The Best Drug-Free Ways to Get Your Exercise

Though there are numerous sports that people with allergies can enjoy, doctors usually recommend that their patients first medicate themselves with antihistamines or nasal steroids before beginning their workouts. But what do you do if you prefer a natural, drug-free approach?

Simple: Think swimming or walking.

For those people who are unwilling to use medication, swimming and walking are the two exercises that are least likely to cause problems, says Harold Nelson, M.D., senior staff physician at the National Jewish Medical and Research Center in Denver. "When you walk, you should obviously breathe through your nose because that greatly protects your lungs."

If you get your doctor's okay and decide to give swimming a try, but you don't own your own pool, insist on a few free laps before plunking your money down for time in a public pool. That way, you can monitor your symptoms in the new environment. Also, be sure to visit the pool on several different occasions, including soon after the water has been chlorinated. "The twitchier people's lungs are, the more likely they are to be bothered by chlorine," Dr. Nelson cautions. "But it's usually not a problem."

Laboratory at Brigham and Children's Hospital in Boston studied 16,862 children ages 9 to 14, they found that obese boys were more than twice as likely as the thinnest boys to have asthma. Obese girls were 1½ times more likely to be asthmatic.

In addition, an analysis of 85,991 nurses in the Nurses' Health Study showed that women who had gained more than 55 pounds since age 18 were nearly five times as likely to develop adult-onset asthma as women whose weight stayed the same.

Until recently, studies failed to establish similar links between obesity and allergy in men. But a University of Oklahoma study of 11,846 men showed that the heaviest men were more than three times as likely to have asthma as the thinnest men.

Experts disagree over which comes first: the obesity or the asthma.

"Obesity in itself would not trigger asthma, because asthma is an immunologic disorder," Dr. Sublett notes. "There's not enough research to determine a cause and effect."

While acknowledging that more research is needed, the authors who examined the Nurses' Health Study offered several possible reasons why being overweight increases the risk of asthma.

• Smaller airways. Since excess weight constricts the chest wall, it reduces airway size and airflow.

• Shallower breathing. Since overweight people often have sedentary lifestyles, they take relatively few deep, cleansing breaths. Incomplete breathing is associated with increased airway "twitchiness."

• More time indoors. Since sedentary people spend more time indoors, they could have greater exposure to such asthma triggers as mold, dust mites, cockroaches, and animal dander.

• Stomach problems. Obesity is a risk factor for gastroesophageal reflux disease (GERD), which is an important risk factor for adult-onset asthma.

Whatever the final answer to this chicken-and-egg question might be, the verdict on exercise itself is clear: It's good for people with allergies, and they should be doing a lot more of it.

"If you're in good cardiovascular shape, you're going to have a lot more tolerance to your environment," Dr. Sublett says.

Get the Green Light

If you have allergies and want to get in shape, how do you get started?

First, experts say, you have to take care of the following preliminaries.

Get tested. If you don't know what's triggering your allergies, you can't take steps to avoid them. The only reliable way to identify such triggers is to get a skin, blood, or patch test at a doctor's office. If you have asthma, you should also get a baseline pulmonary-function test.

By the numbers

22.4
Percentage of U.S. athletes with asthma at the 1998 Winter Olympics

11.4
Percentage of U.S. athletes with asthma who won medals at the 1998 Winter Olympics

17.8
Percentage of U.S. athletes without asthma who won medals at the 1998 Winter Olympics

Get a physical. A complete exam will determine whether you have heart disease, arthritis, or other conditions that can limit your ability to exercise.

Exercise Caution If You Have Asthma

Though becoming physically fit has obvious benefits for everyone, people with asthma need to be aware that exercise alone doesn't appear to actually stabilize or reverse the underlying disease.

"I don't think there's any good evidence that you can improve asthma with exercise," says Harold Nelson, M.D., senior staff physician at the National Jewish Medical and Research Center in Denver. Indeed, a 3-year study of 58 patients with asthma who completed a 10-week exercise class showed that exercise did not improve asthma symptoms, breath-test scores, or reactivity to al-

Identifying the Impostors

Suppose you have been diagnosed with exercise-induced asthma and have been prescribed an asthma inhaler—but you don't feel any better when you take a couple of puffs on the playing field. Does this mean that you have an even more serious condition?

Probably not, says Miles Weinberger, M.D., director of the pediatric allergy and pulmonary division at the University of Iowa College of Medicine in Iowa City. In fact, you might not even have asthma. "If you have no other history consistent with asthma, and you don't get an immediate and impressive response from your inhaler, it's time to be suspicious," he says.

Dr. Weinberger conducted a yearlong study of 32 patients—8 girls and 24 boys, ages 8 to 18—who had been diagnosed with exercise-induced asthma. He measured their breathing and other vital signs as they exercised on treadmills and found that only 4 of them had coughing and wheezing. Seventeen of them had completely normal lung functions.

From such research, Dr. Weinberger identified the following "pseudo exercise-induced asthma syndromes," all of which are essentially benign.

Exercise-induced hyperventilation. This condition causes rapid breathing, chest tightness, and shortness of breath. But it doesn't produce asthma's trademark symptom: wheezing. "When you hyperventilate, you're not in fact having any obstruction to the airflow, which you get with asthma," notes Dr. Weinberger.

lergenic substances. Patients who continued to exercise at least once a week did, however, demonstrate significantly better cardiovascular conditioning.

If you have asthma, you'll first need to get your symptoms under control before you begin an exercise program. That means no coughing or breathlessness at night, early in the morning, or after exercise. And certainly no acute attacks that send you to the hospital. In most cases, this can be accom-plished with the use of medication, but one out of three people may also need allergy shots on a regular basis.

Your doctor will probably recommend that you premedicate before exercise with short-acting beta-agonists or inhaled non-steroidal anti-inflammatory drugs such as cromolyn (Intal) and nedocromil (Tilade). A long-acting beta-agonist, such as salmeterol (Serevent), may be used if you exercise every day.

Exercise-induced vocal-cord dysfunction. This syndrome causes shortness of breath as well. "Your vocal cords are supposed to work automatically by getting out of the way when you want to take a deep breath, then relaxing when you let the air out," Dr. Weinberger says. "What happens in some people is that the vocal cords close instead of open, which creates an obstruction in the upper airway flow." Although this paradoxical condition can be frightening, it's not life-threatening. "A speech therapist can provide help to these people by teaching them how to voluntarily control their vocal cords to keep them open," says Dr. Weinberger.

Hitting the wall. When people reach the limits of their physical abilities, they are said to have "hit the wall." The breathing difficulties that result can mimic exercise-induced asthma.

Dr. Weinberger typically advises his patients with one of these asthma impersonators to stop using their inhalers, relax, and learn how to pace themselves. "Shortness of breath produces anxiety," he says. "Once we tell them, 'Look, nothing bad is going on, you're not getting asthma, you're not going to end up in an ER,' it eliminates the anxiety."

If you think you might have one of these syndromes, get a treadmill-exercise test at a doctor's office. Generally, a pulmonologist (lung specialist) will conduct this test by taking your breath measurements after 10 minutes of brisk treadmill walking.

The "right" medication depends on the severity of your asthma. If it's moderate to severe, leukotriene modifiers and inhaled corticosteroids can be effective "controller" medications and should be taken regularly, but they can't relieve an acute attack. Long-acting beta-agonists seem to be most effective for the prevention of symptoms, although they can produce such side effects as rapid heart rate and increased blood pres-

She Beat Asthma to Become "First Lady" of Track and Field

Born in 1962, Jacqueline Joyner-Kersee was named after President John F. Kennedy's wife because her grandmother figured she would grow up to be "first lady" of something.

Unfortunately, her grim, impoverished hometown—East St. Louis, Illinois—was hardly Camelot. "Jackie" Joyner-Kersee grew up in a ramshackle house across the street from a liquor store and a pool hall. Despite the environment, Joyner-Kersee's mother, Mary—who died of a rare form of meningitis at age 37—saw to it that her daughter steered clear of alcohol, drugs, and boys, and started her on the road to becoming "first lady" of track and field.

Joyner-Kersee went on to dominate the heptathlon, a demanding seven-event competition that measures speed, strength, and stamina. Between 1984 and 1996, she won six Olympic medals—including gold medals in the heptathlon and long jump—making her the most decorated woman in U.S. track and field history. Such was her athletic prowess that she appeared on the cover of *Sports Illustrated* under the headline "Super Woman."

Privately, however, she didn't always feel so super. During her late teens, she had learned from her doctors that she had asthma, but she refused to accept the diagnosis. "I lived in denial," she says. "When you're a young person growing up, you're always told, 'If you have asthma, you can't do anything.' I just knew there was no way I could have it. I shouldn't be able to run at all."

Although she was prescribed inhalers to prevent asthma attacks as well as other inhalers to relieve acute attacks, she used them only periodically. "I would take my medications on a regular basis and feel great," she says. "Then I wouldn't take them and would find myself sick again."

During a 1987 drill, Joyner-Kersee experienced a wake-up call: an asthma at-

sure in some people. If your asthma is mild, however, the inhaled nonsteroidal anti-inflammatory drugs can effectively prevent exercise-induced asthma with minimal side effects. But these are only general guidelines.

Since asthma is such a variable disease, only your doctor can tell you what regimen is right for you, and the process could still involve some trial and error. In the end, however, you should be able to find a med-

tack that left her in the hospital. From that moment on, she was determined to respect asthma as seriously as she respected her athletic opponents.

"I knew in my heart that asthma was getting the best of me and that I wouldn't be able to run anymore," she says. "So I had to discipline myself, take my medicine, and work with my doctor as I work with my coach."

She now keeps her condition under control with a long-acting beta-agonist (Serevent) and an inhaled corticosteroid (Flovent). She takes two puffs of each, morning and evening. For emergencies, she uses a short-acting beta-agonist (Ventolin). To keep on top of her asthma, she measures her breathing with a peak-flow meter. If the levels are low, it's an early sign that an asthma attack is on the way, and she can take steps to prevent it.

She has also learned to avoid her most common asthma triggers: grass pollen, mold, peanuts, and shellfish. In addition, she eats a nutritious diet, drinks plenty of water, and practices deep-breathing exercises. "I keep my body in the best shape possible," she says.

Since retiring from competition in 1998, Joyner-Kersee has kept busy as a motivational speaker, director of her own sports-marketing firm, and leader of the JJK Community Foundation, which helps disadvantaged youth.

Hoping to reach out to others with asthma, she's also a member of the Asthma All-Stars, a group of elite athletes that includes Olympic swimmer Amy Van Dyken and football star Jerome Bettis. Their message: People with asthma can live without limits.

Although Joyner-Kersee acknowledges that asthma is part of who she is, she refuses to let it slow her down. Through careful management, she has mastered the disease so completely that she doesn't even consider it to be a handicap.

"I've come a long way," she says.

ication that works for you. "The medicine is so good now that everybody should be able to exercise however they like," Dr. Nelson says. "Their disease shouldn't be dictating to them."

Take Stock

Assuming your doctor tells you that you're good to go, how do you choose an allergy-friendly exercise program?

First, think hard about the activities you'd like to do. Here are some questions you should ask yourself.

Where can I find the time? "You have to fit exercise into your schedule the same way you fit in brushing your teeth," Dr. Randolph says. "It has to become second nature."

How can I make it fun? "You have to make it attractive," Dr. Randolph says. Home exercise is good, he notes, because it allows people to exercise in familiar surroundings

Breathing Exercises

The art of breathing has been taught for thousands of years. Breathing is thought to be the bridge between body and mind. When your mind is calm, your respirations are deep and slow. But when your mind is tense, they are more rapid and shallow. That's why learning to breathe properly calms the mind and helps the body. Clinical evidence shows that proper breathing can improve conditions ranging from asthma to heart disease.

Breathing exercises are tools that can help you learn how to inhale and exhale properly. Do the following exercises a few times daily, especially when you're feeling tense or anxious. Within the first few days, you should notice a change for the better in your breathing. You could monitor your progress with a peak-flow meter. Your breathing capacity should increase in a few months.

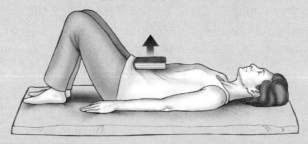

1. Simple belly breathing. Lie down on a mat or blanket on the floor. Keep your legs slightly apart. Place a book on your stomach, with the binding just touching the bottom curve of your rib cage. Inhale through your nose, unless

while watching TV or listening to music.

How can I keep it simple? "Americans like to have it easy," Dr. Randolph says. "A stationary bike or treadmill makes exercise easy to do."

How can I make it pay off? "You have to make it rewarding," Dr. Randolph says. "There has to be an incentive for you to do this." His suggestion: Once a week, allow yourself a treat you wouldn't ordinarily eat as a reward for meeting your exercise goals.

Get Active

Now comes the fun part: choosing an exercise. Until recently, people with allergies—especially exercise-induced asthma—had few choices: swimming and maybe walking.

"Swimming is the best tolerated exercise for people with asthma," Dr. Nelson says. "It's the perfect setting because the water is warm and the air is fully saturated with water vapor."

you find it hard to do so because of a cold or sinusitis. While breathing through your nose, imagine that you are actually drawing air in from the back of your throat, not just your nostrils. This should feel almost as if you are drawing air from an internal source. As you inhale, try to lift the book as high as you can with your stomach muscles. Try to keep your chest motionless. As you exhale, use the same belly muscles to squeeze all of the air out of your lungs. As you push the air out, the book will lower. When you've nearly reached the end of your breath, begin to hum. You'll notice that you still have enough air left to hum for several heartbeats. Do this exercise slowly, so that you are taking only about four full breaths per minute.

2. Pursed-lips breathing. For this next exercise, you can stand, sit, or lie down. Draw in a belly breath. When you exhale, purse your lips firmly and exhale as forcefully as you can, as if you were blowing out a giant candle. By pursing your lips this way, you produce a controlled, powerful stream of air.

In general, the best exercise environment is warm and humid. The worst environment is cold and dry. That's why allergists once warned patients against such activities as ice-skating and cross-country skiing.

Today, however, the prevailing attitude is that people with allergies, even those with asthma, can do whatever they want. But there is a catch: To ward off symptoms of allergic rhinitis, patients are told to premedicate with antihistamines, nasal steroids, or nasal sodium cromolyn. And, as already noted, people with asthma will need to premedicate with a drug chosen specifically to match the severity of their symptoms.

Indoor Exercise: Some Insider Tips

By exercising indoors, you can avoid the most notorious allergy triggers, especially pollen and pollution. But you can't automatically assume that an indoor environment is okay.

The Best and Worst Sports

If you have allergies, choosing the right sport might seem to be as problematic as choosing the right car. But you can find a sport that will provide you with years of dependable "service" if you follow a few guidelines.

In general, sports that require continuous activity are more likely to trigger symptoms than sports that require intermittent activity. When you go for a long-distance run, for example, you're not only inhaling vast amounts of air that might contain large amounts of pollen, mold, and other allergenic substances but also bypassing your body's natural filtering and humidification system, your nose.

Since running and other endurance sports force you to breathe through your mouth, you can start experiencing asthma symptoms in as little as 6 minutes, says Harold Nelson, M.D., senior staff physician at the National Jewish Medical and Research Center in Denver.

Although swimming is a continuous activity, it's good for people with allergies because it's practiced in a warm, humid atmosphere in a horizontal position that may help mobilize mucus from the bottom of your lungs.

With the exception of swimming, however, stop-and-go sports are the best bets for people with allergies. "Tennis would be very good because you rarely play a point that lasts as long as 6 minutes," Dr. Nelson says.

Check out the following list to find out which sports are the best—and the worst—for people with allergies.

Often, indoor air is even worse than outdoor air because it contains high concentrations of mold, animal dander, dust mite parts, cockroach parts, cigarette smoke, and other chemical irritants. "Exercising indoors would seem to be preferable, especially if you have air-conditioning," Dr. Randolph says. "But that's only if you've created a relatively allergen-free environment."

That means doing things like plugging leaks in faucets and pipes to prevent mold growth; encasing pillows, mattresses, and box springs to contain dust mites; and banishing indoor smoking.

It also means finding new homes for any pets to which you are allergic. (For tips on reducing allergens if getting rid of your pet is just not an option, see Pet Allergy on page 356.) Since animal dander can stay airborne for weeks or even months, exercising in a dander-contaminated house makes about as much sense as performing aerobics in a ragweed patch.

Although it might cause some short-term

Best Sports	Worst Sports
Baseball	Aerobics (high intensity)
Bicycling (low or moderate intensity)	Basketball
Bowling	Bicycling (high intensity)
Boxing	Cross-country skiing
Downhill skiing	Field hockey
Football	Ice hockey
Golf	Ice-skating
Gymnastics	Long-distance running
Handball	Rugby
Isometrics	Soccer
Karate	
Racquetball	
Sprinting and other short-intensity track-and-field events	
Stationary biking (low or moderate intensity)	
Surfing	
Swimming	
Tennis	
Walking (low or moderate intensity)	
Water polo	
Weight training	
Wrestling	

pain, finding your pet a new home is essential to your long-term health. You must reduce your total allergic load so you can handle the extra stress of exercising. If you don't control your environment, your environment will control you.

"Do anything you can to reduce the allergic load," Dr. Sublett emphasizes. "If you can reduce those day-to-day exposures, you'll have a greater level of tolerance for other exposures."

Once you've created an allergen-free environment, your next step is to further reduce your risk of developing exercise-induced asthma or other symptoms by following these general precautions. With them, you can feel free to exercise at an intensity that suits your fitness level. Your goal should be to exercise at least ½ hour a day, 5 days a week, Dr. Sublett advises.

• Avoid exercise if you have an upper-respiratory viral infection. It increases your susceptibility to exercise-induced asthma.

• Premedicate. Many different medication regimens are recommended for the prevention of exercise-induced asthma, but Dr. Randolph says that one of the simplest and most effective is taking two puffs from a beta-agonist inhaler, such as albuterol (Proventil), 15 minutes before exercise.

• Drink plenty of fluids, especially before exercising. This prevents dehydration, which can be especially bad for people with allergies since it thickens mucus in the lungs.

Timing Is Everything

Conventional wisdom has it that the worst time to exercise outdoors is the early morning because that's when pollen counts are highest. Not so, says Harold Nelson, M.D., senior staff physician at the National Jewish Medical and Research Center in Denver.

While it's true that ragweed plants drop their pollen right after sunrise, it takes time for the pollen to dry out and waft into the air. "Ragweed pollen counts begin to rise at about nine in the morning and peak about noon," Dr. Nelson says.

As for grasses, they don't pollinate until afternoon. "By the time grass pollen gets to the cities, it's about suppertime," notes Dr. Nelson.

Here's a breakdown of the best times to exercise outdoors, depending on your allergy triggers.

• If you're allergic to ragweed, exercise early in the morning or after work.

• If grass pollen is your allergy trigger, the best time to exercise is early in the morning or during your lunch hour.

• If you're allergic to molds, there is no best time to exercise. Dry-spore molds are most active during the day, while forest molds are most active at night.

The Allergy-Free Exercise Plan

If you have allergies, it's certainly worth taking an average of 30 minutes a day to boost your cardiovascular system with exercise. Walking will help your body use the oxygen you take in more efficiently. With your doctor's okay, here's a program that just about anyone can follow, courtesy of Elaine Ward, managing director of the North American Racewalking Foundation in Pasadena, California.

For each exercise session, begin with at least 5 minutes of easy walking and a few minutes of stretching to warm up. And at the end of your walk, repeat the easy walking and stretching to cool down. By the end of the session, you should feel mildly tired, but not exhausted. Rest at least 2 days during each week and, if you need to, skip a day or scale back on the number of minutes.

Each day, you'll be walking in one of the following styles.

- Tempo or long: Walk at a moderate pace that's brisk enough to get your heart pumping but won't leave you out of breath.
- Intervals: Walk for 5 minutes at a moderate pace, then speed up for 1 minute. Repeat for the total time.
- One-minute count: Walk for 5 minutes at a moderate pace, then count the number of steps you take for 1 minute. Repeat for the total time. As you get faster, the number of steps will increase.

	Day 1 Tempo	**Day 2** Intervals	**Day 3** Long	**Day 4** Tempo	**Day 5** 1-Minute Count
Week 1	15 min.	20 min.	30 min.	15 min.	20 min.
Week 2	20 min.	25 min.	30 min.	20 min.	25 min.
Week 3	15 min.	25 min.	30 min.	15 min.	25 min.
Week 4	20 min.	25 min.	35 min.	20 min.	25 min.

- Perform warmup exercises. A warmup helps your lungs gradually adjust to increased demands. You can try running in place for 2 minutes or sprinting for 20 seconds. Forcing your lungs to instantly respond to the demands of exercise increases the risk of exercise-induced asthma.

- Breathe through your nose. This naturally filters out pollutants, irritants, and allergens. It also warms and moistens the air before it reaches your lungs.

- Cool down. Stretching or doing light exercise for several minutes after your workout may prevent the sudden changes in lung temperature that often trigger a post-workout attack of exercise-induced asthma.

- Know your limits. Although people with

allergies don't necessarily need to exercise less intensely than other people, they do need to be more cautious. "You just have to be really tuned in to yourself," Dr. Sublett says. "Don't push beyond your limits."

Finally, though a gym might seem to be an ideal place to exercise if you have allergies, don't sign any membership papers until you've had an opportunity to give the place a good look-over, and even more important, a good "smell-over." Your nose will alert you to the presence of mold, cleansers, perfumes, and other allergens and irritants.

If the gym's air seems okay, ask the manager for a few on-the-house workouts. By spreading your workouts over several days, you'll know if the gym is harboring such allergens as dust mites, which thrive in areas of high humidity where there's an abundance of sloughed-off human skin. Find another gym if the workouts leave you sneezy and wheezy.

Outside Exercise: Outwit Allergies in the Great Outdoors

If you have asthma, allergic rhinitis, or other allergies, you can still exercise outside on most days.

To get the most out of your workouts,

heed the following all-natural tips. Also, remember to follow the same premedication, warmup, and cooldown guidelines you follow for indoor exercise.

• Avoid exercising near busy roads. Not only will you inhale more vehicle exhaust, but you'll also be exposed to more road dust, which according to one study contains allergens from 20 different sources.

• Judge exercise intensity with a "talk test." As long as you can carry on a conversation while exercising, you're not pushing yourself too hard. Slow down if you feel dizzy or faint.

• Don a dust mask when necessary. It'll keep those nasty particles from pestering your airways during pollen season. And during cold weather, a dust mask will help warm the cold, dry air that sets off asthma attacks. Forget about wearing a cotton or wool scarf. They release fibers that irritate twitchy lungs.

There are times when you shouldn't exercise outdoors. Stay inside on high-pollen days when the count is higher than 1,000 and on days when temperatures are over 90°F or below zero. And avoid outdoor exercise during pollution alerts. In one study, people with asthma who were exposed to ozone experienced a 9 percent drop in lung function and displayed higher reactivity to other allergens.

Allergy-Free
STRESS BUSTERS

IF YOU PUT STRESS on trial for causing allergies, it might beat the rap on a technicality. But even the most lenient jury would find it guilty of being an accomplice.

Strictly speaking, of course, your immune system's overreaction to certain allergens causes allergies. But stress acts as the explosives expert in the allergy gang. It may not actually cause the attack, but it blows the safe open to allow the allergens to do their dirty work.

Stress can bring on asthma attacks, and some experts believe it probably exacerbates nearly every kind of allergy. It increases the adrenal gland's production of cortisol and spurs the sympathetic nervous system to make more epinephrine and norepinephrine. An oversupply of these hormones cuts your immune system's effectiveness.

Suppose you get in the way of some pollen being carried on a gentle summer breeze. When the pollen enters your nose, an SOS signal is immediately telegraphed to your brain, which orders a calibrated response—perhaps three sneezes and a small rush of mucus to eject the foreign invader. The calibration ought to be within bounds: big enough to do the job, small enough to trigger only as many defenses as are necessary.

When stress is involved, though, things can start to go haywire. Stress lowers the level of cyclic adenosine monophosphate (cAMP), a neurotransmitter that keeps air passageways open and prevents the brain from ordering a nuke-the-allergens response. As a result of these lowered levels of cAMP, your brain is not able to send adequate amounts of antibodies to combat the invading substance. That's why anything that significantly lowers stress might also lower allergic reactions. In fact, it's possible to completely "unlearn" the tendency to allergic reaction.

Stress comes at us from several angles, of course. Its sources can include people, debts owed to "Soprano" associates, leaky life rafts, bad sandwiches—you name it. These stressors act on your central nervous system. And anything capable of doing that can cause alterations in immunity.

Whenever stress levels decrease, benefits accrue across the board—not just in reducing allergies but also in overall life satisfaction. To take advantage of these benefits, check out the following 10 approaches to reducing stress. They've been helpful to many millions of Americans. Chances are that one or more of them could become a rewarding part of your life.

Biofeedback

Our conscious minds often overlook valuable data coming from our various body parts. These messages include little things like "This knee hurts whenever it bends too much" or "Shoulder muscle strands are tightening."

Our bodies deserve some help in getting their internal memos through to our heads. One technique for doing just that is biofeedback. With the use of an electronic monitoring device, messages from various parts of the body are brought up to a conscious level. From that vantage point, we can do something constructive about them.

In terms of stress and allergies, biofeed-back helps us learn when and where our bodies are storing stress. The more stress we release, and the more we unlearn habits of storing stress, the less we're likely to suffer from allergies. This is especially true about the stress felt when allergy symptoms kick in.

Biofeedback typically uses electronic devices to monitor heart rate, muscle tension, brain waves, or other indicators of a person's emotional and physical states. Contracted muscles transmit more electricity, so a device that measures muscle tension can squeal on a stress-harboring body part. The person hooked up to the device then consciously relaxes the appropriate muscles. Science has shown that when our muscles are relaxed, especially our face muscles, we are less capable of feeling anxiety. So the awareness that biofeedback provides pays off in peace of mind as well as allergy relief.

Fortunately, you don't have to invest in electronic gadgetry to get some of the benefits of biofeedback. A mirror will do just fine. The following exercise is recommended by Naras Bhat, M.D., founder and medical director of Cybernetix Medical Institute in Concord, California.

Stand in front of a mirror with your chest and belly exposed. Take a breath and watch to see where you expand as you inhale. Thoracic breathing, which means your chest is doing most of the work, shows stress, and it also traps stale air in your lungs. It's easy to identify because your chest will expand when you inhale.

Consciously shift to belly breathing. The mirror will show you whether you have it right when you see your belly expand as you inhale.

When you get your body to stop sending distress signals, your mind will refocus and reclaim a sense of control. After a few practice sessions, you'll learn how to consciously control your reactions. Then, when allergies or asthma attack, simply ask yourself to breathe from your belly. The attack may be significantly reduced in severity. Eventually, attacks should become less frequent as well. "We can't escape allergens or other stressors," says Dr. Bhat, a biofeedback and immunology practitioner for 26 years, "but we can unlearn our reactivity."

Cognitive Reframing

Country folks have a saying: "It ain't what you eat, it's how you chew it." In other words, how you handle an experience often determines how it will feel.

Cognitive reframing is a psychological technique that validates that bit of wisdom. Its stress-busting potential makes it particularly interesting for those who have allergies.

It's a simple, commonsense concept: You exchange unpleasant, negative thoughts for useful, positive ones. Since being upset often makes allergy symptoms worse, handling stress better could result in fewer allergy problems overall. That's why many self-help books, some of them bestsellers, have been based on cognitive reframing. For a basic sense of how cognitive reframing works, try this exercise recommended by Ken Leight, Ph.D., a licensed clinical psychologist and cognitive-behavioral psychotherapist with New Roads Behavioral Health Group in Linwood, New Jersey.

Think of a time recently when you felt bad. Describe the situation briefly, but specifically, in writing. Write down the emotions you had and how powerful they felt. Now write out another way to view the experience. Make this viewpoint something you can believe, but this time be kinder to whoever (or whatever) you thought was at fault. See if you can be more flexible, less angry, less concerned about shame.

Suppose, for example, that your husband didn't notice your new haircut. Your first reaction might be anger, and you might say to yourself, "He never pays attention to me." Now, try to think of an alternate reason for this behavior. Perhaps he is so worried about how the two of you will make the mortgage payment this month that it's taking all of his attention. Or perhaps his picture of you, as the lovely woman he married, is so strongly ingrained in his mind that your image is unchangeable.

Compare your new take on the situation with how you reacted when it happened. Ask yourself how you now feel. Worse?

Slightly better? Much better? Chances are, you'll feel better. Why? Because you've reclaimed a sense of control over a difficult emotion. Plus, you've allowed yourself to consider different scenarios in which you're not the offended party, but the ultimate benefactor.

"Finally," Dr. Leight adds, "imagine that you're actually in that situation again but having these more positive thoughts (with an intention to really believe them)."

For millions of people, exercises like the one above have been a pathway to happier, healthier lives. For deeper, more directed results, find a therapist in your area who is trained in cognitive reframing. He can speed your progress with trained observations and thought-provoking questions to assist you in reducing stress.

How you react to your allergies can also determine how you feel and, ultimately, how much you suffer, claims Dr. Leight. In a vicious cycle, your thoughts can create stressful feelings that aggravate or perpetuate allergic symptoms. Rather than thinking "this is awful" or stubbornly persevering in a stressful or environmentally sensitive situation, cultivate the ability to think calmly and adaptively and in ways that promote greater peace of mind. For example, a more positive way to react to your allergies would be: "I may be having an allergy attack, but I don't need to be stressed. In fact, I have many ways in which I can relax and a variety of options for controlling my allergy symptoms."

Guided Visualization

Think about this statement: Imagination can make allergy symptoms disappear.

Sound like wishful thinking? Well, guided visualization has made believers out of many doctors and patients. This technique works through the profound connection between the healing systems of the body: the immune, the hormonal, and the nervous systems. These systems are connected to the brain's capacity to produce images. "Imagery is the control language of the housekeeping system of the body," says David Bresler, Ph.D., codirector of the Academy for Guided Imagery in Mill Valley, California, and former director of the UCLA Pain Control Unit. The academy has trained more than 30,000 health care professionals and offers local referrals at (800) 726-2070.

Guided imagery is nothing new. Some cultures believe that the images someone visualizes will shape that person's experience of reality. Further, these cultures believe that people can consciously sharpen these images to their own liking and cause reality to follow suit, hence controlling their own destinies.

According to Dr. Bresler, allergies are rooted in early trauma. As a result, the body often overacts, producing allergic symptoms.

How powerful are images in triggering allergic reactions? Many people who are allergic to roses will, if shown a fake rose, kick into a sneezing fit. But that's not really surprising: A fear-inducing cause-and-effect relationship, repeated often enough, is very significant to the mind. Fear tends to make the mind clench, ordering overreaction to a given stimulus. Guided imagery is a very effective way to reduce such anxiety and fear.

To try out the effects of guided visualization on your allergy symptoms, try the following exercise from Dr. Bresler.

"When you feel an allergy attack coming on, close your eyes and take a very deep breath in through your nose," Dr. Bresler advises. "Slowly breathe out through your mouth. Inhale again, and as you exhale, allow all the tension to let go.

"Now, imagine there's a ball of pure energy or white light that starts in your lower abdomen. As you inhale, imagine it rising up the front of your body to your forehead. As you exhale, imagine it going down your spine, down your legs, and into the ground. Circulate this ball of energy around for a few minutes, draining away any tension, tightness, pain, or discomfort into the ground. If any part of your body is still feeling the effects of the allergy, send the ball of energy to it as you inhale, and as you exhale, send all of the allergy symptoms down your spine, down your legs, and into the ground. Repeat this cycle until you feel more comfortable," he says.

Humor Therapy

Really intense laughter makes us react in some very funny ways. One response is to lift our shoulders high and project them forward. Another is to raise our hands and cover our chests, stomachs, or faces. Still another is to rock backward. Or to bend over double.

Imagine these postures with no smiles or laughter in the scene. They are basically attitudes of defense. We react that way because humor is really a kind of assault; it's intent on turning our sense of things upside down. But it's an attack that makes us feel better. When we laugh, we let our guard down for a moment. A feeling of relief usually ensues.

At the same time, a sense of humor arms us against the disappointments, absurdities, and pains of life.

What does this have to do with allergies? Well, allergies are a defensive overreaction to allergens and other stressors. So, the theory goes, if we can tickle ourselves into defenselessness, we might experience less-severe allergy symptoms. For many people, that theory works.

"One of the best ways to handle stress is to laugh your way out of it," says Joel Goodman, Ed.D. "Humor is a very powerful and delightful way of heading off stress. Good things happen inside. Respiration and circulation get a boost. More oxygen enters the blood. Stress-related hormones decrease. Clearer thinking returns."

Dr. Goodman is the director of The Humor Project in Saratoga Springs, New York, which holds conferences and workshops on humor and supplies humor consultants to corporations from AT&T to ZiffDavis Media. You can contact The Humor Project online at its Web site www.HumorProject.com. "Eighty percent of the people who attend our conferences report that they have a good sense of humor, but 98 percent admit that they can't tell a joke to save their lives," he notes.

Instead of trying to become a stand-up comic, just ask yourself what makes you laugh. Start assembling a personal collection of books, videos, cartoons, toys, and props. Have smile-coaxing items such as smiley-face balls or a Laugh-Aide box to keep handy both at work and at home. Chances are, something of their spirit will filter into your approach to life, and that will lessen your stress.

It's important, Dr. Goodman adds, that you use humor as an ally, not as a weapon. Put-down humor tends to spark retaliation or withdrawal. It's preferable to laugh *with* other people rather than *at* them.

Hypnosis

Does the word *hypnosis* conjure a picture of a nightclub hypnotist making people do silly things to amuse the audience?

Well, you're not alone. But today's practitioners, who often prefer to call it hypnotherapy, want us to know better. It isn't about relinquishing your will. It's only a deeper form of relaxation, an altered state of consciousness, says Reg Sheldrick, Ph.D., president of the American Guild of Hypnotherapy in Kenner, Louisiana.

Hypnosis has been used to heal various illnesses since ancient times. In ancient Greece, for example, people feeling under the weather could strap on their sandals and walk to a healing temple, where a physician might treat them by inducing a trance state and implanting a therapeutic suggestion. The modern revival of clinical interest in hypnosis dates to 1955, when the British Medical Association recommended the undertaking of serious studies. It wasn't until 1962, when researchers conducted a 6-month treatment period, which was reinforced by the patients' daily auto-hypnosis (self-hypnosis) regimen, that promising results could finally be verified.

Research suggests that self-administered hypnosis therapy oriented toward relaxation may be an effective treatment for asthma, especially in children. Some studies have shown that this approach results in reductions in the severity of asthma symptoms and in the number of emergency room visits. Although data suggest that hypnosis is an effective treatment for asthma, more studies need to be completed before doctors can unequivocally endorse hypnosis as a treatment for asthma. Researchers are optimistic about the connection, however, and refer to hypnosis as a powerful technique.

"It's important to know that only about 20 percent of us are highly likely to achieve a trance state," says Andrew Weil, M.D., director of the program in integrative medicine and clinical professor of medicine at the University of Arizona College of Medicine in Tucson. "Another 20 percent, though, will barely respond at all. Hypnosis will affect the rest of us to some degree between those extremes."

Dr. Sheldrick, however, reports 80 percent success in teaching the people he works with to achieve a deep state of self-hypnosis. He adds that learning self-hypnosis is easy and that it's a valuable technique in combating allergy symptoms. So when you begin to feel allergy symptoms coming, place yourself into a hypnotic state and give yourself suggestions to stay calm and relaxed. Dr. Sheldrick teaches his clients to enter hypnosis by giving them a simple suggestion: "Take a deep breath. Exhale. On your second breath, put your right hand on your left shoulder. Speaking only to yourself, address yourself by your first name, telling yourself to be calm and relaxed."

For example, if you feel pollen tickling dangerously inside your nose, or if you react to perfumes and someone wearing a quarter-cup of Chanel just walked close by, quietly anchor your hand on your shoulder and silently call yourself by name, adding, "Be calm and relaxed." Keep repeating your self-instruction in time with your breathing until you feel calmer. This technique can be done almost anywhere, any time you feel allergies coming on. A hypnotist can offer special techniques that are tailored to the situations that trigger stress for you.

Journaling

Over time, negative feelings can undermine your immune system. But before you can change negative feelings and thought processes, you need to clearly identify them. And the best way to do that is to put it in writing. Believe it or not, keeping a journal can help in the fight against allergies.

Researchers at North Dakota State University in Fargo randomly assigned a group of people with asthma or rheumatoid arthritis to write regularly about the most stressful experience in their lives or about emotionally neutral topics. After 4 months, 47 percent of those who wrote about the most stressful event in their lives showed greater improvement and reduced symptoms of their illnesses. Of the people who wrote only about emotionally neutral topics, only 24.3 percent showed improvement.

In another study, people who had recently lost their jobs were asked to write down their deepest feelings regarding unemployment. Another group wrote only about their job-seeking plans. Eight months later, the first group was twice as successful in finding new jobs.

Clearly, expressing deep feelings is a first step toward sorting them out. That alone relieves stress, and it can also lead to doing something constructive about those feelings.

If you'd like to try journaling, here are some guidelines: Set a realistic schedule for your writing and stick to it. When you

Fascinating
fact!

write, keep the verbal flow going no matter what. No one else will see your writing, so why worry about grammar or punctuation, or even about making perfect sense? It's important to open the reservoir of feelings and write about them regularly. If you do, your allergy symptoms will significantly improve.

Massage

Getting a massage is one of life's great pleasures. It's also one of the best ways to rub stress out of your system. Apparently, more and more people are catching on to its benefits: Massage has now become the second most popular alternative healing practice in America. In fact, insurance plans will sometimes even pay for physician-ordered massage.

"Research shows that the rhythmic pressure of massage lowers heart rate and blood pressure while improving blood circulation," says Dr. Weil. It also carries oxygen and nutrients to the cells and removes waste products such as lactic acid, which causes muscle cramps.

In a groundbreaking study, 40 prematurely born infants were divided into two groups. One group received a gentle 15-minute massage three times a day, while the other group received no special treatment. Babies in the first group gained almost 50 percent more weight, became more responsive, and were able to leave the hospital 6 days earlier than babies in the second group.

Another study, conducted at the Touch Research Institute at the University of Miami School of Medicine in 1998, examined the potential of massage in 32 children with asthma. Though the youngest children seemed to benefit most, anxiety and stress-related hormone levels decreased immediately for children of various ages. Measures of airflow improved significantly as well.

Be aware that many states require no licensing or examinations for massage therapists. Before hiring a massage therapist, ask what accreditation or training the person has. Both the Commission on Massage Training Accreditation and the National Certification Board of Therapeutic Massage and Bodywork hold high standards. The American Massage Therapy Association helps people find qualified massage therapists for its more than 42,000 members nationwide. They can be contacted at (888) 843-2682.

Of course, one of the greatest benefits of massage is the fact that you can take matters into your own hands, so to speak. Following are some do-it-yourself massage techniques that you can use anywhere for symptom relief.

During an asthma attack, lightly tap your fingertips in a circle around your sternum

(1a), suggests Denise Borrelli, Ph.D., vice president of the American Massage Therapy Association in Evanston, Illinois. Then, using a light, flat-handed stroke, push downward from your sternum, along the left side of your body, toward your stomach (1b).

For sinus headaches, says Dr. Borrelli, place your hands on the base of your skull on your occipital ridge and move your thumbs in deep circles where your neck muscles meet your head (2a). Then place all four fingertips from each hand at the midline of your forehead. Pull them with a spreading motion out to the sides of your forehead (2b). Repeat this motion over your cheekbones. Next, do flat-handed strokes, starting where your ears and neck meet and going straight down to your collarbone (2c).

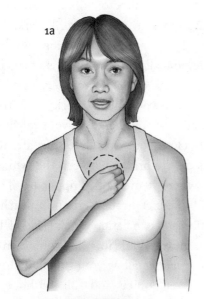

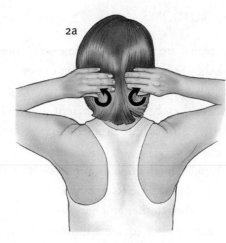

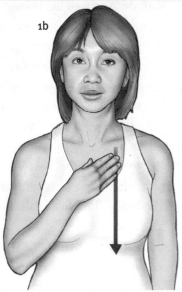

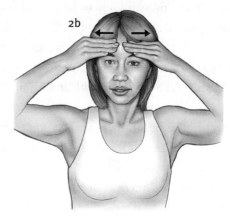

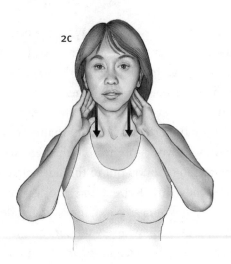

2c

Meditation

Our brains are problem-solving machines. And they're quite good at what they do, generally speaking. But when they get overstressed, they become inefficient. It's then that they can become problem-*causing* machines.

Think of meditation as a reset button. It gives the brain time to rest, so it can come back to work fresher and happier. Research has documented that meditation can decrease blood pressure, lower heart and respiratory rates, and increase bloodflow. All of these signal relaxation, which can help keep allergies at bay.

Meditation is easily learned, and it's up to you whether you want to view it as a religious practice or simply as a relaxation technique. Classes are offered by many schools and yoga centers, and books and tapes on the subject are widely available.

Meditation works by gently focusing one's attention on a single object. This object of meditation can be as simple as your breathing or a mantra—a word, short phrase, or sounds.

"Anyone can meditate, even if it's only for 1 minute," says Leonard Perlmutter, founder and director of the American Meditation Institute in Averill Park, New York. "For a simple breathing-awareness meditation, all you have to do is sit in a firm straight-back chair or cross-legged on the floor with your head, neck, and trunk straight. Rest your hands on your thighs and gently close your eyes. Let your attention focus on the bridge between the two nostrils, where it meets the upper lip. Then, with full concentration, attend to each inhalation and exhalation for a period of 1, 2, or 3 minutes. While focusing your attention in this manner, allow your breathing to become even, quiet, and full, without any pauses or sounds. As thoughts appear, witness and honor them without getting involved and quickly redirect your attention back to your breathing. When practiced daily, this simple breathing-awareness meditation creates physical, mental, and emotional benefits, which enhance one's overall sense of well-being."

According to Perlmutter, Eastern traditions see the breath as the physical manifestation of the mind. Therefore, calming the breathing calms the mind.

Meditating with a mantra is just as simple. You can invent your own, or you can use favorite words from whatever traditions you may embrace. The role of the mantra is to deflect anxiety and agitation, leading the mind toward peaceful thought.

Social Involvement

Because social connection is a terrific buffer against stress, being friendly aids in the fight against allergies. Indeed, scientists know that having a social support system—a mostly harmonious network of family, friends, and associates—is an all-around predictor of good health.

In one study, 276 people were interviewed to learn how many close social ties they had. They were then injected with a cold-causing virus. Subjects with six or more close social ties were only one-fourth as likely to catch a cold as those with three or less. The pattern held true overall: More social ties equaled less illness. Scientists theorize that the decreased stress levels that come with a strong social support system lead to a stronger immune system and better resistance to infectious disease. It's possible, then, that this increased functioning of the immune system can help the body better fight off allergens.

How should you go about increasing your social connectedness? Reflect on the things that naturally interest you, then go wherever people with the same interests are likely to congregate, suggests Bruce S. Rabin, M.D., Ph.D., professor of pathology and psychiatry at the University of Pittsburgh School of Medicine and author of the book *Stress, Immune Function, and Health*.

"Use your common interest to break the ice," Dr. Rabin advises. "It may seem difficult at first, but if other people care about the same things, that could be the basis of a connection."

The bulletin boards of local libraries are always a nexus for folks who want to meet and talk about or act on their specialized interests. So are local museums, coffeehouses, and schools. Beyond that, there are clubs, societies, publications, the Internet, and regional get-togethers for practically every field of interest under the sun.

In addition, many special-interest magazines have regular columns about upcoming events all around the country. When you embrace what (and whom) you love in life, your social connections expand naturally—and keep you healthier all the while.

12

Millions of Americans who regularly practice yoga

Yoga

When something lasts five millenia, it's a good bet that it's more than a fad. Yoga has done that. It's also gaining great popularity in America right now, with many athletes, including some entire sports teams, using yoga as part of their physical conditioning routines.

The payoff most associated with yoga is flexibility. But two other benefits are equally important: stability and strength. Yoga aims for an ideal balance of these three benefits and of all the various parts and systems of the body with one another. It also aims to make the mind a clear, calm observer of the body's movements and processes.

The best-known aspect of yoga is its system of postures, called *asanas*. There are also breathing techniques, called *pranayamas*. These relax and strengthen the diaphragm, the muscle wall between the lungs and the digestive tract, which often stores tension.

For relief of allergy or asthma symptoms, try the following technique, shared by Michele Franey of Egg Harbor Township, New Jersey, a highly regarded instructor with 20 years of experience.

"First, stack some bolster pillows or tightly rolled blankets against a wall. Lie back against them, well-supported, at about a 45-degree angle to the floor, your head resting back but higher than your chest. Let your knees bend outward and bring your feet together sole to sole, heels drawn in close to your pelvis. A heavy object placed in front of your toes will help you hold the position. If your legs don't touch the floor, support them with pillows. Let your arms rest softly beside your body, pillows beneath them for support. The palms of your hands should be turned up. Have someone gently and briefly press your shoulders back to open and lift your chest.

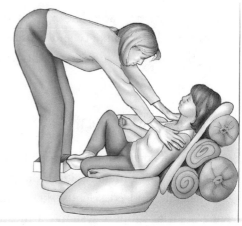

This yoga breathing technique can help open the air passageways.

"This calming position can be held for up to ½ hour. It helps the chest widen and all air passageways open. The diaphragm, abdominal, and pelvic muscles can fully relax, and the lungs can expand slowly. Mucus or phlegm can drain. If coughing or sneezing occurs, sit up until it passes, then relax back again," says Franey.

Yoga is best learned from a qualified instructor. Try to attend a variety of classes. Most teachers will let you observe for free or participate for a small fee. Always tell the teacher about your allergies or asthma and problem areas you may have, such as a sore back or neck.

Mind what your body tells you, especially when it signals pain. Yoga rewards patient, gradual improvement. Remember that it's not a competition to see who is most flexible. Rather, yoga is a health-promoting practice you can do for yourself. Maybe that's the secret behind 5,000 years of popularity.

The Allergy-Free CHILD

YOU WOULD DO ANYTHING to protect them. If you could, you would roll up your sleeves and take on each and every one of their enemies yourself. But when your children's foes are millions of tiny particles, you may find yourself with your hands tied behind your back.

You can't see them, but you've probably witnessed the effects that dust mites, pollen, and pet dander can have. They run rampant through your child's immune system, leaving rashes, a runny nose, and a wheezy chest in their path. Despite our best counterattacks, allergies to these substances and others are assaulting our children in ever-increasing numbers.

Not even the most knowledgeable allergists can tell you exactly why children's allergies are increasing. Some possible theories include an increased use of vaccinations and antibiotics, which may kill off "good" bacteria as well as "bad," and improved hygiene,

which may hinder the natural development of children's immune systems. In addition, sedentary lifestyles increase children's exposure to indoor allergens, since they're more likely to hunker down in front of a TV or computer screen and breathe stale air than to enjoy a sunny day outdoors. And the obesity associated with this sedentary lifestyle has been linked to increased asthma rates in children.

It may be a long time before doctors can explain why allergy rates are soaring, but that's what allergy rates indeed are doing, especially among our children. In Western countries, the frequency of allergic diseases has doubled in the past 25 years. In the United States alone, 20 to 25 percent of children have some form of allergy, and nearly five million children now have asthma. What's a parent to do?

While you can't prevent your children from getting allergies in the first place, you can take steps to delay or reduce the odds. And here's good news: You can start making a difference even before they're born.

Where Did They Come From?

Before we talk about how to delay allergy, let's take a look at how your children get allergies in the first place. Even this is not an easy question to answer, but three major factors seem to contribute to allergy development: genetics, exposure to allergens, and exposure to nonallergic factors.

No matter how hard you try, you can't change your children's genes. But when it comes to your children's allergies, you do have one thing in your favor: What you're

The Hygiene Hypothesis

The prescription your allergist probably gives when it comes to delaying allergy in infants is avoidance. Avoid food allergens, avoid environmental allergens, and maybe—just maybe—your child will grow up happy, healthy, and allergy-free.

Recent studies, however, have been coming ever closer to proving the validity of the so-called hygiene hypothesis. This is the notion that by cleaning our children constantly, discouraging them from getting dirty, pumping them full of antibiotics every time they get sick, and using antibacterial soaps, we're not allowing their immune systems to fully develop. And as the theory goes, this Westernized lifestyle makes them more susceptible to allergic conditions.

Studies testing the relevance of the hygiene hypothesis have covered a vast range of subjects. Several have shown that children raised on farms around animals have lower levels of allergy and asthma than their urban counterparts. Others have indicated the same low levels among children exposed to pets, day care, and older siblings.

These study results, while fascinating, should not cause a shift in your attitude about your child's exposure to allergens. While some allergens may help infants develop immunity, little work has been done on determining how much exposure is enough and what the proper methods are of exposing your child in the first place. "It's not something that's absolute for every child, and there are bound to be some glaring exceptions," says Dennis Ownby, M.D., professor of pediatrics at the Medical College of Georgia in Augusta. "Certainly, if multiple studies continue to show the same things, there will in all likelihood be a shift in our understanding and thinking about this." In the meantime, however, it's best to heed the advice of your allergist and establish a low-allergen environment for your young one.

The Family Tree of Allergies

You know the old saying about how you can't choose your relatives? Well, when it comes to allergies, some children may wish they could. Unfortunately, those tiny strands of DNA in your cells are the major factor that will determine whether or not your child gets allergies. The statement below shows what kind of risk of developing allergies your child may face.

If _____ has/have allergies, then the chances of the child having allergies is ____.
one parent . . . 20 to 40 percent
both parents . . . 40 to 60 percent
a sibling . . . 25 to 35 percent
nobody . . . 5 to 15 percent

allergic to is not necessarily what your children will be allergic to. You pass on a general *tendency* to develop allergies, not a specific allergy. So if you have asthma to ragweed and your spouse has hives to animal dander, it's possible that your child will have eczema to corn.

Gender (males typically have a higher rate of allergy than females), early exposure to viruses, and tobacco smoke can all play a role in the development of allergies as well. Other than your child's gender, these factors are something that you as a parent can influence.

• Delaying Allergies

Before your child is born, you can take some positive steps to reduce the likelihood that your baby will have allergies. And after your child's arrival, you can use several strategies to reduce your infant's risk. The most important? Breastfeeding

during the first few months after your child is born.

Pregnancy Tips

• Even if you smoked before pregnancy, now's the time to stub those butts in the ashtray. Exposure to tobacco smoke increases children's wheeziness in infancy, which in turn increases their risk of developing asthma later in life.

• Peanuts might be a food to avoid. "I've had patients whose mothers consumed peanuts during pregnancy, and they come out of the womb sensitized to peanuts before they've even eaten one," says Michael Zacharisen, M.D., assistant professor of pediatrics and medicine at the Medical College of Wisconsin in Milwaukee.

Infancy Tips

• If you are physically able, breastfeeding for 4 to 6 months is a major key to helping your child reduce the risk of allergy. Six months of breastfeeding—or even longer—is ideal because by then, your baby's immune system and digestive tract are better developed.

• Even if you're breastfeeding, your child can still be exposed to allergenic foods through your breast milk, so you might want to steer clear of foods such as cow's milk, eggs, and peanuts, particularly if allergies run in your family. A diet high in saturated fat has also been linked to allergy in infants, so try to limit your visits to fast-food restaurants.

• Many infant formulas are composed primarily of cow's milk or soy, two well-known allergens to children. If you feel that your infant is in a high-risk group for getting allergies, choose a hypoallergenic formula instead, such as Alimentum, Nutramigen, or Good Start.

• Limit your child's exposure to colds and other childhood viruses. "Children are more exposed to viral infections," says Farhad Imani, Ph.D., assistant professor of medicine at the Johns Hopkins University in Baltimore, "and their immune systems are not fully developed yet, so the viruses can sway naive cells to respond in ways they wouldn't respond in adults." Dr. Imani discovered that when human B cells (cells that recognize and attack intruders) were exposed to common viruses in the lab, they actually became cells that produced immunoglobulin E (an allergic antibody).

When Allergies Strike

Despite your best efforts, preventing your children from developing allergies can be tricky. Sometimes, the pull of their genetic makeup can be just too strong to overcome, and allergies will run their course no matter

An Allergy-Free Pregnancy

Your allergic condition during pregnancy can be about as unpredictable as a new baby's crying: Sometimes it gets worse, sometimes it gets better, and sometimes it goes away completely. Unfortunately, patients with severe asthma will most likely find their asthma symptoms getting worse.

Maternal allergies, particularly asthma, slightly increase the risk of infant mortality, low birth weight, and preterm birth. Fortunately, you can reduce any health concerns by following your doctor's allergy advice. Several drugs used to treat asthma and allergies have been found to be safe during pregnancy. As long as immunotherapy was started long before pregnancy, continuing it during pregnancy has also been shown to be safe. Talk to your doctor about your options.

how hard you try to stop them. This is absolutely *not* something that you should feel guilty about. With proper management of their asthma and allergy symptoms, your children will go on to live healthy and normal lives.

But before you can effectively manage your child's allergic symptoms, you need to understand a few unique aspects of allergies in children. Childhood allergies are sometimes difficult to self-diagnose because symptoms—and even the conditions themselves—can change as a child grows older.

Known as the atopic march, this evolution of allergic symptoms varies greatly from patient to patient. About one-third of patients will get better and one-third of them will get worse. The rest will essentially march in place—meaning that their symptoms neither subside nor intensify.

Doctors can use clues from the atopic march, however, to seek out and fight an allergic condition in children before it happens. "We know that allergies like hay fever frequently precede asthma, so it's important to intervene early when we see allergic symptoms, in the hope of diminishing a future of asthma," says Dr. Zacharisen.

Fighting Food Allergies

Whereas children usually need two or three pollen seasons to develop allergic rhinitis (hay fever), they often become sensitized to particular foods before they're even born.

"These early indications of immune responses to allergens are not necessarily harmful, but they may reflect the maturation of the immune system," says Dr. Zacharisen. In fact, food allergies are so prevalent that 6 to 8 percent of kids under age 3 get them.

Unfortunately, any type of food can cause an allergic reaction, but six suspects shoulder most of the blame: cow's milk, eggs, peanuts, wheat, soy, and tree nuts. Tree nuts refer to the traditional nuts, which include walnuts, almonds, pecans, filberts, and pistachios—in contrast to those that are not really nuts, such as peanuts (legumes), water chestnuts (vegetables), and coconut. These six evildoers account for 90 percent of food reactions. And of these, cow's milk is the leading offender by a landslide. The good news is that most children will outgrow their allergies to milk, eggs, wheat, and soy by age 10. On the other hand, a peanut or tree nut allergy is typically lifelong, says Dr. Zacharisen.

Most of the time, if your child is allergic, he will react within the first 2 months of life with gastrointestinal disorders. The most common symptom is chronic diarrhea, but other symptoms your child may experience include vomiting, colic, and—paradoxically—constipation, to name a few. "If a child has a reaction to a food, it tends to happen within minutes to up to 2 hours after the child eats the food," says Anne Muñoz-Furlong, founder and president of the

Food Allergy and Anaphylaxis Network in Fairfax, Virginia.

Second to gastrointestinal disorders, be sure to look for problems in the respiratory system. Coughing, congestion, asthma, and wheezing are all common. "Respiratory symptoms can accompany a food-allergic reaction, but as isolated symptoms, they would be very uncommon," says David Skoner, M.D., chief of allergy and immunology at Children's Hospital of Pittsburgh. "More often, you see them accompany diarrhea or vomiting." Children with food allergies can also develop problems of the skin, including eczema and hives.

Read on to discover some practical tips on how to deal with your child's food allergies.

• **Managing Childhood Food Allergies**

To effectively manage your child's food allergies, you first need to identify which foods trigger the allergic symptoms and then become vigilant about eliminating these from your child's diet.

• If you think that your child may be at high risk for developing food allergies, try a food introduction schedule. (For details of one expert's plan, see "Healthy Foods for a Healthy Baby.")

Healthy Foods for a Healthy Baby

After 6 months of exclusive breastfeeding, your infant's immune system and gastrointestinal tract should be mature enough to handle some solid foods. If your baby has a high chance of getting a food allergy, however, the opportunity for this condition to strike is greatest as you begin this process.

Introduce the solid foods into your baby's diet in small amounts, one at a time. Be sure to wait for 5 to 7 days before adding each new food. If your infant reacts to a food with sneezing, rashes, diarrhea, or a behavioral change, consult your pediatrician.

Michael Traub, N.D., is a naturopathic physician in Kailua Kona, Hawaii, who has worked with many children with food allergies. Below is his recommended calendar of foods, and the times when they should be introduced into your child's diet.

• **6 months:** carrots, squash, yams, broccoli, cauliflower, zucchini, Jerusalem artichokes, sprouts. Foods should be cooked, mashed, mixed with water, and given in servings of 1 to 2 tablespoons a day.

• **7½ months:** kiwifruit, pears, prunes, cherries, bananas, blackberries, and apple-

• Watch your child carefully during the first years of life to see if any gastrointestinal, respiratory, or skin-related symptoms occur after eating. If you happen to see these symptoms in your child, keep a record of them. "What you need to do is keep a diary of what you feed your child, what time you feed him it, and what type of reaction you're seeing, so you'll have something to show your doctor," says Muñoz-Furlong.

• The only proven therapy for food allergies is strict avoidance of the allergenic food. Once your doctor has determined what that food might be, cut the food out of your child's diet and replace it with something that provides similar nutrition.

• Become a regular label reader. Sometimes, even the brands you've known for years can change their ingredients without telling you. Be sure to read the labels each and every time you buy a product. And even then, reading the label might not be enough. "You also must learn the ways that these common foods, such as milk and eggs, can appear on the label," Muñoz-Furlong says. "For milk, it might be curds or whey or casein. For eggs, it might be albumin. These are the names that a parent needs to know to look out for these types of foods." (For more information on ingredient listings, see Food Allergies and Intolerances on page 278.)

sauce. Two to 3 tablespoons of any of these fruits a day, cooked, is sufficient. Be sure that these foods are amply mashed or strained so that they're not choking hazards.

• **9 months:** sweet potatoes, cabbage, oatmeal, papaya, potatoes, blueberries, lima beans, string beans, nectarines, peaches, split pea soup, plums, and beets. Serve 2 to 4 tablespoons of any of these a day, chopping into small pieces any that may pose a choking hazard. At 9 months, you can also include rice or oat cereal mixed with water or breast milk.

• **12 months:** acorn squash, barley, chard, yogurt, parsnips, asparagus, avocado, egg yolk, rice, quinoa, barley, and buckwheat. Four to 10 tablespoons a day. At this point, you can also serve beans, spinach, peas, and raw fruits.

• **18 months:** lamb, greens, kelp, eggplant, rye, chicken, rutabaga, fish, buckwheat, and spinach

• **21 months:** eggs, turkey, wheat, Cornish hen, beef liver, pineapple, oranges, brewer's yeast, goat's milk, and cow's milk

• **2 to 3 years:** clams, soy, cottage cheese, lentils, tomato, cheese, beef

• Beware of high-risk situations, such as restaurants, sleep-overs, or school. Restaurants are one place where you'll need to be extremely careful. "You really want to be conservative in what you order and stay away from desserts and sauces," says Muñoz-Furlong. "Ask lots of questions about surprise ingredients and be specific." At a friend's house or at school, talk to the other parent, the teacher, or the principal about your child's food allergy and make sure they know how to deal with it.

• Organize your kitchen, pantry, and refrigerator so that allergenic foods will be out of the reach of small hands.

• If you use a particular kitchen utensil on an allergenic food, make sure you clean it thoroughly before using it to prepare something for your child with allergies.

• Food allergy is one of the most common causes of anaphylaxis, so you'll want to have special precautions in place if your child is at risk for this condition. (For more information, see Anaphylaxis on page 211.)

• Oftentimes, food allergy will provoke asthma, allergic rhinitis, and skin allergy symptoms. To prevent and treat those particular conditions, see the tips in the following sections.

The Skinny on Your Child's Skin Problems

The word *eczema* is a derivative of the Greek word *ekzein*, which means "to boil out." Doesn't sound very pleasant, does it?

If your infant happens to suffer from eczema, however, you'll soon realize why this not-so-pleasant term is used to describe this chronically recurring symptom of atopic dermatitis. Itchy, bubbly, and crusty, this rashlike condition usually appears in early infancy. Ninety-five percent of the time, the condition will surface by age 2, if it's going to surface at all.

While the allergens that cause rhinitis and asthma are pretty clear-cut, nobody is really sure why children get atopic dermatitis. Dust mites, pollen, and foods all play a role in the development of eczema, but those roles remain fairly unclear. "We've discovered that there are about 20 genes responsible for the expression of eczema," explains Vincent S. Beltrani, M.D., associate clinical professor of dermatology at Columbia-Presbyterian Medical Center in New York City. "That's why no two cases of eczema are ever alike." One thing that is clear is that 10 to 15 percent of babies suffer from it in varying degrees. Infant eczema typically appears in patterns on the cheeks, chin, arms, and legs.

Luckily, eczema tends to go away as a child ages—only an estimated 5 percent of schoolchildren and 2 percent of adults have it. For older children whose eczema persists, however, it appears in the areas of the body that are most accessible to scratching fingernails, such as behind the knees and ears and inside the elbows, ankles, and buttocks. Here, the itchy patches become rough and pebbled and grow worse when the areas become sweaty. "Instead of being bubbly and thin, it's thick and scratched to death," says Dr. Beltrani. "Some people literally scratch off the surface of their skin."

Unfortunately, childhood eczema is a pretty good sign that your child will have a future of allergic conditions. An estimated 33 percent of children with atopic dermatitis go on to develop asthma, and 25 percent get allergic rhinitis. "It's one early physical indicator of a predisposition toward allergy," says Dr. Zacharisen. But if your infant's skin starts "boiling out," don't panic. Just follow the steps below.

• Easing Childhood Eczema

Avoidance of those things that trigger your child's eczema goes a long way in managing the condition. In addition, because of the intense itching associated with eczema, it may be difficult to keep your child from scratching. By limiting scratching, however, you can help the eczema to heal.

• Dust mites, pollen, and certain foods may play a role in atopic dermatitis. Try to identify the irritating allergen with the help of your doctor, and then keep your child out of contact with that allergen.

• Certain nonallergic irritants such as soaps, wool, synthetic fabrics, or other types of clothing can make already developed dermatitis worse. Make sure that your child avoids contact with these irritants, and choose clothing and bedding fabrics that breathe, like cotton.

• Overheating and sweating are common triggers of childhood eczema. Watch your child carefully for symptoms and scratching after he has been exercising or playing outside.

Things That Make Bumps in the Night

If you look at your child's skin and see a scaly, itchy rash, eczema is the likely cause. If you see red, raised individual blotches all over his skin, however, it's probably urticaria, or hives. The distinction is important because whereas eczema is usually associated with environmental allergens, an allergic reaction to food or drugs causes hives. In children, a viral illness is another common cause. In about 15 percent of people with hives, pressure, heat, cold, sunlight, or another physical factor causes the hives to appear.

An urticaria attack usually lasts only a few days, but chronic cases can last for months and even years. Usually, the hives are treated with a course of oral antihistamines, or corticosteroids if that is found to be ineffective. (For more information about urticaria, see Symptom Solver: Skin Problems on page 411.)

• One commonly associated symptom of all forms of atopics is dry skin. Creams and ointments can often be helpful in keeping skin moist. "There is no miracle cream," says Dr. Beltrani. "Anything they like they can use, as long as it's cosmetically acceptable." Test a drop on the skin first, as sensitivities can occur. (For more information, see Symptom Solver: Skin Problems on page 411.)

• Try to discourage your child from scratching his eczema. The eczema will more readily appear where the skin is broken, and scratching will heighten the chance of that occurring. Instead, try a cold compress like an ice pack wrapped in a thin towel to relieve and prevent itchiness.

• Itchiness can be so severe at times that children will unconsciously scratch themselves at night. Having your child wear cotton mittens can reduce the harsh effects of nighttime scratching.

• Soaking in a lukewarm bath for 5 to 10 minutes a day helps clear the skin of any irritants. Just be sure to pat dry and moisturize your child thoroughly with a cream or ointment immediately after the bath.

• Topical corticosteroid creams are the main treatment prescribed for childhood atopic dermatitis. Generally, a low dose (like a 1 percent hydrocortisone cream) is used on the face, and a higher dose can be used on other areas of the body. But be sure your doctor is very clear with you about what creams should be used and when you should use them. Some primary care physicians prescribe clotrimazole (Lotrisone), a high-potency steroid cream, more than any other, while specialists tend to not prescribe it at all.

The physicians that oppose its use contend there is danger in administering such a high-potency steroid to a child experiencing this chronic condition. The result could be permanent skin damage, as children that are prone to this condition have skin that is thin and more susceptible to damage, says Dr. Beltrani. Ask questions to make sure your child has the right cream for the job.

• Applying corticosteroids to moist skin immediately after bathing is the best way to get the full effect of the medication.

• Tacrolimus (Protopic) is another drug that you may want to ask your doctor about. Ordinarily used to help the body accept transplanted organs, tacrolimus has shown great promise in treating atopic dermatitis in children, without the serious side effects of corticosteroid creams, says Dr. Beltrani.

Halting Childhood Allergic Rhinitis

Sniffling, sneezing, coughing, and hacking—America's parents may be hearing these sounds of sickness all too frequently. Allergic rhinitis is known to affect 20 percent of the U.S. population, but among children, that number may be as high as 42 percent. The fallout in the United States alone is a $6 billion medical bill served up annually. It's not a fun proposition, and having a home or yard full of allergen enemies can make it even less enjoyable for you and your child.

Allergic rhinitis—your doctor's fancy word for the runny nose and watery eyes of hay fever—typically digs its hooks into children around age 10 but rarely before age 3. That's because it takes a few pollen seasons for the allergic sensitivities to develop. Children can develop hay fever symptoms to seasonal allergens (grass and plant pollen), perennial allergens (dust mites, mold, and animal dander), or food.

One thing that may help you determine if your child has allergic rhinitis is the presence of an "allergic look." Children with rhinitis develop certain characteristics in re-

sponse to their symptoms, like an overbite from gasping to get more air, allergic "shiners" (dark circles around the eyes), and a crease on the nose caused by frequent rubbing. These signals are not present in all children, but they're a dead giveaway that something is wrong if they are present. See the illustrations on page 313 for examples of the allergic look.

An allergic look is an obvious indication of allergic rhinitis or sinus problems in a child. One side effect of rhinitis, however, is not so obvious and can be detrimental to your child's health. Otitis media is an infection of the middle ear, and it usually affects children between 6 and 24 months old. The tricky thing about otitis media is that it sometimes causes no pain, but it can lead to

The Common Cold . . . or Allergies?

If your child is sneezing and sniffling through childhood, you may encounter a common dilemma: Is it allergic rhinitis (hay fever), or is it a cold? Young children have so many colds (from 6 to 12 a year) that sometimes it's tough to tell if it's allergies or a virus causing the sniffles. David Skoner, M.D., chief of allergy and immunology at Children's Hospital of Pittsburgh, offers up a few ways you can determine if it's a cold or allergies.

	Colds	Allergic Rhinitis
Duration:	3 to 5 days (rarely more than 10)	2 to 3 weeks (or more)
Nose Symptoms:	Colored or cloudy discharge Stuffiness	Clear, waterlike discharge Sneezing and itchiness
Other Symptoms:	Sore throat, fever Muscle aches and pains	Red, itchy eyes

This chart may help, but the symptoms of colds and allergic rhinitis can often be so similar that you should let a pediatrician make the final call.

hearing loss and even learning problems if you don't catch it early.

As the theory goes, the mucus and inflammation generated during a bout of allergic rhinitis can block the eustachian tube, the thin tunnel connecting the back of the nose to the middle ear, which leads to otitis media. "We think that viruses probably cause ear disease," says Dr. Skoner, "but allergies give you a higher risk to get the ear disease, and you're going to see a lot of ear disease in allergic kids because of that." If your infant has numerous colds or rhinitis, be sure to talk to your pediatrician about otitis media.

For any other concerns about your child's rhinitis symptoms and for tools to ease his discomfort, check out the following tips.

• Reducing the Symptoms of Childhood Rhinitis

Work with your child's doctor to identify preventive measures to reduce your child's rhinitis symptoms and to find the best medications for your child's unique situation.

• As early as infancy, your child may exhibit symptoms of rhinitis. Watch closely for signs and be wary of any ear problems or frequent colds. These might be indicative of an allergy problem. The earlier you can catch rhinitis in the act, the better.

• If your child shows the symptoms of rhinitis before age 3, ask your pediatrician or allergist if a particular food might be the cause. Airborne allergens typically don't cause rhinitis until age 3.

• If your young child does develop rhinitis to airborne allergens, the first step is to do your best to eliminate the offending allergen from your household. (For more information, see The Allergy-Free Home on page 73 and Pet Allergy on page 356.)

• Before you talk to your doctor about a prescription antihistamine, be sure to try all the preventive measures first. Many of the side effects of rhinitis medications have a greater effect on children than on adults.

• The symptoms of allergic rhinitis may impair your child's performance at school, but the sleepiness caused by antihistamines like diphenhydramine (Benadryl) and chlorpheniramine (Chlor-Trimeton) could make things even worse. Ask your doctor about one of the nonsedating or less-sedating antihistamines like loratadine (Claritin), fexofenadine (Allegra), or cetirizine (Zyrtec). Most of these drugs are now approved in syrup form for even 2-year-olds.

• To tackle congestion, your doctor may prescribe a decongestant as well. For convenience, antihistamines and decongestants are sometimes combined in one pill (Claritin-D or Allegra-D, for example). The side effects of decongestants are also more likely to cause problems in children than adults, so use them cautiously, and be sure you use a dose recommended for children.

• For severe cases, doctors will sometimes prescribe a corticosteroid spray to relieve the stuffy nose, irritation, and discomfort of allergic rhinitis. At one time, researchers were concerned that some nasal sprays (popular brand names include Flonase, Nasonex, and Rhinocort) stunted growth, but these concerns have appeared only in rare cases. Ask your doctor if you're worried about your child's prescription nasal spray.

• Concerns over growth reduction appear to be more legitimate with corticosteroids in a pill form, such as betamethasone, cortisone, and prednisone. If your child's prescription involves oral corticosteroids, express your concerns to your doctor. Still, there may be no other alternative. Despite such adverse effects as weight gain, high blood sugar, and increased blood pressure, oral corticosteroids may be the lesser of two evils since the consequences of uncontrolled allergy can be even worse.

• Cromolyn nasal sprays (like Children's NasalCrom, NasalCrom) may offer a good alternative to corticosteroid nasal sprays without the unwanted side effects.

• Most of the time, red, itchy eyes, known as allergic conjunctivitis, go hand in hand with allergic rhinitis. (For tips on treating this condition, see Symptom Solver: Eye Problems on page 426.)

• Immunotherapy may be an appropriate treatment for older children with allergic rhinitis symptoms. A typical course of immunotherapy usually involves getting an "allergy shot" every 1 to 6 weeks for about 3 to 5 years. Not only can immunotherapy effectively knock out allergic rhinitis symptoms for a number of years after treatment is stopped, it can even permanently end symptoms in some instances. "Of all the allergy therapy we have, this comes the closest to a cure," says Dr. Skoner. While immunotherapy is considered safe, you need to be aware that there is the possibility that it could bring on anaphylaxis. Because of this, your child will need to wait in the doctor's office for at least 20 minutes after each treatment.

Attacking Your Child's Asthma

In the classic William Golding novel *Lord of the Flies*, Piggy's asthma is symbolic of his physical weakness, making him a hapless victim to the other boys on the island.

Luckily, modern medicine has made sure that your child with asthma does not have to meet the same fate as Piggy. In fact, researchers found that 44 of the 196 U.S. athletes competing in the Winter Olympics in 1998 had clinical asthma, and 5 of them went on to win medals.

How did these athletes go from wheezing to winning? All it takes is a good doctor and the right asthma-management plan. While there's no guarantee that your children with asthma will go on to become Olympic athletes, there's no reason they can't.

Understanding asthma starts with understanding the changes that take place inside the body. Three major changes—inflammation, excess mucus, and the tightening of smooth muscle bands—cause the airways to close up, and soon your children may feel as if they were breathing through drinking straws. An estimated 75 to 85 percent of the time, an allergy is either the leading or a contributing cause of the asthma attack.

Fortunately, you do have weapons to help you deal with the source of wheezy lungs.

• Alleviating Childhood Asthma

Asthma is a serious condition, so it's important that you work closely with a doctor to manage your child's symptoms. Check out the following strategies.

• Like allergic rhinitis, food often triggers allergic asthma symptoms in infancy, and environmental allergens (pollen, dust mites, dander, and mold) can cause asthma in early childhood. If you suspect that your child is allergic to a food or environmental allergen, do your best to limit his exposure to it.

• Irritants such as smoke, perfumes, household cleaners, cold air, and dust can cause nonallergic asthma. Try to keep irritants like these away from your at-risk child. In particular, avoid smoking around your infant.

• A recent study has indicated that stress in the primary caregiver (usually the mother) is related to subsequent wheezing among infants and also may be related to the later development of asthma. "Stress may be another factor or adjunct, just as viral infections or indoor pollution allergens, which prime the immune system in a way that increases the chances of developing asthma,"

says Rosalind J. Wright, M.D., instructor of medicine at Harvard Medical School and lead researcher on the study. Such findings may suggest that future asthma interventions should, in part, focus on supporting families and reducing stress, particularly in early childhood, she says.

• About 80 percent of children with asthma develop symptoms before age 5. Watch for some of the signals. Parents should listen for a slight cough that gradually becomes more pronounced. They also should be aware that a bout of flu or a sinus infection can intensify a child's allergic symptoms.

• Pay close attention to the snacks your child munches on. Research indicates that snacks high in trans fats can cause wheezing and asthma. (For more information on fatty snacks and healthy snack alternatives, see "Know Your Enemy.")

• Shut off the video games and get your child outside and moving. Recent research has linked obesity and increasingly inactive lifestyles to a rise in asthma, and aerobic exercise just might be the best way to fight it. Just make sure that your child always warms up and cools down before and after exercise routines, stays hydrated, and has asthma medication close at hand at all times. Swimming is a highly recommended exercise for children with asthma because the moist, warm air prevents airway obstruction.

• Often, allergen avoidance alone cannot tame the symptoms of asthma. If you've seen the early symptoms of asthma in your child, you should see a doctor about an individual asthma-management plan.

• Asthma is often a tricky diagnosis to make because it can appear in many different ways with many different symptoms. To help your doctor make the best diagnosis, keep a diary on the length, frequency, and severity of your child's symptoms. Also be

Know Your Enemy

Parents should be careful when they purchase snack foods for children who have allergies to milk or eggs. Why? Because milk and eggs are disguised in many forms, says Debby Demory-Luce, R.D., Ph.D., with the USDA/ARS Children's Nutrition Research Center at Baylor College of Medicine in Houston. She suggests getting familiar with the lists here. These ingredients, which appear in popular snack foods, could translate into problems for the milk- or egg-sensitive child.

For Milk	For Eggs
Milk solids	Vitellin
Milk protein	Egg solids, white, yolk
Lactic acid	Globulin
Lactose ("lact")	Oxomucin
Whey	Ovomucoid ("ovo")
Curds	Mayonnaise
Caseinates (all forms)	Albumin
Rennet	Simplesse
Sodium lactate	
Butterfat	
Nondairy (defined as less than ½% milk by weight)	
Artificial butter flavor	

"If there is a question about a snack food and what it contains, call the manufacturer or just be cautious and avoid that snack food all together," says Dr. Demory-Luce.

While these children need to eliminate some dairy products from their diet, parents can substitute many calcium-rich snack foods. Dr. Demory-Luce suggests slices of fresh fruit and vegetables served them with milk-free dips and fortified rice milk; almonds; calcium-fortified juice and milk-free muffins made with diced carrots or dried fruits; calcium-fortified vegetable juice and pudding made with fortified soy milk; or fruit slushies made with fortified soy milk and fresh fruit. "I encourage parents to be adventurous and to try to modify recipes to meet their child's needs," says Dr. Demory-Luce.

sure to give the doctor information on the child's allergic history, the family's allergic history, the frequency and symptoms of the child's illnesses, and possible exposures to irritants and allergens.

• To stop an asthma attack before it even has a chance to start, look for early warning signs in your child. Besides coughing or wheezing, kids often will experience changes in appearance or mood and complain about how they feel. All of these may be signs of an impending asthma attack.

• The primary medication prescribed to children with asthma is some form of inhaler. (For more information, see "All about Inhalers.")

• Another way to manage asthma symptoms is with a peak-flow meter, which measures breathing ability. Generally, a doctor will establish a child's baseline reading on the peak-flow meter, and then a parent can take measurements once a day

All about Inhalers

Trying to understand the different types of asthma medications, the different devices for using the medications, and the different times when each should be taken might leave *you* breathless and gasping for answers. Here's a quick and easy guide to inhalers of all shapes and sizes.

Types of Medication

Bronchodilators. Used primarily as a rescue medication, bronchodilators immediately open the lungs up at the surge of an asthma attack. Common product names are Proventil, Ventolin, Maxair, and Tornalate.

Corticosteroids. Corticosteroids such as Vanceril, Beclovent, Aerobid, Azmacort, Flovent, and Pulmicort are common asthma medications. Unlike bronchodilators, which "rescue" people from an asthma attack, corticosteroids are used on a daily basis to prevent attacks from happening in the first place. The effects of inhaled corticosteroids on the growth of children have been controversial. Discuss this risk with your doctor.

Cromolyn-based inhalers. Intal and Tilade, two cromolyn-based inhalers, are not as strong as corticosteroids, but they also pose less risk for adverse side effects.

Types of Inhalers

Dry-powder inhalers. A new form of inhaler preferred by some people is the dry-powder inhaler. Some common asthma medications are available in dry-to make sure the lungs are functioning at a suitable level. A drop in the peak-flow reading can indicate an oncoming asthma attack, giving a parent plenty of time to intervene.

• A new type of pill medication known as a leukotriene antagonist has been successful in controlling asthma in many patients. In most cases, these medications (some brand names are Singulair and Accolate) are safe for children 2 years old or older.

• If nothing else seems to be helping, you may want to ask an allergist about immunotherapy. Studies show that a lengthy course of allergy shots can reduce asthma symptoms to the point where some patients can safely cut back on their asthma medications.

• Children with asthma often have a reduction in saliva flow and increased stomach acid reflux as a result of their inhaler use. As a result, they may be more at

powder form, but not all of them. A dry-powder inhaler can be advantageous because you don't have to time your breathing with the activation of the inhaler as with a metered-dose inhaler; the dry-powder inhaler releases medicine as you breathe.

Metered-dose inhalers. This is the most common type of inhaler, and it's probably the one you're most familiar with. It consists of a metal cylinder nestled inside a plastic tube that lets out a burst of medication when you push down on it. To use this inhaler, hold it a few inches away from your mouth and activate it shortly after starting a deep breath. Then hold it in your lungs for 10 seconds, exhale, and wash your mouth out thoroughly after you're done.

Nebulizers. People with severe asthma may need to use a nebulizer, a small machine that creates a mist of one of the bronchodilator medications. Nebulizers, however, are used less and less frequently these days because they are expensive, inefficient, and dangerous if used improperly.

Spacers. For young children or people who have trouble timing their breath with their metered-dose inhaler, a spacer can be helpful. A spacer is just a long plastic tube. The spacer goes on one end of the inhaler, and your mouth goes on the other end. Once the inhaler is activated, you can breathe the medicine out of the spacer when you wish. For children under 5, a spacer combined with an attached face mask is a good way to make sure the appropriate amount of medication is inhaled.

risk for gingivitis and cavities. Luckily, a child can help reverse the effects of asthma medications on teeth by rinsing with water four times a day.

The Best Natural Remedies for Your Children's Allergies

If your child is diagnosed with allergies, you'll need to work closely with your doctor to find the best possible treatment options. While conventional medicine offers a variety of prescription and over-the-counter medications, alternative medicine has its own range of natural remedies for treating and relieving allergies. But are these remedies safe for kids? According to Mark Stengler, N.D., a naturopathic and homeopathic physician in La Jolla, California, many of them are. For detailed instructions on use and dose for all these herbs and supplements, contact a licensed herbalist or alternative practitioner.

For allergic rhinitis, Dr. Stengler recommends the following nutritional and herbal supplements: nettle, quercetin, grape seed extract, flaxseed oil, astragalus, and licorice root.

Dr. Stengler suggests these supplements for asthma: licorice root, flaxseed oil, vitamin C, grape seed extract, quercetin, and magnesium.

For skin problems, Dr. Stengler recommends these natural remedies: vitamin C; burdock root; creams containing chickweed, calendula, or chamomile; vitamin E oil; and an oatmeal bath.

Always talk to a practitioner about your choice of natural supplements and remedies. Ask about possible side effects when used alone or in combination with other medication, herbs, or supplements, because the reactions may be different for your child. If children follow their doctors' diet and supplement recommendations, they should notice improvement over the course of 2 to 4 weeks.

Allergies at School

Sure, it's pretty easy to monitor your kids' allergy and asthma symptoms when they're hanging around the homestead. But what about during the other 8 hours of the day, when they're at school?

Without a doubt, allergies can hamper your children's school performance. Asthma and rhinitis alone account for around 10 million missed school days a year. And even when your children are at school, medication side effects, lack of sleep, or a general sense of fatigue from allergy symptoms can prevent them from giving classes all they've got.

Whether it's in the lunchroom, the classroom, or the gym, schools pose a unique set of circumstances for the child with allergies or asthma, says Dr. Zacharisen, who offers the following advice for parents of children with allergies.

• Dealing with Allergies at School

• With your allergist, work out a school management plan that describes the symptoms to monitor in your child and how to intervene. An asthma-management plan should include asthma triggers, emergency contact information, signs of an asthma emergency, and the proper steps to take in case of an emergency.

• Make sure your child is taking the prescribed daily maintenance medication. This will help prevent problems at school. In addition, be certain that your child's emergency medication (be it an inhaler or an EpiPen) is readily available at school. Discuss proper use of the medication with the school nurse and any teachers who supervise your child during the day.

• If your child has food allergies, pack his lunch every day, and make sure he is aware of the danger of trading foods. Also, inform teachers and administrators of the concerns in case of class celebrations or field trips.

• If your child has exercise-induced asthma, inform the physical education teacher about his symptoms and what to do in the case of an emergency. Tell the teacher that your child should be a full participant in activities but at times may need to take it a little slower than the other children.

• Learning disabilities may be a result of a lack of alertness caused by asthma-related sleep deprivation. If your child is having such problems, talk to your physician about your child's asthma-management plan.

Allergies in Adolescence

Once upon a time, getting your children to take their asthma medication was easy. All you had to do was ask nicely, and it was as good as taken. Then they became teenagers. Now, it's a war just to get them to sit and eat with the family, much less take their asthma medication. Teenagers have reached the time in their lives when they want to assert their independence, and as a result, getting them to comply with their asthma-management plan is not easy.

Tragically, an estimated three to six times more teenagers die of asthma-related causes than children ages 5 to 10, and the major reason is that teens just aren't taking their medicine. Luckily, you as a parent can make a difference. "Mom or Dad tend to clump 'Did you take your medicine?' with 'Did you clean your room?' or 'Did you take out the garbage?' At this point, the teen has tuned them out and doesn't even hear what they're saying," says Renee Theodorakis, M.A., director of adolescent services for the Asthma and Allergy Foundation of America in Washington, D.C. "The way Mom and Dad ask the question needs to change."

In some ways, your doctor can also help with compliance by prescribing the right medicines. Your teen might find it more socially acceptable to take a pill than to rely on an inhaler.

PART FOUR

Allergy-Free
ACTION PLANS

Are You
ALLERGIC?

To find out if you have allergies, take this quick and easy quiz. Simply add up the number of points that apply to each question to which you answer yes.

Do you have hay fever symptoms such as sneezing, watery nasal drainage, and nasal itchiness? (4 points) . . . . Y N

Do you have chronic nasal congestion, postnasal drip, or both? (3 points) . . Y N

Do you have sinus problems—frequent "colds" or headaches? (2 points) . . . Y N

Do your eyes itch, water, get red, or swell? (4 points) . . . . Y N

Do you have asthma (wheezing), a tight chest, or a chronic cough? (1 point) . Y N

Do you have skin problems such as eczema, hives, or itching? (2 points) . . . Y N

Do you have indigestion, bloating, diarrhea, or constipation? (1 point) . . . . . . Y N

Do you have chronic fatigue or tiredness? (4 points) . . . . Y N

Are your symptoms seasonal only—or worse seasonally? (4 points) . . . . Y N

Do your symptoms change when you go indoors or outdoors? (3 points) . . . Y N

Are your symptoms worse in parks or grassy areas? (4 points) . . . . Y N

Are your symptoms worse in the bedroom, after going to bed, or in the morning when you get up? (2 points) . . . . Y N

Are your symptoms worse when you come into contact with dust when vacuuming or cleaning around thick carpeting, heavy drapes, and so on? (4 points) . . . . Y N

Are your symptoms worse around animals? (2 points) . . . . Y N

Do you have any blood relatives with allergies: one or both parents, brothers or sisters, or children? (6 points) . . . . Y N

If you scored less than 7, it's unlikely you have allergies.
If you scored between 8 and 12, it's possible you have allergies.
If you scored between 13 and 30, it's probable you have allergies.
If you scored more than 31, it's very likely you have allergies.

Learn to Dodge
Allergic Woes from
HEAD TO TOES

ALLERGY ALMOST SEEMS too bland and mundane a word to describe all the types of trouble this condition can cause.

Headache. Now that's a title that sums up the problem. And *heartburn* certainly conveys the sting of that fiery ailment.

But what does the term *allergy* describe? How do you feel when you have an allergy? What happens to you?

As it turns out, those simple questions have complex answers. Because when you try to define the word *allergy*, you'll find that it's an umbrella term that covers a pack of problems.

This section showcases more than a dozen of the most common allergy-related maladies, from allergic rhinitis (also known as hay fever) to allergies from insect stings and bites. (For information about the most common general allergy symptoms, such as sneezing, coughing, and itchy skin, turn to part 5.)

In each chapter, you'll learn to recognize the signs of the condition and discover just how swirls of allergy-related cells and chemicals deep in your body can lead to those unpleasant symptoms.

Most important, each chapter contains an Action Plan of tools and tactics, recommended by leading allergy experts in America and beyond, that's specially designed to help you break free from each of these conditions or avoid them in the first place.

While you'll most likely head for the conditions that you know or suspect you have, you may find the other chapters helpful, too. Some of the information may confirm your suspicions. Some may surprise you, since people who have one kind of allergy often have others. And some may save your life.

For example:

• Did you know that carrying a simple pen-size device—and knowing how to use it—is the single best way to handle an attack of anaphylaxis? This full-body allergic reaction can be terrifying in its swiftness and severity, as you itch maddeningly and struggle to breathe through a tight throat. It's often caused by eating an allergenic food, sometimes even the merest trace. By learning how to recognize its symptoms and using that pen-size injection of epinephrine, you give yourself a good shot at surviving the episode.

• Did you know that asthma can be managed most effectively by using a combination of natural therapies and prescription drugs? This breath-taking disease can suck the quality of life right out of your days and nights as you struggle with lungs that are tight, inflamed, and gummy with mucus. But when you use a careful mix of conventional medications backed up with alternative approaches, you can breathe a sigh of relief.

• Did you know that stinging insects such as yellow jackets, fire ants, and wasps aren't the only bugs that can cause allergic problems? Cockroaches and dust mites, which leave behind a shower of allergens in many of our homes, are widespread triggers of asthma and allergic rhinitis. You can learn how to strengthen your body's ability to cope with these harmful insects—or terminate them before they bother you.

• Did you know that thousands of consumer products are made from a product that gives many Americans allergic fits? The culprit is latex, and a bad encounter with the stuff in a balloon, condom, or even a pair of panty hose can leave a sensitized person with an itchy rash, a runny nose, or worse. We'll tell you how to keep this stuff away from you and how to help yourself if some slips through your defenses.

From allergies to your cat and dog to allergies to less obvious triggers such as mold, nickel, and drugs, the following chapters will provide you with all the clues you need to become an allergy supersleuth. After all, uncovering what triggers your allergies is the first step in defeating them.

ANAPHYLAXIS

YOU MAY HAVE SEEN an episode of *ER* or another medical drama where a patient suddenly went into anaphylactic shock. Indeed, for sheer drama, few medical conditions can beat anaphylaxis. But if the reaction is happening to you or someone you love, forget trying to be a hero. Get to a real emergency room—fast.

Anaphylaxis is what's known as a systemic reaction, during which exposure to an allergen triggers an allergic response throughout your body rather than just near the site, such as what usually occurs with an insect sting. Unfortunately, it doesn't take much to trigger this body-wide allergic response. A single peanut or a tiny yellow jacket sting can set off the reaction.

During an anaphylactic attack, a rush of chemicals—histamines, leukotrienes, and prostaglandins—is released in an attempt by the body to defend itself. These chemicals are produced by basophils, which are found in the blood, and mast cells, which are found throughout the body, including the skin, nose, and gastrointestinal tract. Anaphylaxis can produce a wide range of symptoms because of the extensive presence of these defensive cells.

Anaphylaxis may sometimes affect many organs, such as the throat, lungs, blood vessels, and intestines, or it may affect only one or two. During an anaphylactic attack, the histamine and other chemicals released by your body may:

• Produce widespread itching, welts, and hives on your skin

• Cause blood vessels to become leaky, resulting in a drop in blood pressure, swelling of your skin, and fluid in your lungs

• Bring the circulation of your blood and oxygen to a near-standstill as your blood pressure drops

• Make it difficult or impossible to breathe as your tongue and throat swell up and your lungs go into asthmatic spasms

• Trigger nausea, vomiting, and diarrhea as your gastrointestinal system goes haywire

Anaphylaxis can strike within seconds or minutes of exposure to an allergen. Or it may sneak up slowly, with symptoms delayed up to 2 hours from the time of exposure. Initial symptoms may even disappear, then return full-force within 4 to 12 hours.

According to Anthony Szema, M.D., assistant professor of medicine and surgery and director of the Allergy and Asthma Center at the State University of New York at Stony Brook, factors that increase your risk of death from anaphylaxis include uncontrolled asthma, prescription beta-blocker use, cardiovascular disease (atherosclerosis), your age (if 45 or older), and not having an EpiPen with you or not using it in time.

What Anaphylaxis Feels Like

Because so many strange things are suddenly happening to you all at once, anaphylaxis usually feels as scary as it is, notes Susan Dunmire, M.D., associate professor of emergency medicine at the University of Pittsburgh School of Medicine.

"It's a terrifying feeling," Dr. Dunmire says. "You may become flushed, and your skin may become quite itchy and red. The frightening thing is that you begin to feel swelling in your mouth and throat, and then you begin to feel you're having difficulty taking a full breath. You may feel like you're

Anaphylaxis, Drawn and Quartered

Anaphylaxis is an allergic reaction that can trigger reactions all over your body. Here is a list of the ways it can affect the various systems in the body.

Cardiovascular: Light-headedness, feeling faint, loss of consciousness (known as syncope), heart palpitations

Upper respiratory: Nasal congestion, sneezing, difficulty swallowing

Lower airway obstruction: Coughing, wheezing

Skin: Welts or hives, swelling of the skin (particularly in the face and around the lips and tongue), flushing

Gastrointestinal: Bloating, nausea, vomiting, diarrhea, cramps

Elsewhere: Metallic taste in the mouth, cramping of the uterus during pregnancy, sudden need to urinate

suffocating. As your blood pressure drops, you feel dizzy and sweaty and become pale."

Your body is not kidding: Anaphylaxis can kill by suffocation.

While some of the symptoms of anaphylaxis may appear ambiguous on paper, when you have it, you generally know it.

"Usually, it is obvious. The onset of most

Epinephrine and Emergencies

If you have had an anaphylactic reaction, your allergist should prescribe a self-administered syringe of epinephrine for emergency use if anaphylaxis recurs. It's a good idea to have a syringe available in your home, car, and workplace.

Two versions that are available include the EpiPen Auto-Injector, a spring-loaded hypodermic needle for adults, and the EpiPen Jr., a self-injecting version for children.

The EpiPen is simple to use and needs only 3 pounds of force to trigger the spring injection mechanism. Be careful not to trigger it accidentally, and do not inject it near a bone—only into the thigh.

Patients, their family members, and close friends should know how to use an EpiPen in an emergency and should ask the patient's permission first. Some states (but not all) have Good Samaritan laws protecting people who administer EpiPens for others.

Experts recommend that EpiPens—and training in their use—should be more widely available, such as in schools, in malls, and on group camping or bicycling trips. Talk to an allergist about getting an EpiPen if you are in charge of such a group.

To use an EpiPen:
1. Pull off the gray safety cap.
2. Place the black tip on the thigh, at a right angle to the leg, through clothing if necessary.
3. Push quickly against the thigh.
4. Hold in place several seconds, then remove and discard.
5. Massage the injection area for 10 seconds.

An EpiPen can take 10 to 20 minutes to reach full effect, and the benefits generally last 60 to 90 minutes. Use that time to get to an emergency room. In severe cases where there is no response to the EpiPen injection after 10 minutes and medical help has not arrived, you can give a second injection, if one is available.

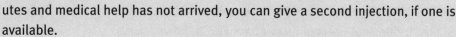

anaphylaxis is fairly rapid," reports Dr. Dunmire. "Start worrying when the person says, 'I don't feel well. My whole body feels weird.'"

While people can recover from anaphylaxis on their own, and anaphylaxis is usually not fatal, you have no way of knowing this at the onset, warns David B. K. Golden, M.D., associate professor of medicine at the Johns Hopkins University in Baltimore who specializes in research into anaphylaxis and insect sting allergies. So anaphylaxis should always be treated as a medical emergency.

What to Do during an Anaphylactic Reaction

While there are many conditions that respond successfully to natural self-care remedies, anaphylaxis is not one of them. If you experience the severe symptoms described earlier, you need to dial 911, or the emergency number for your community, immediately for help. Do not attempt to drive yourself to the emergency room. And if you have experienced this most severe of allergic reactions in the past and been seen by a doctor for it, it is time to give yourself the emergency shot of epinephrine that he prescribed for exactly these repeat occurrences.

"It is critical to use epinephrine as quickly as possible. It's the only thing that will slow or stop the anaphylactic reaction," says Dr. Golden.

Although epinephrine is available only by prescription, you make it naturally in your adrenal gland, especially when you are under stress. In fact, epinephrine is just another name for adrenaline.

An injection of epinephrine feels like the jolt you would get from drinking a hundred

Is Pretreatment a Possibility for Anaphylaxis?

In certain cases, you may be able to "pretreat" yourself with antihistamines and prescription drugs if you know that you may be exposed to a trigger of anaphylaxis. This treatment would typically begin about 12 hours in advance.

Pretreatment is not always advisable, however, because the antihistamines may mask early symptoms of anaphylaxis. You should always talk to your doctor before using antihistamines as pretreatment.

For exercise-induced anaphylaxis, your doctor will probably recommend that you pretreat with antihistamines before exercise and that you begin your daily workout gradually. But for severe anaphylactic reactions, workouts are out.

Pretreatment is sometimes used before medical procedures that could trigger anaphylaxis. It does not prevent latex anaphylaxis, however.

cups of coffee, says Dr. Golden. It will leave you with a headache for perhaps a half-hour, but it is safe for most people.

Another key drug for treating anaphylaxis is diphenhydramine hydrochloride, the generic name for the over-the-counter antihistamine Benadryl. Benadryl works more slowly than epinephrine and will help reduce minor symptoms, such as itching and hives, but not the symptoms that could kill you. Because people with severe anaphylaxis are prone to vomiting, however, it may not be a good time to take pills.

The Best Ways to Protect Yourself

The best way to avoid a trip to the emergency room is to not get anaphylaxis. The trick is to identify your allergies and learn to avoid the allergens that trigger them. This means talking to an allergist even after you have recovered from a relatively mild anaphylactic reaction.

Sound obvious?

A study of people who had insect sting anaphylaxis found it is not.

"You'd be amazed how many people have this condition and don't go to the hospital," says Dr. Golden. He found that 90 percent of adults didn't even tell their doctors about their anaphylactic reactions.

This can be a potentially dangerous mistake. If you have had anaphylaxis in the past, the odds are you will have it again. A study of 380 anaphylaxis patients found

that while 25 percent had just one episode, 18 percent had two episodes, and 57 percent had three or more. The severity of symptoms can vary with each attack.

So take charge of your health: Be sure to tell your doctor about any allergic reaction you've experienced, especially if you had the symptoms of anaphylaxis in the past.

In addition to medical testing, your doctor or allergist may ask you to keep a diary to help identify the cause of your symptoms. Once the allergens have been identified, he will work with you to avoid them. This can be tricky, since allergens may appear in products you wouldn't suspect. If you are allergic to a food or drug, for example, throw out anything containing the culprit. Don't forget to weed through your cupboards, refrigerator, medicine chests, and drawers.

Also be sure that your conversation with your doctor includes a discussion about the best treatment options that are available to you. Dr. Golden has found that doctors sometimes don't tell their patients about all of the treatments available, such as venom immunotherapy.

Immunotherapy can reduce the risk of fatal anaphylaxis from insect stings to nearly zero. But there is a risk: If too much is given too soon, the allergy shots used to desensitize you can actually trigger anaphylaxis. If you and your doctor do decide that venom immunotherapy is right for you, you'll need to plan on staying in the doctor's office for a while after your treatment for observation because of this risk.

In addition to venom immunotherapy, new treatments are constantly being developed. "See your doctor on a regular basis, in case there's some new form of treatment that might be beneficial to you," Dr. Golden advises. Your doctor can help you weigh your options and find out what treatments are right for you.

The Anaphylaxis Enigma

Your odds of experiencing anaphylaxis over the course of your lifetime are about one in a hundred. "Unfortunately, you cannot always predict when you might experience an attack," says Lori Kagy, M.D., a physician in Little Rock, Arkansas.

There are two reasons for this unpredictability. First, the cause cannot always be identified, even with allergy testing. "This is the case about one-third of the time, and it appears to be more common in women," Dr. Kagy notes.

Second, many cases of anaphylaxis are not due to allergies. These are sometimes called anaphylactoid reactions, though the body's response is virtually identical to allergic anaphylaxis and potentially just as deadly. Drugs and exercise can cause non-allergic anaphylaxis. There may be no warning prior to an anaphylactoid reaction because you do not need previous exposure to become sensitized, as with an allergy. Even when allergies are to blame, you may not know that you have become sensitized.

The moral of the anaphylaxis story, then, is to get immediate medical treatment if you ever feel the symptoms of anaphylaxis coming on. You may be embarrassed if you call 911 and your symptoms turn out to be an innocent case of the hives, but at least you'll be alive.

Where's the Risk?

Researchers at the University of Tennessee College of Medicine in Memphis analyzed the probable causes of nonfatal anaphylaxis in 266 patients. Their findings:

- No identifiable cause: 37 percent
- Foods, spices, and food additives (about half of these were peanuts and crustaceans): 34 percent
- Medications (about half of these were nonsteroidal anti-inflammatory drugs, or NSAIDs): 20 percent
- Exercise: 7 percent
- Insect bites: 1.5 percent
- Hormonal changes: less than 1 percent

Anaphylaxis
ACTION PLAN

The keys to surviving anaphylaxis are using an EpiPen quickly and calling 911 immediately. Ambulance paramedics are usually well-equipped to handle anaphylaxis. "They can basically have the patient treated by the time they get to the emergency room," says Dr. Dunmire. Some places, however, do not allow paramedics to administer epinephrine.

Early Warnings

The earliest symptoms of anaphylaxis often appear on the skin. Body-wide hives or itching is a sign of a systemic allergic reaction that can develop into anaphylaxis, so you should call 911. In addition to body-wide hives, call 911 if you experience the following, which suggest a body-wide anaphylactic re-action.

- Itching or tingling, possibly in the groin or armpits, palms, soles of the feet, lips, or scalp.
- Flushing (warmth and redness)
- Feeling of impending doom, often caused by a drop in blood pressure or difficulty breathing
- Hay fever–like symptoms, including runny nose and sneezing

Red Alert

The most serious warning signs of anaphylaxis are difficulty breathing and a drop in blood pressure, indicated by severe dizziness. Call 911 immediately if the following symptoms appear.

- "Lump" in the throat or throat tightness
- Difficulty swallowing and hoarseness
- High-pitched wheezing around the throat or neck when trying to inhale (from trying to get air past the swelling)
- Wheezing or whistling sound from difficulty exhaling—and slow exhaling
- Chest tightness
- Light-headedness
- Fainting

Causes of Anaphylaxis

It can be daunting to look at a list of the many things that could trigger anaphylaxis. Being informed, however, could mean the difference between life and death.

Food

Food is the most common cause of anaphylaxis, at least outside of hospitals. Reactions can become progressively more severe with subsequent exposure to a food allergen. Common food allergens include:

- Peanuts
- Shellfish such as shrimp, clams, lobsters, and crabs
- Fish
- Cow's milk
- Hen's eggs
- Tree nuts, such as walnuts, almonds, pecans, cashews, hazelnuts, and Brazil nuts
- Soy
- Wheat

   In addition, beware of food additives such as sulfites, especially if you have severe asthma. Sulfites are found in red wine, dried fruits and vegetables, potato products, and pickles.

Insects

Stinging insect venom can cause anaphylaxis, depending on the amount of venom from a sting or number of stings. The most common insect allergies are:

- Yellow jackets
- Fire ants
- Paper wasps
- Hornets
- Honeybees

Drugs

More than 500,000 serious allergic reactions to drugs occur in hospitals in the United States each year. Penicillin-type antibiotics alone are blamed for more than 5,000 deaths each year, about 75 percent of the deaths from anaphylaxis. Another 900 deaths are caused by dyes used during radiology exams. Insulin anaphylaxis sometimes occurs in pregnant women with gestational diabetes who receive intermittent insulin. Allergists can test for penicillin and insulin allergies. Testing for sensitivity to other drugs is not very accurate.

Medications that can cause anaphylaxis include:

- Penicillin and related antibiotics, such as amoxicillin
- Seizure and antiarrhythmia medications
- Nonsteroidal anti-inflammatory drugs (NSAIDs), such as aspirin and ibuprofen
- Muscle relaxants
- Vaccines
- Radiology dyes
- Antihypertensives
- Insulin
- Blood products

Allergic reactions to vaccines are not always due to a sensitivity to eggs. Rather, the gelatin or yeast sometimes used to culture the vaccine typically is the culprit.

Latex

Latex can cause anaphylaxis. The greatest danger occurs when latex is in contact with moist areas of the body or with internal surfaces during surgery, because the allergen is readily absorbed into the body. It can be triggered by:

- Latex gloves and food contaminated by latex gloves
- Latex condoms
- Balloons
- Bananas, chestnuts, and other foods that cross-react with latex allergy

Exercise

Exercise can trigger anaphylaxis, even in people with no preexisting allergies or asthma. Eating 3 to 4 hours before exercising increases the risk, as does taking aspirin or other NSAIDs, but it may be triggered merely by brisk walking or bicycling.

Nonallergic Anaphylaxis Causes

Triggers of anaphylactoid responses include:

- Narcotics—opiate painkillers, including codeine, morphine, and meperidine hydrochloride
- Aspirin and other NSAIDs
- Blood and blood product transfusions
- Food additives

Until Help Arrives

If you believe anaphylaxis is occurring and you have an EpiPen, use it—and the sooner the better. Be aware, though, that an EpiPen only buys time. Use it to get to an emergency room, even if the symptoms appear to have cleared up.

If you are with someone who appears to be having an anaphylactic reaction and he doesn't have an EpiPen, perform the following steps as necessary until help arrives.

- Have the person lie down and elevate his legs and feet about 12 inches.
- Try to keep the person relaxed.
- If the person vomits, turn him on his side to clear the airway. And if he's unconscious, sweep your finger through his mouth, but not into his throat.
- Watch to make sure that he continues breathing, and perform rescue breathing if he stops.
- Because of airway swelling, rescue breathing may be difficult, but do your best. To help a child, seal your mouth over his nose and mouth.
- If there also is no pulse, perform full CPR.

When It's Not Anaphylaxis

The most common mimic of anaphylaxis is a vasovagal response—fainting in response to a fright—particularly when it follows an injection. As with an anaphylactic reaction, its symptoms are light-headedness or fainting. When the person lies down, however, the symptoms begin to subside within 5 minutes, and they disappear within 30. If the person also has hives and itching, this is a clue that it is not a vasovagal response.

An internal hemorrhage can also cause light-headedness and a weak pulse but would not cause difficulty breathing. It is still a medical emergency, however.

A heart attack can produce shortness of breath and chest pain. But these same symptoms can be signs of anaphylaxis, especially in middle-aged or older people.

Finally, niacin vitamin supplements can also cause body-wide flushing and tingling. Remember, an anaphylactic reaction is serious. If you suspect that you are experiencing anaphylaxis, regardless of symptoms, seek immediate medical attention.

In the Ambulance

Paramedics can confirm whether anaphylaxis is occurring by checking blood pressure and testing for heart arrhythmias.

To treat anaphylaxis, they might administer injections of epinephrine; injections of an antihistamine such as diphenhydramine (Benadryl); intravenous fluids, which will help to bring blood pressure up; and oxygen, to compensate for obstructed airways.

In the Hospital Emergency Room

Doctors will begin or continue all of the procedures used in the ambulance as long as necessary. In addition, they might take a blood sample for later diagnosis to look for the chemical tryptase, a marker of anaphylaxis.

For severe cases, you should remain under observation for 4 to 6 hours after your initial symptoms. Milder cases may require less time in the ER.

In addition to the epinephrine, doctors may give you antihistamines, typically diphenhydramine (Benadryl), primarily to reduce skin reactions. If you had a severe reaction, you might also be given corticosteroids to reduce the swelling of the skin that occurs later. You could also be given bronchodilators to improve your breathing.

After the ER

Symptoms may reappear, typically within 4 to 6 hours after the attack, but possibly up to 2 days later. Because of all the medications you were given in the hospital, though, the rebound symptoms may be minor. If in doubt about the severity of the symptoms you're experiencing, call your doctor or 911. You may also have some occasional dizziness. Angioedema, or swelling of your skin, especially in the face, can last a few days.

In the future, always have epinephrine handy. Ask your doctor to prescribe enough EpiPens so that you'll have one anywhere you go—your home, car, workplace, and so on. In addition, post emergency numbers on the refrigerator and teach your children to call 911. You should also wear a medical identification bracelet and keep a medical information card in your wallet.

ASTHMA

THINK OF YOUR LOWER AIRWAYS as an upside-down tree: Air moves down a trunk (your windpipe), which splits into two big branches (the right and left bronchi). These large airways then subdivide even further into progressively smaller branches and twigs, the smallest of which are called bronchioles. Your lungs contain about eight million of these bronchioles.

Clustered at the end of each bronchiole, like the buds of a tree, are millions of tiny air sacs, which are called alveoli. This is where oxygen is transferred to your bloodstream. Your lungs contain about 300 million alveoli.

When you breathe in normally, you create a partial vacuum by unconsciously contracting and flattening your diaphragm. Air enters your lungs so effortlessly that you don't give it a second thought.

If you have asthma, however, your "tree" fills with "sap." One minute you're breathing normally. The next minute it feels as though someone has poured wet cement into your lungs. It's so hard to breathe that you might as well be sucking in air through a straw.

What is responsible for this *Rhapsody in Blech*? Biology.

People with asthma have a more pro-inflammatory immune system, experts say. Or, to put it another way, they have sensitive immune systems that often overreact, causing inflammation in certain organ systems.

So just as people with allergic rhinitis (hay fever) have "twitchy" sinuses and people with eczema have "twitchy" skin, people with asthma have "twitchy" lungs. Since they're hyperreactive to things in the environment, their lungs easily become inflamed and congested.

The difference is that asthma, unlike

most other allergic conditions, can be fatal. "Asthma can kill," says Betty Wray, M.D., interim dean of the Medical College of Georgia School of Medicine in Augusta and past president of the American College of Allergy, Asthma, and Immunology. "In the 1960s and 1970s, we rarely saw deaths or even hospital admissions. But for unknown reasons, over the past 15 years the prevalence and mortality have increased."

Here's what happens during an asthma attack.

1. **Inflammation.** In response to an asthma trigger, mast cells, the immune cells in your bronchioles, release histamine and other inflammatory chemicals. This causes the bronchioles to swell from the *inside*. As your passageways become narrower, it becomes increasingly difficult to breathe in and out.

2. **Constriction.** At the same time your passageways become inflamed, the muscles that circle the *outside* of your bronchioles become tighter. As they squeeze the bronchioles like a tight rubber band, your passageways become even narrower.

3. **Mucus production.** As the chemical assault continues, your lungs respond by making more mucus than usual. As it plugs up your already-narrow passageways, you develop wheezing, coughing, and chest tightness.

Many people with asthma find it more difficult to exhale than to inhale. That's because air gets trapped in obstructed airways. Even people with mild asthma can trap al-

Why Asthma Makes It Hard to Breathe

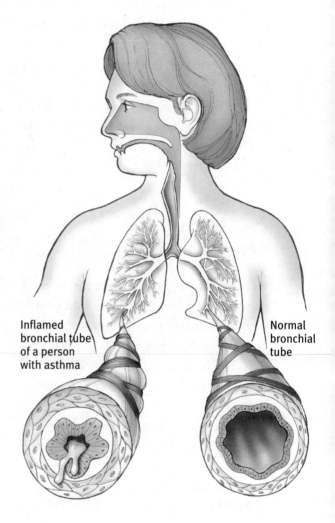

Inflamed bronchial tube of a person with asthma

Normal bronchial tube

Air enters the respiratory system from the nose and mouth and travels through the bronchial tubes. In a person with asthma, the muscles of the bronchial tubes tighten and thicken, and the air passages become inflamed and filled with mucus, making it difficult for air to move. In a person without asthma, the muscles around the bronchial tubes are relaxed and the tissue is thin, allowing for easy airflow.

most 2 liters of air—as much as in an empty 2-liter bottle.

Sometimes, asthma attacks subside within 30 to 90 minutes without treatment, only to reappear a few hours later. More often, though, they just get worse. Without proper treatment, an asthma attack can last for hours or even days.

This is the essence of life with asthma. When your asthma is out of control, you never know when the next attack will strike or how long it will last.

Clearing the Air of Asthma Myths

As if managing your symptoms weren't enough, you may have to deal with people who tell you that your symptoms are psychosomatic. You may be warned that prescription drugs are addictive, and you may be told to get by with an over-the-counter drug.

Such advice is outdated and dangerous since it can prevent you from seeking the care that can control your asthma.

So let's set the record straight.

Asthma is a real disease. Like diabetes and arthritis, asthma is a chronic *physical* illness, not an emotional one, although stress can make the symptoms worse and may sometimes even trigger them.

Asthma drugs aren't addictive. You can't get hooked on any of them. The fact that asthma symptoms return or worsen when medications are stopped reflects the benefits of the drugs, not a physical dependence like that seen with narcotics.

Over-the-counter asthma drugs aren't as effective as prescription medications. Nonprescription bronchodilators and tablets are less effective than prescription bronchodilators and may have serious side effects at low doses.

Fewer than one-third of pharmacists participating in a national survey even recommend such products. Although these drugs may make you feel better, they do not treat the underlying process that can cause potentially permanent injury to your lungs over time.

The sad truth is that asthma is a serious disease that demands serious attention. Consider these sobering statistics.

Asthma is widespread. Each year it affects more than 15 million Americans, including 5 million children.

Asthma is deadly. It results in 1.8 million emergency room visits, 500,000 hospitalizations, and more than 5,000 deaths every year.

Asthma is expensive. Each year it results in 9 million lost workdays and 10 million lost schooldays.

The annual cost to society is an estimated $14.5 billion.

And it's getting worse.

Some 22 million Americans will have asthma by the year 2010 if current trends continue, according to the Pew Environmental Health Commission and the Johns

Hopkins University School of Public Health in Baltimore.

That means asthma will strike 1 out of every 14 Americans and affect 1 out of every 5 families.

By 2020, some 29 million Americans will have asthma.

If you have asthma, you know how drastically it can affect every aspect of your life, including your psychological health. One study shows that nearly half of asthma patients have symptoms of depression. Another study shows that asthma seriously affects most patients' sex lives. Nearly 16 percent of the study participants reported moderate limitation in their sexual functioning. Another 19 percent reported that their disease prevents them from having sex at all.

Early Treatment Is Essential

Until the late 1980s, asthma was thought to be primarily a disease of congestion, so the goal of treatment was to open up clogged airways with bronchodilators. Gradually, however, researchers began to understand that the underlying cause of asthma is chronic inflammation. So in 1997, the National Heart, Lung, and Blood Institute issued updated guidelines that recommended early and aggressive use of anti-inflammatory drugs, especially inhaled corticosteroids.

"It is absolutely critical to intervene early in life, if possible, before you even become symptomatic," says Donald Leung, M.D., head of pediatric allergy and immunology at the National Jewish Medical and Research

Asthma Remedies through the Ages

Some of the remedies used to treat asthma throughout history are as odd as they are diverse. For example, ancient Greek doctors told asthma patients to wear bags around their necks containing a stinky root from a plant in the carrot family.

During the 19th century, American doctors actually encouraged patients to take up smoking. Among the "healing" substances that were rolled into cigarettes or stuffed into pipes: tobacco, nitrate powders, and jimsonweed, a plant containing a toxic alkaloid.

A century ago, patients also relied on "secret" asthma formulas, many of which contained alcohol, cocaine, and morphine.

Perhaps the most prescient of historic healers, however, was Moses Maimonides, a 12th-century rabbi and physician. His recommendations included striving for moderation in food, drink, sleep, and sexual activity; avoiding polluted city environments; and eating lots of chicken soup.

Center in Denver and editor of the *Journal of Allergy and Clinical Immunology.* "Once you become symptomatic, it's like the tip of an iceberg." Dr. Leung recommends visiting the allergist or pulmonary doctor for pulmonary function tests.

Since asthma is a highly variable disease, it's graded by four categories.

Mild intermittent. Symptoms occur less than two times a week, and nighttime symptoms occur less than two times a month. Flare-ups are brief, lasting from a few hours to a few days.

Mild persistent. Symptoms occur more than two times a week but less often than once a day. Nighttime symptoms occur more than two times a month. Flare-ups may affect daily activities.

Moderate persistent. Symptoms occur daily, and nighttime symptoms occur more than once a week. Flare-ups occur more than twice a week, may last for days, and may affect daily activities.

Severe persistent. Symptoms are continuous, limiting physical activity and interfering with normal activities.

Over time, uncontrolled asthma can cause a destructive condition called airway remodeling. Continued assaults by inflammatory chemicals cause the lung tissue to thicken and lose its ability to clear away the mucus. In some instances, these changes are irreversible.

In people without asthma, lung function peaks at about age 20, then gradually declines.

"People with asthma never reach that peak at age 20," Dr. Leung says. "After age 20, they actually have an accelerated decline in their lung function."

Famous People with Asthma

If you have asthma, you have something in common with many high achievers. Here's a list of famous people from various arenas who have had to deal with asthma.

- Entertainers: film director Martin Scorsese, rocker Alice Cooper, folk singer Judy Collins, actress-singer Liza Minnelli, symphony conductor/composer Leonard Bernstein, and actress Elizabeth Taylor
- Authors: John Updike, Charles Dickens, and Henry Ward Beecher
- Athletes: track star Jackie Joyner-Kersee, swimmers Kurt Grote and Amy Van Dyken, basketball player Dennis Rodman, football player Jerome "The Bus" Bettis, diver Greg Louganis, and baseball Hall-of-Famer Jim "Catfish" Hunter
- Politician: Calvin Coolidge, 30th president of the United States (since "Silent Cal" distrusted doctors, he relied on patent medicines and even closed himself off in a room filled with chlorine vapor in a futile attempt to relieve his asthma)

The worst form of asthma, status asthmaticus, results in a severe airflow obstruction that is life-threatening. About 1 percent of all asthma attacks are this severe. People with this condition cannot lie down or speak in more than monosyllables. They often die of respiratory failure.

Who Gets Asthma?

Like other allergic conditions, asthma is strongly influenced by heredity. If one of your parents has allergies or asthma, your odds of getting asthma are 25 percent. If both parents have allergies or asthma, your odds of getting asthma rise to 50 percent.

"There are probably more than 20 genes that are involved in allergy," Dr. Leung says.

But many environmental factors are involved, too. They include:

• Parental smoking. Infants who live with a mother who smokes are twice as likely to get asthma as those who have a nonsmoking mother. Living with a dad who smokes increases the risk even more.

• Premature birth. Preemies are four times more likely to develop asthma than full-term babies.

• Other allergies. About 80 percent of children who have asthma also have another allergic condition such as allergic rhinitis or eczema.

• Viral infections. Many young children develop asthma after a bout of a respiratory virus, especially the respiratory syncytial virus (RSV). Many adults experience worse asthma after a bout of bronchitis or pneumonia.

Other environmental factors that are believed to play a role in asthma include socioeconomic status, family size, and geography. Low income, small families, and urban living seem to raise the risk of asthma. On the other hand, if you were born and raised on a farm, you may have a lower risk.

• Age of Onset

About half of children with asthma display symptoms by age 4. About one-half to two-thirds of children with asthma eventually "outgrow" it. The other one-third, however, either stay the same or get worse. In addition, about 40 percent of children who outgrow asthma will have some symptom-free years then relapse and have asthma again, Dr. Wray says.

Age plays a strong role in the kind of asthma that people develop. People under age 50 tend to have allergic asthma. Their disease is caused by immune system reactions to well-defined allergy triggers such as pollen and mold. People over 50, on the other hand, tend to have nonallergic asthma. In many cases, the patient's history often reveals what is causing the asthma.

About 5 to 15 percent of asthma patients have what's called aspirin-sensitive asthma, which means that they are susceptible to attacks after taking aspirin and other nonsteroidal anti-inflammatory drugs (NSAIDs).

• **The Lifestyle Connection**

Although indoor exposure to dust mites, cockroaches, mice, and animal dander is associated with asthma, that alone cannot account for the astonishing rise in the number of asthma cases.

Researchers suspect that the real culprit might be recent changes in the so-called Western lifestyle. Among them: more time spent indoors with TVs, videos, and computers; poor nutrition; less exercise; and increasing obesity.

In children and adolescents, there's a stronger link between asthma and obesity among girls than among boys. In adults, obesity is considered a major risk factor for the development of asthma in both men and women.

Weight gain in adulthood is especially risky. One study found that nurses who gained more than 25 kilograms (about 55 pounds) since age 18 were almost five times as likely to develop asthma as nurses whose weight remained stable.

Obstructive sleep apnea is characterized by episodes in which breathing stops during sleep. It is a common consequence of obesity and is also strongly associated with adult-onset asthma.

Although anyone of any age can develop asthma, the disease is not an equal-opportunity offender. Statistics show that asthma may be linked to the following factors.

• Age. Of the more than 15 million Americans who have asthma, 10.5 million are under age 45. In 1992, the prevalence of asthma in Americans under age 18 was 6.1 percent, the highest of any age group.

• Gender. About 6 million U.S. women under age 45 suffer from asthma, compared to just 4.5 million U.S. men in the same age group. Statistics from 1992 reported that young men under age 18 had a high asthma prevalence of 7.2 percent, compared to young women in the same age group who had a prevalence of 5 percent.

• Geography. More Americans living in the Northeast (61.8 cases per 1,000 people) have had asthma than people in the Midwest (56.6 cases), South (51.8 cases), and West (52.9 cases).

• Income. Recent statistics report that households with an annual income between $10,000 and $20,000 have the highest number of asthma cases (80.5 cases per 1,000 people).

• Ethnic group. There are approximately 56.9 asthma cases per 1,000 for Whites under 45 years compared to 76.6 cases for Blacks in the same age group. A 1993 study also found that Black children and young adults are three to four times more likely than Whites to be hospitalized for asthma and are four to six times more likely to die of the disease.

What Are the Symptoms of Asthma?

If you think that wheezing is the most common asthma symptom, think again. It's coughing.

Asthma-related coughing can vary. It can be dry and nonproductive, but it also can be wet and very productive.

Many adults live in a state of denial about their coughing. They become so accustomed to it that they don't think of it as a problem, let alone as an asthma symptom. Here are three other telltale symptoms of asthma.

Wheezing. This is the familiar high-pitched whistling sound that results from air that is moving in and out of congested airways. Wheezing can range from a soft noise at the end of an exhalation to a loud rasp that occurs during inhalation and exhalation.

Note: If wheezing stops during the middle of an asthma attack, it's usually a sign that the airways are totally blocked. The person is typically in great distress and should be taken immediately to the emergency room.

Hyperventilation. Adults normally breathe 10 to 20 times a minute. To find out what's normal for you, count your breaths for a minute when your asthma is under good control. During an asthma attack, people typically breathe much faster than the normal rate.

Note: If breathing slows down during an asthma attack, it's usually a sign that the episode is severe and the person should be rushed to the emergency room.

Chest or neck tightness. Children with asthma often suck in their chests so deeply that their ribs show. In adults, such tightness more often involves the neck muscles. As they struggle to get more air into their lungs, their necks bulge. If this occurs, the person should see the doctor immediately or go to the emergency room.

How Is Asthma Diagnosed?

For such a common disease, asthma is tough to diagnose. Since asthma is similar to many other lung conditions, it's often misdiagnosed. In as many as 75 percent of men who have smoked, doctors initially diagnose asthma symptoms as chronic bronchitis or emphysema.

"Many doctors, especially those in primary care, do a poor job of diagnosing asthma," says Jay Portnoy, M.D., chief of allergy, asthma, and immunology at Children's Mercy Hospitals and Clinics in Kansas City, Missouri. "They call it bronchitis and prescribe antibiotics." For people who have asthma, this presents a double whammy: Their asthma doesn't improve, and they become susceptible to antibiotic-resistant germs.

"When you look at people who die from asthma, a lot of them were inadequately treated," Dr. Portnoy says.

Even when doctors know it's asthma, they sometimes say it's a chest cold, a wheezing problem, or RADS (reactive airways dysfunction syndrome, an airway sensitivity that often develops after inhaling an irritant chemical in toxic concentrations) in order to avoid worrying the patient. Although patients might be treated with asthma medications, such a hazy diagnosis is a disservice to them because it prevents them from seeking useful information about their disease. As a result, it's important to find a doctor who is knowledgeable about asthma and is not working under the false assumption that asthma is a disease that "dares not speak its name."

You should seek out a definitive diagnosis if you experience any of the following symptoms.

• Shortness of breath at any time of day or night
• Wheezing
• Coughing up phlegm, especially if it's discolored or blood-streaked
• Persistent cough
• Chest tightness or pain

In the doctor's office, an asthma workup usually consists of the following:

Medical history. You'll be asked if you've experienced respiratory symptoms before. Often, patients report that they've had frequent episodes of "bronchitis" since childhood. Asthma is a prime suspect if you've been diagnosed with bronchitis or pneumonia more than once in any given year. You'll also be asked if you experience respiratory symptoms during hay fever season, while exercising, or following vigorous outbursts of laughing or crying.

Masqueraders of Asthma

In adults, many nonasthmatic conditions can mimic the symptoms of asthma. That's why taking the time to get a proper diagnosis with a pulmonary function test is so essential.

The following is a list of medical conditions that share similar symptoms with asthma.

• Upper airway diseases: allergic rhinitis (hay fever) with associated cough, vocal cord dysfunction
• Large airways obstruction: enlarged lymph nodes or tumor, narrowing of the large airways (tracheal or bronchial stenosis), chronic obstructive pulmonary disease, chronic bronchitis
• Small airways obstruction: cystic fibrosis, heart disease, congestive heart failure, pulmonary infiltration with eosinophilia (coarse, round, granular cells), pulmonary embolism (blood clot)
• Other causes: recurrent cough not due to asthma, swallowing difficulties, gastro-esophageal reflux disease (GERD), cough caused by medications

Physical exam. Your doctor will listen to your breathing with a stethoscope. You may also undergo a chest x-ray or CAT scan to determine whether you have asthma or some other condition. If your doctor is really up to speed, he will screen you for allergic bronchopulmonary aspergillosis, a fungal infection that often accompanies asthma.

Lung function tests. Your doctor may ask you to blow into a spirometer, a device that measures forced expiratory volume (FEV). You'll perform the test before and after using an inhaled bronchodilator such as albuterol (Airet). If your FEV score is at least 12 percent better after using the bronchodilator, it's almost certain that you have asthma. If the results are inconclusive, you may be asked to take a methacholine (Provocholine) challenge test. In people with asthma, this substance causes wheezing. In people without asthma, it doesn't.

Allergen testing. Since allergies are closely associated with asthma, you may be asked to take a skin-prick test or blood test to see if you're allergic to pollen, dust mites, or other substances. If you can identify what triggers your asthma, you can take steps to avoid it. (For more information about allergy testing, see Hay Fever on page 307.)

• Differential Diagnosis #1: Occupational Asthma

Between 5 and 10 percent of American adults with asthma develop the disease from on-the-job exposure to allergens and irritants. Offending substances range from wood dusts (especially cedar and hardwoods) to accidental exposure to such gases as chlorine and sulfur dioxide to cereal grains and powders.

Here are other common triggers and the workers at highest risk of developing occupational asthma because of them.

• Animals/animal dander: farmers, veterinarians, laboratory personnel
• Shellfish: shellfish farmers and processors
• Wood and vegetable products: carpenters, woodworkers, grain handlers, bakers, food process workers, printers
• Enzymes: bakers, nurses, detergent-industry workers, pharmaceutical employees, plastics workers
• Amines: shellac, rubber, lacquer handlers; photographers; solderers; chemists; chemical manufacturers; fur dyers
• Anhydrides: paint, plastics, electronics, epoxy resin, chemical manufacturers
• Diisocyanates: polyurethane, plastics, varnish, foam, foundry, rubber manufacturers, spray painters
• Fluxes: electronics workers, metal joiners
• Latex: health care and rubber-industry workers
• Metals and metal salts: hard metal, electroplating workers; printers; tanners; diamond polishers; platinum refiners; hard-metal grinders; solderers; locksmiths
• Other chemicals: chemical, reactive dye, resin, glove manufacturers; meat wrappers; chemical packagers; refrigeration, textile industry, health care workers; hairdressers

For more information about occupational asthma, see The Allergy-Free Workplace on page 111.

• Differential Diagnosis #2: Exercise-Induced Asthma

Some 80 to 90 percent of people with chronic asthma have exercise-induced asthma. But people with asthma aren't the only ones who get exercise-induced asthma. While about 7 percent of Americans have asthma, an estimated 11 percent of Americans have exercise-induced asthma. That means 4 percent of Americans experience asthma *only* when they exercise.

If you have this problem, you experience wheezing, chest tightness, coughing, or chest pain within 5 to 20 minutes after commencing vigorous exercise. You're especially likely to develop such symptoms when you exercise in cold, dry air.

Exercise-induced asthma is diagnosed by medical history and breathing tests to ensure that the problem isn't chronic asthma. Fortunately, most exercise-induced asthma can be easily prevented.

Although exercise can be problematic for anyone with asthma, doctors emphatically say it's the one asthma trigger you *should not* avoid.

"If you exercise regularly and get in good cardiovascular shape, you're going to have a lot more tolerance to things in the environment and just do better in general," says James Sublett, M.D., national medical director of Vivra Asthma and Allergy, a network of clinics headquartered in Louisville.

Prevention strategies and medical treatments for exercise-induced asthma are described in this chapter. (For more information about the best ways to exercise if you have asthma, see The Allergy-Free Exercise Plan on page 159.)

• Differential Diagnosis #3: Cough-Variant Asthma

In some people with asthma, cough is the only symptom. They don't wheeze, they have normal lung function tests, and their peak-flow scores don't improve after using a bronchodilator.

So what's the problem? They still have underlying inflammation that's damaging their lungs.

Most people with cough-variant asthma have short, high-pitched, nonproductive coughs. Others, however, have low-pitched, productive coughs. Many patients cough several times a minute, which prevents them from getting a good night's sleep.

Treatment with inhaled or oral corticosteroids usually clears up the underlying inflammation and stops the cough.

• Differential Diagnosis #4: Chronic Asthmatic Bronchitis

Sometimes, asthma and bronchitis coexist in a nasty condition called chronic asthmatic bronchitis.

THE HIDDEN CONNECTION

Uncommon Asthma Triggers

Sometimes an asthma attack can be set off by an unlikely trigger. Most people know that, for example, dust mites can cause problems, but did you know that irritants such as the sulfites in salad dressings and dried fruits can trigger an attack?

Following is a list of some little-known asthma triggers.

- Perfumes, scented soaps, and deodorants
- Food additives, especially sulfites or metabisulfite preservatives used in wine, beer, juices, salad dressings, and dried fruits
- Mice
- Pine resin from Christmas trees
- Goose droppings
- Lady beetles
- Cocaine and heroin
- Hormone-replacement therapy. (Postmenopausal women typically have a lower risk of asthma, but the landmark Nurses' Health Study shows that estrogen-only *and* estrogen-progestin formulas increase the risk of asthma.)

It most commonly affects people who are middle-aged or older and who have a long history of cigarette smoking. Symptoms include the wheezing and shortness of breath typical of asthma and the coughing spells and thick-mucus production typical of bronchitis.

People with chronic asthmatic bronchitis are at higher risk of developing more serious lung diseases and infections as well as cardiovascular problems.

In addition to standard asthma medications, treatments include smoking cessation, decongestants, and, in severe cases, supplemental oxygen.

What Triggers Asthma?

Fighting asthma might seem overwhelming when you consider that the place where you spend 90 percent of your time—indoors—contains more than 2,000 possible asthma triggers.

Yet the task isn't quite as daunting as it may seem. Despite the huge number of *possible* triggers, some people with asthma react only to one or a few allergic triggers, such as dust mites that lurk in bedding. In fact, many researchers believe that dust mites, which like the Western lifestyle as much as we do, are a *major* asthma trigger. As evidence, they point to research showing that previous mite-free New Guinea experienced an increase of asthma cases after the introduction of mite-infested Western blankets.

Unfortunately, people who have asthma also can respond to a multitude of nonallergic irritants such as the sulfites in wine and beer.

Harold Nelson, M.D., senior staff physician at the National Jewish Medical and Research Center in Denver, attributes this to the innate "twitchiness" of asthma patients' lungs. "The problem with sulfites is that they break down into sulfur dioxide," he says. "The twitchier that people's lungs are, the more apt they are to respond to sulfur dioxide."

But there's no predicting who will respond to what. "Asthmatics vary in their response to irritants," Dr. Nelson says.

Here are some of the most common allergic and nonallergic triggers that can set off an asthma attack: respiratory tract infections including viral head colds and acute bronchitis; dust mites; pollens from trees, grasses, and weeds; animal dander from furry pets; feathers from pet birds; insect parts from cockroaches and some flies; foods such as shellfish, peanuts, and cow's milk; molds; cigarette smoke; fireplace smoke, woodstove smoke, and kerosene-heater smoke.

Also included in the list of triggers are sleep (in people with asthma, the nighttime airway narrowing that most people experience is exaggerated); household irritants such as car exhaust, paints, cleaning solvents, bleaches, detergents, furniture polish, and insecticides; exercise; crying, laughing, or yelling (which may trigger a form of ex-

The Trouble with Fragrances

Comedians have gotten lots of laughs out of the notion of "fragrance-free zones." But if you're one of the many people who react to perfumes, colognes, and hair sprays, a fragrance-free zone probably sounds like heaven.

If your perfume-wearing friends have ever accused you of being a hypochondriac, here's proof that your symptoms aren't all in your head:

When researchers at the Tulane University Medical Center in New Orleans studied 77 people with asthma in a laboratory setting, they found that 38 different fragrances caused reactions. The top 6 were Red, White Diamonds, Giorgio, Charlie, Opium, and Poison.

ercise-induced asthma); cold air; weather changes such as fog and smog; and cooking odors.

Allergy to food proteins also can cause an asthma attack. One study shows that people with asthma who react to dust mites and cockroaches also react to shrimp.

Conventional Medical Treatment Is Essential

As much as we'd like to recommend an all-natural regimen for asthma treatment, that would be irresponsible. Asthma is such a serious disease that not even the most alternative-minded doctors recommend switching from a conventional action plan to an exclusively alternative one.

Although they believe that natural interventions in diet, nutrition, and stress reduction can make a huge difference in your quality of life, doctors who practice alternative medicine say that such interventions should *complement* but not replace conventional care.

Many conventionally trained doctors discourage the use of herbs as a primary treatment. Some, however, such as Robert Rountree, M.D., a holistic physician in Boulder, Colorado, and coauthor of *Immunotics*, do use herbs to treat their asthma patients. But Dr. Rountree is quite selective about it. "I use alternative medicine as a complement to conventional therapies in almost all of my patients with asthma. If at all possible, I try to get patients

off chronic medications. But if a patient has moderate to severe asthma, I use conventional medication as the primary approach and then use herbs and vitamins to keep the drug dosage as low as possible and to minimize the drug side effects," he explains.

When patients need daily medication to control their asthma, Dr. Rountree recommends placing them on a conventional medication such as salmeterol (Serevent), rather than a potentially risky herb such as ephedra. "Serevent is a great drug," Dr. Rountree says. "If you have a chronic problem that's really socked in, what's wrong with the drugs?"

In fact, it should be noted that today's asthma drugs are more safe and effective than they were a generation ago. "Patients have never had as many therapeutic choices," says Robert Nathan, M.D., associate clinical professor of medicine at the University of Colorado Health Sciences Center in Denver and an allergy practitioner in Colorado Springs. "There's been an explosion in the number of drugs used to treat allergies and asthma."

Evidence shows that these drugs save lives. Consider what happened in Israel between 1991 and 1995. As sales of inhaled corticosteroids went up, asthma deaths went down, bucking a trend found in most other Westernized countries.

Conversely, exclusive reliance on self-treatments can be life-threatening. A study published in the *Journal of Allergy and Clinical Immunology* found that adults who treated their asthma with herbal remedies were 2½ times as likely as adults using conventional treatments to end up in a hospital. Adults who treated their asthma with coffee or black tea fared even worse. They were nearly 3 times as likely to be hospitalized.

The Integrated Approach

While you should never rely solely on natural remedies to treat your asthma, that doesn't mean your only recourse is to follow a conventional drug regimen. There are dozens of additional things that you can do—ranging from dietary changes to stress reduction—that can improve your asthma, reduce your reliance on conventional drugs, and make you feel better. "I've been treating asthma for 20 years with natural remedies," Dr. Rountree says. "Most of my patients do quite well with this approach."

Remember, you don't have to be a slave to your asthma. With proper management, you can break those bonds and enjoy a life of asthma *freedom*. That means:

• No major or minor symptoms, including wheezing, coughing, shortness of breath, and chest tightness

• Sleeping through the night without symptoms

• No more sick days from work or school because of asthma

• Full participation in physical activities

• Little or no side effects from asthma medicine

Working with Your Doctor

If this is the first time that you've consulted a doctor about your asthma, you need to work with him to establish a written action plan. Since asthma is such a variable disease, such plans vary from patient to patient. But every plan should include a list of your asthma triggers and ways to avoid them, a schedule for taking the medications that control inflammation and prevent asthma attacks, and detailed instructions on what to do when you experience symptoms. Most important, your doctor will give you step-by-step instructions on what to do during an emergency.

Here are the questions that you'll need to answer in order to develop an effective emergency plan.

• What are the signs that tell you to seek care quickly?

• What should you do if your medicines don't seem to be working?

• Where should you go to get care quickly?

• Should you call your doctor first or go to the emergency room?

• What should you do if you have an asthma emergency very late at night?

Before every doctor visit, you need to determine whether or not your asthma is under control. Write down any questions or concerns you have, including any that seem trivial. In order to fine-tune your action plan, your doctor will need as much information as possible.

To get the greatest benefit from your action plan, you will need to learn to identify the early warning signs of an oncoming asthma attack. Check the following list for the three warning signs you experience most often before an attack. When you experience them in the future, follow your asthma action plan.

- A drop in your peak-flow reading
- Chronic cough, especially at night
- Difficult or fast breathing
- Chest tightness or discomfort
- Becoming short of breath more easily than usual
- Itchy, scratchy, or sore throat
- A tendency to rub or stroke your throat
- Fatigue
- Sneezing
- Runny nose
- Feeling that your head is stopped up
- Headache
- Fever
- Restlessness

Is Your Asthma Under Control?

Answer yes or no to the following questions. Do this just before each doctor's visit.

In the past 2 weeks . . .

1. Have you coughed, wheezed, felt short of breath, or had chest tightness . . .
   During the day? Y N
   At night, causing you to wake up? Y N
   During or soon after exercise? Y N
2. Have you needed more quick-relief medicine than usual? Y N
3. Has your asthma kept you from doing anything you wanted to do? Y N
   If yes, what was it? _____
4. Have your asthma medicines caused you any problems, like shakiness, sore throat, or upset stomach? Y N

In the past few months . . .

5. Have you missed work or school because of your asthma? Y N
6. Have you gone to the emergency room or the hospital because of your asthma? Y N

What Your Answers Mean

All "no" answers: Your asthma is under control.

One or more "yes" answers: Your action plan needs adjustment.

- Itchy, watery, or glassy eyes
- A change of color in your face
- Dark circles under your eyes

Conventional Asthma Treatments

Conventional doctors can choose from a wide array of treatment options to help their patients with asthma. Some of these options include the avoidance of allergy triggers, the use of a peak-flow meter to monitor lung capacity, and various prescription drugs.

• Environmental Control

Most doctors—conventional and alternative—recommend that people with asthma clean up their "nests," starting with the bedroom. That means eliminating or reducing the following allergy triggers: animal dander, dust mites, cockroaches, pollen and outdoor mold, indoor mold, tobacco smoke, and indoor/outdoor pollutants and irritants. (For specific remediation advice, see The Allergy-Free Home on page 73.)

Since many people with asthma are sensitive to weather changes, pollen, and pollution, doctors advise them to check the weather forecast, pollen count, and smog index, and refrain from outdoor activity when conditions are likely to cause asthma attacks.

Indoors, try to maintain a constant temperature and humidity. When pollen, smog, and outdoor humidity are high, keep windows closed and run the air conditioner while inside the house or in the car.

Doctors also recommend aggressive steps to control other causes of asthma.

Allergic rhinitis. Standard treatments include intranasal corticosteroids, oral non-sedating antihistamines, and antihistamine-decongestant combinations. (For more information, see Hay Fever on page 307.)

Rhinosinusitis. You may need medical measures to promote drainage. (For more information, see Sinusitis on page 381.)

Respiratory infections. Viral respiratory infections are the most common cause of asthma symptoms. As a result, all patients with persistent asthma are advised to get annual flu shots unless they have a severe systemic sensitivity to eggs.

Gastroesophageal reflux disease (GERD). Avoid eating or drinking anything 3 hours before going to bed. Avoid caffeine, alcohol, and chocolate. Elevate the head of your bed 6 to 8 inches. Drug therapy may be necessary.

Obstructive sleep apnea. Consider weight reduction. Use a nasal continuous positive airway pressure (CPAP) machine during sleep. The machine is helpful because it forces air across the barrier created by the back of the tongue that blocks the airway. Research shows that nasal CPAP machines improve lung function in people with asthma and sleep disorders. CPAP machines are available through a doctor's prescription at most medical supply stores.

Aspirin sensitivity. Avoid aspirin, and know the risks of using other nonsteroidal anti-inflammatory drugs. Recent research shows that some patients improve with oral aspirin desensitization.

Sulfite sensitivity. Avoid foods processed with sulfites, including processed potatoes, dried fruit, shrimp, wine, and beer.

Beta-blockers. Avoid using these drugs in any form, including eyedrops. Consider alternative drugs such as acetazolamide (Diamox) and pilocarpine (Salagen).

• Peak-Flow Meters

A peak-flow meter is an inexpensive plastic device that measures your lung capacity. For many patients, it's an essential tool for managing their asthma more effectively at home.

No matter what kind of asthma you have, a peak-flow meter gives you an objective warning of an impending attack. This is especially important if you're one of the many people with asthma who brush off early symptoms as "nothing important." By using a peak-flow meter, you give yourself a window of opportunity to stop an asthma attack before it becomes serious.

First, you must determine your personal best peak-flow number. Here's how.

Measure your peak flow each day for 2 to 3 weeks during a period when your asthma is under good control.

1. Move the marker to the bottom of the scale, stand or sit up straight, and take a deep breath. Hold your breath while you place the mouthpiece in your mouth, between your teeth. Blow out as hard and fast as you can and write down the number you get.

2. Take a daily measurement between noon and 2:00 P.M. Also measure yourself immediately after using a quick-relief medication or at any other time your doctor suggests. Write down every number.

3. Your personal best is the highest peak-flow number you had during the 2 to 3 weeks.

Next, calculate your peak-flow zones, which correspond to the colors of a traffic light.

Green zone. Meaning that you're at 80 to 100 percent of your personal best, this zone signals good control. Take your usual daily long-term control medicines, if any. Keep taking these medicines even when you are in the yellow or red zones.

Yellow zone. At this level, you're performing 50 to 70 percent of your personal best, signaling caution: Your asthma is getting worse. Add quick-relief medicines such as short-acting beta$_2$-agonists. You might need to increase other medicines as directed by your doctor.

Red zone. When you're in this zone, you're performing below 50 percent of your personal best. This signals a medical alert. Add or increase quick-relief medicines and call your doctor immediately.

Once you know your peak-flow zones, make peak-flow monitoring part of your daily routine. Take your score every

(continued on page 242)

The Ups and Downs of Asthma Medications

Following is a list of the medications most commonly prescribed for asthma and their benefits and drawbacks. If you have concerns about any drugs that you are taking for your asthma after studying this chart, discuss them with your doctor.

In addition, many new asthma medications are expected to be introduced within

Class of Allergy Drug	Example of Drug	Benefits
Inhaled corticosteroids	Fluticasone (Flovent)	Most potent and effective long-term, anti-inflammatory medications currently available. They improve symptoms and pulmonary function, reduce the need for quick-relief medications, and have fewer side effects than oral corticosteroids.
Anti-inflammatory inhalants	Cromolyn (Intal)	A nonsteroidal alternative to low doses of inhaled corticosteroids, especially in the treatment of mild persistent asthma. They improve symptoms and pulmonary function, reduce the need for quick-relief medications, and have a good safety profile. They also can be used on an as-needed basis to prevent symptoms caused by expected exposure to allergens, cold air, and exercise.
Leukotriene modifiers	Zafirlukast (Accolate)	Improve symptoms and pulmonary function and reduce the need for quick-relief medications. May be considered as an alternative therapy to low doses of inhaled corticosteroids in mild persistent asthma, but their exact role in therapy has yet to be determined
Short-acting beta$_2$-agonists	Albuterol (Airet)	Relaxes bronchial smooth muscle, usually opening up airways within 5 to 10 minutes. Therapy of choice for relieving acute symptoms and preventing exercise-induced asthma
Long-acting beta$_2$-agonists	Salmeterol (Serevent)	Relax bronchial smooth muscle, reduce need for quick-relief medication, help prevent exercise-induced asthma. Often used with inhaled corticosteroids to control symptoms, especially nighttime symptoms
Bronchodilators	Theophylline (Accurbron)	An alternative but not preferred stand-alone therapy for persistent asthma. Can control nighttime symptoms
Oral corticosteroids	Prednisone (Deltasone)	Broad, anti-inflammatory effects
Anticholinergics	Ipratropium (Atrovent)	Alternative for those who cannot tolerate the effects of beta$_2$-agonists. Treatment of choice for asthma in patients receiving beta-blockers

the next decade. Among the most promising are drugs that block production of the allergy antibody immunoglobulin E (IgE). These drugs may have to be taken indefinitely and could be very expensive. A study of one such drug, Xolair, showed that it helped people with asthma decrease or discontinue their use of corticosteroids.

Drawbacks

Local reactions include cough, loss of voice, and oral thrush (candidiasis). Long-term risks include osteoporosis, especially in postmenopausal women, and increased intraocular pressure and cataracts in older adults. To counteract these effects, people are often instructed to take supplemental calcium and vitamin D or go on hormone-replacement therapy. Adrenal suppression can affect patients who take high doses. Although some studies have found that inhaled corticosteroids suppress growth in children, at least one study has found that they do not affect children's final adult height.

May provide an added benefit to inhaled corticosteroids

Depending on the drug, risks include elevated liver enzymes, poor absorption when taken with food, and adverse interactions with other drugs, especially theophylline (Accurbron) and warfarin (Coumadin). In rare instances, these drugs are associated with Churg-Strauss syndrome.

In adults, the most common side effects are rapid heartbeat, jitteriness, shaky hands, and restlessness. These can be especially pronounced in older patients with ischemic heart disease.

Should not be used to treat acute symptoms. In some patients, continuous therapy becomes less effective.

Absorption varies depending on age, diet, and usage of other medications. Side effects include nausea, insomnia, hyperactivity, cardiovascular effects, tremors. Theophylline (Accurbron) can adversely react with oral contraceptives, antibiotics including ciprofloxacin (Cipro) and erythromycin (E-Mycin), H2-antagonists including cimetidine (Tagamet), and epinephrine (EpiPen) and may also exacerbate underlying heart conditions.

Because of their poor safety profile, they're considered treatments of last resort. Among their many adverse effects are confusion, agitation, and changes in glucose metabolism. *Note:* If you take these drugs for more than 10 days, you'll need to go off them gradually. Stopping them all at once can be life-threatening.

Adverse effects include headache, dizziness, nervousness, dry mouth, and cough.

morning when you wake up *before* taking any asthma medications. Also take your score during an asthma attack and after taking medication for an asthma attack. This can tell you how well your medication is working. Finally, if you use two different peak-flow meters (for example, if you have one for home and another for work), make sure that they're the same brand.

To measure your progress, keep a peak-flow diary. Your doctor should be able to provide you with one. The diary should contain blanks for you to fill in the following information.

• Your peak-flow scores
• A checklist of asthma medicines you've taken
• A record of triggers and symptoms
• Any other pertinent information

When you go to see the doctor, always bring your peak-flow meter and peak-flow diary.

• Pharmacotherapy

"With aggressive care, we can control asthma very well," says Martha White, M.D., director of research at the Institute for Asthma and Allergy in Washington, D.C. "It's not the slightest bit uncommon for us to see a patient who has a history of going to the emergency room three or four times a year. When you put them on a good asthma-management program, however, the emergency room becomes a thing of the past."

The gold-standard treatment, Dr. White says, is inhaled corticosteroids. That's be-

cause they have proven to be the single most effective drug in controlling the underlying cause of asthma: inflammation. (Because many side effects are associated with oral corticosteroids, doctors usually prescribe them as a last resort.)

Note: These drugs are *not* the same as the anabolic steroids that are used by some athletes to build muscle. In fact, they were first derived from extracts of animal adrenal glands.

Although inhaled corticosteroids have the potential to cause side effects, they're considered safe at recommended dosages, says Dr. White.

To be effective, they must be used every day, and they must be used properly.

Since they don't provide immediate relief, however, patients often stop taking them. Studies show that the dismal adherence rate—less than 50 percent—may be at least partly responsible for the epidemic of asthma deaths. "The problem is that most people continue to treat allergic diseases episodically," Dr. Nathan says. "They start to feel better, stop taking their drugs, and only start them again when the symptoms reach a certain level."

In mild cases of asthma, nonsteroidal drugs such as cromolyn and nedocromil can be used to control inflammation. Cromolyn is derived from the herb khellin, which comes from a Mediterranean plant. Some alternative-minded doctors prefer cromolyn over inhaled corticosteroids because it has almost no side effects. "For allergic asthma, one of the safest and best drugs is inhaled cromolyn (Intal)," says Andrew Weil, M.D., director of the program in integrative medicine and clinical professor of medicine at the University of Arizona College of Medicine in Tucson. To open up clogged airways, doctors also commonly prescribe bronchodilators—usually beta$_2$-agonists. These are available in two forms: short-acting (to treat asthma attacks) and long-acting (to prevent asthma attacks).

Since it's most effective to direct the medication to the scene of the crime—your lungs—most of today's asthma drugs are delivered by inhalation. Exceptions are leukotriene modifiers, anticholinergics, theophylline (Accurbron), and oral corticosteroids.

Recommended drug interventions depend on the severity of your asthma.

Mild intermittent. No daily medication needed. If you use a quick-relief bronchodilator more than twice a week, however, you may need to start long-term control therapy.

Mild persistent. You may be prescribed one daily long-term control medication.

Moderate persistent. Inhaled corticosteroids, with or without additional long-term control medications, may be prescribed to you.

Severe persistent. You may take multiple long-term control medications, including high-dose inhaled corticosteroids and, if needed, oral corticosteroids.

Finally, know that just because you've been prescribed a daily drug regimen, that doesn't necessarily mean you have to stay on it for life.

If your asthma has been well-controlled for 2 to 3 months, you can—under your doctor's supervision—gradually decrease the dose, frequency, or number of medications you take. After another 2 to 3 months, you should return to your doctor for a reevaluation.

If you're using inhaled corticosteroids, some doctors suggest reducing the dose by 25 percent every 2 to 3 months to determine the lowest dose required to control symptoms.

Note: If you have persistent asthma, you'll probably need to stay on medication to suppress the underlying inflammation and prevent airway remodeling.

• Inhalation Devices

Inhalation devices are the most efficient way to deliver asthma medication directly to your lungs. They come in several different varieties.

Metered-dose inhaler (MDI). Designed for adults, MDI's deliver beta$_2$-agonists, corticosteroids, cromolyn, nedocromil, and anticholinergics. They consist of a metal canister, which is placed in a plastic housing. When the canister is depressed, the medicine sprays from the housing's mouthpiece.

MDI with spacer/holding chamber. Designed for people age 5 and above, it's easier to use than a standard MDI and less likely to misdirect the spray onto your face. Since it lowers the risk of thrush and other side effects, it's recommended for all patients who use inhaled corticosteroids. Children under age 5 usually use it with a face mask.

Breath-actuated MDI. This device is designed for people age 12 and above who have difficulty triggering a puff while inhaling.

Dry-powder inhaler (DPI). Designed for people age 4 and above, it releases a fine powder into your lungs as you inhale. The advantage is that it gets the medicine where

Use Your Inhaler Correctly

The most efficient way to get asthma medication into your lungs is with an inhaler. If you haven't used one before, though, it's important that you familiarize yourself with the technique *before* an emergency situation arises. First, take off the cap and shake the inhaler. Breathe out all the way. Hold your inhaler the way your doctor recommended (see illustrations A, B, and C).

As you start breathing in slowly through your mouth, press down on the inhaler one time. (If you use a holding chamber, first press down on the inhaler. Within 5 seconds, begin to breathe in slowly.) Keep breathing in slowly as deeply as you can. Hold your breath as you count to 10 slowly. For inhaled quick-relief medicine (beta$_2$-agonists), wait about 1 minute between puffs. There is no need to wait between puffs for other medicines.

A

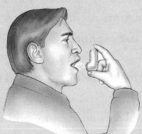

One way your doctor may have suggested you use your inhaler is to hold it 1 to 2 inches in front of your mouth (about the width of two fingers). Push down on the canister and inhale the medication.

B

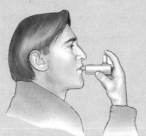

A second way your doctor may have told you to use your inhaler is with a spacer. These come in many shapes.

C

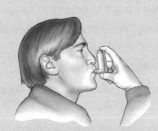

The third way your doctor may have told you to use your inhaler is to put it in your mouth. Do not do this with steroids.

it belongs—your lungs. The disadvantage is that it takes effort.

Nebulizer. Designed for people of any age who cannot use an MDI with a spacer/holding chamber, this machine delivers an ultrafine mist containing $beta_2$-agonists, cromolyn, or anticholinergics. Nebulizers are especially useful for infants, young children, elderly patients, and anyone in the midst of a moderate to severe attack.

If you're prescribed an inhalation device, you want to get the biggest possible benefit out of the lowest possible dose. To do that, proper technique is essential.

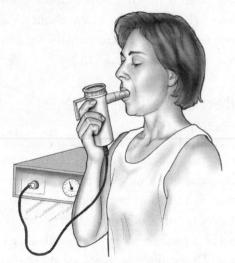

Compression nebulizers are machines that provide a mist containing $beta_2$-agonists, cromolyn, or anticholinergics. They're helpful for anyone who can't use a metered-dose inhaler with a spacer, such as infants, young children, and elderly patients.

Make it a routine. Take your medicine at the same time that you do some other daily activity, such as when you eat a meal or brush your teeth. Tape a written reminder to your refrigerator or bathroom mirror.

Don't leave home without it. Your quick-relief bronchodilator, that is. If you experience symptoms away from home, it can spare you lots of misery—or even save your life.

Do leave your other inhalers at home. Many people with asthma get into trouble because they mix up their quick-relief medications with their long-term controller medications. To avoid confusion, keep your inhaled corticosteroids, long-acting $beta_2$-agonists, and other medications in a place that'll remind you to use them twice a day, such as next to your toothbrush.

Easy does it. Overuse of bronchodilator drugs increases the risk of toxic drug levels, irregular heartbeat, and seizures. The maximum daily use of a bronchodilator is two puffs every 4 to 6 hours. If you need to use one more frequently, see your doctor. You may need a more effective medication.

Gargle to prevent side effects. After using an inhaled corticosteroid, gargle with water to wash away the medicine and prevent mouth irritations and oral yeast infections (thrush).

Keep it clean. If you see any powder where the medicine sprays out, it's time to clean the housing. Remove the metal canister, then rinse the mouthpiece and cap with warm water. Let them dry overnight.

Know when to replace the canister. Calculate the life span of each canister by dividing the number of puffs it contains by the number of puffs you take each day. For example, if it contains 200 puffs and you take 8 per day, it should last 25 days. Write the replacement date on your canister.

• Strategies for Preventing Exercise-Induced Asthma

Since most people with asthma develop symptoms from vigorous exercise, conventional doctors recommend the following interventions. Check with your doctor to see which of these might be right for you.

Short-acting beta$_2$-agonists. Take two to four puffs no more than 30 minutes before exercise, or use as directed by your doctor. If possible, use the inhaler immediately before exercise. It prevents symptoms for 2 to 3 hours.

Cromolyn or nedocromil. Take two to four puffs no more than 30 minutes before exercise, or use as directed by your doctor. If possible, use immediately before exercise. It prevents symptoms for 1 to 2 hours.

Long-acting beta$_2$-agonists. Take two puffs from a metered-dose inhaler or one puff from a dry-powder inhaler at least 30 minutes before exercise or use as directed by your doctor. It prevents symptoms for 10 to 12 hours.

Leukotriene modifiers. Take a pill at least 2 hours before exercise, or use as directed by your doctor. It prevents symptoms for up to 24 hours.

• Immunotherapy

Allergy shots can help relieve your asthma if you fall into any of these categories:

• You need to use asthma medications only during certain seasons of the year and have a demonstrated pollen allergy.

• You have asthma year-round and have a demonstrated allergy to dust mites.

• Your asthma medications are either ineffective or cause too many side effects.

• Your asthma is caused by a pet that you are not willing to give away.

• You have difficult-to-control asthma and allergic rhinitis that leave you feeling unwell most days.

Note: If conventional allergy shots don't work, you can try the various immunotherapies offered by environmental-medicine doctors. (For more information about these therapies, see The Environmental-Medicine View of Allergies on page 33.)

Alternative/Self-Help Treatments

After the federally funded Center for Complementary and Alternative Medicine Research in Asthma began operations at the University of California, Davis, its researchers took on a big homework assignment: Determine the scope of alternative asthma treatments in the United States and identify the ones with the most promise so they can be studied in depth.

Hoping to find sympathetic and knowledgeable health care professionals experienced in using alternative methods, the researchers surveyed subscribers to the respected, peer-reviewed journal *Alternative*

Therapies in Health and Medicine. Their only caveat: Participants had to be actively treating patients with asthma.

They received 564 responses from the following groups.

- Medical doctors: 37 percent
- Alternative/complementary practitioners with doctoral degrees: 27 percent
- Registered nurses: 11 percent
- Acupuncturists: 4 percent
- Unspecified: 18 percent

When asked to rank alternative asthma therapies, the M.D.'s and non-M.D.'s came up with nearly identical Top Nine lists. Here are the therapies that *both* groups rated as most useful.

- Diet
- Environmental control
- Nutritional supplements
- Homeopathy

The Pros and Cons of Steam Inhalation

Since asthma symptoms often improve in a warm, moist environment, such as a swimming pool, you'd think that steam inhalation would make an ideal, natural remedy.

Not necessarily.

For some people with asthma, steam itself is an asthma trigger.

Other people are allergic to the essential oils that are often used for steam inhalation, such as eucalyptus, peppermint, tea tree, rosemary, sage, lemon, and lime essential oils, says Robert Rountree, M.D., a holistic physician in Boulder, Colorado, and coauthor of *Immunotics*.

"If you're not sensitive to those oils, however, they're great," says Dr. Rountree. "They really open you up. Steam vapor inhalation is especially good if you have a lot of thick mucus."

The easiest method is to boil a pot of water, turn off the heat, carefully remove the pan from the stove, drape a towel over your head to keep the vapor in, lean your head forward, and inhale deeply. Just be sure to stay far enough away from the water to avoid burning yourself. Commercially made steamers—some including face masks— are also available from appliance manufacturers such as Remington.

If the essential oils listed above don't do the trick, remember what Mom used to do and add a dollop of Vicks VapoRub to the solution.

To get the moisturizing benefits of steam without the heat, try using a nebulizer and adding a few drops of the essential oils listed above.

"This super-moisturizing mist helps break up the mucus plugs clogging your small airways," Dr. Rountree explains.

- Herbs
- Meditation/prayer
- Mind-body therapy
- Acupuncture
- Detoxification

Since the survey was conducted, the Center for Complementary and Alternative Medicine Research in Asthma has fine-tuned this list. But it still ranks dietary changes, nutritional supplements, and other natural strategies very near the top.

• Lung-Friendly Foods

The next time you sit down to eat dinner, take a second look at what you have on your plate. What you eat can make a big difference in your asthma symptoms. Read on to learn how to eat for better health.

Load up on antioxidant-rich foods. These include dark green, dark yellow, and orange vegetables and fruits, all of which are packed with beta-carotene. They also include selenium-rich fish, lean meat, cereals, and Brazil nuts. When Cornell University researchers studied people with above-average and below-average levels of these antioxidants, they found that the difference in lung function was comparable to the difference between people approximately 4 years apart in age. The design of this study does not prove that consuming more antioxidants would improve lung function, but the results suggest this possibility, which needs to be confirmed in a different kind of study.

Eat an apple a day. When British researchers studied 2,512 middle-aged Welshmen, they found that those who ate at least five apples a week had significantly better lung function than those who ate no apples at all. Researchers theorize that apples are protective—in women as well as men—because they contain high amounts of antioxidants.

Increase intake of "E-foods." Eating foods rich in vitamin E not only improves your antioxidant status but also actually lowers your blood level of the allergy antibody immunoglobin E (IgE), according to a British study of 2,600 adults. The benefits level off at 7 milligrams of vitamin E, about the same amount contained in 1 ounce of dried sunflower seeds. Other good natural sources of vitamin E include vegetable oils, wheat germ, whole cereal grains, fruits, green vegetables, meat, and eggs.

Eat more yogurt. Preliminary research at the University of California, Davis, found that daily consumption of 450 grams of yogurt, almost 2 cups, with live cultures results in a fivefold increase in interferon-gamma. This is important, since interferon-gamma blocks production of IgE.

Drink some coffee. Caffeine belongs to the methylxanthine family of chemicals that help relax smooth muscles in the bronchial tubes. In one large study, adults with asthma who drank two to three cups of coffee daily had 25 percent fewer attacks than non–coffee drinkers. Try this only if you have mild intermittent asthma and have normal pulmonary function tests.

Note: Avoid excessive coffee consumption if you're already using antiasthma drugs or stimulant medications. Check with your doctor or pharmacist to make sure that the amount recommended above is okay for you.

Go fish. Omega-3 fatty acids in fish appear to have an anti-inflammatory effect. Australian researchers have found a lower prevalence of asthma in children who eat lots of fresh, oily fish, while U.S. researchers have found that regular consumption of fish actually improves lung function.

Visit the water cooler. Dehydration probably can trigger or worsen asthma and increase your risk of respiratory infections. Conversely, proper hydration has been shown to lessen exercise-induced asthma. Keep in mind that you can double your benefits by "eating" your water in the form of water-rich fruits and vegetables. An apple and a tomato each contain about 4 ounces of water.

Here's an easy way to calculate the minimum amount of water you need each day: Multiply your weight by 0.04, then multiply the result by 2 to determine the recommended number of cups. (For example, if you weigh 150 pounds, you should get 12 cups a day from all sources.) Generally, the rule of thumb is to drink 8 to 9 cups of water as fluid. Water, milk, juice, decaf coffee and tea, and herbal tea all count toward your fluid quotient.

Make olive oil your favored fat. Polyunsaturated vegetable oils, margarine, and vegetable shortening are all pro-inflammatory. Extra-virgin olive oil isn't. Use it as your main fat.

Watch the trans fats. In 10 European countries, asthma rates are highest in teens who eat the most trans fats in processed food. Since the amounts of trans fats are not listed on food labels, look for clues like "partially hydrogenated oil." Some manufacturers offer trans fat–free versions of the same food. One example: Swiss Miss Fat-Free French Vanilla Hot Cocoa Mix doesn't contain trans fats, but Swiss Miss French Vanilla Hot Cocoa Mix does.

Junk the junk food. Saudi Arabian researchers have found that urban children who eat a junk-food diet similar to that of their Western counterparts have far more asthma than rural children who eat the traditional Saudi diet rich in cow's and goat's milk, rice, vegetables, lamb, chicken, dates, and fruit.

Consider vegetarianism. In one study, 25 asthma patients avoided meat, fish, eggs, dairy products, coffee, ordinary tea, chocolate, sugar, salt, tap water, soybeans, and peas. Foods they ate included lettuce, carrots, beets, onions, celery, cabbage, cauliflower, broccoli, cucumbers, radishes, artichokes, beans, blueberries, strawberries, raspberries, cloudberries, black currants, gooseberries, plums, and pears. After 4 months, 71 percent reported significant improvements. After a year, the number rose to 92 percent. Most were able to reduce or stop asthma medications.

• Vitamins and Minerals

These three supplements should be part of every patient's antiasthma regimen in addition to drug therapy, Dr. Rountree says.

Magnesium. "I put every person with asthma whom I see on magnesium," Dr. Rountree says. This essential mineral is a natural bronchodilator because it relaxes

Reduce Side Effects with Supplements

For relieving symptoms and simply getting your asthma under control, asthma medications are truly a godsend. They aren't without side effects, however. Fortunately, you can combat many of these by getting an adequate intake of certain nutrients.

Vitamin C. Corticosteroids—especially oral and possibly high-dose inhaled—can increase your risk of cataracts. As a result, "I tell all my patients to take at least 500 milligrams of vitamin C. Some take much more," says Marianne Frieri, M.D., Ph.D., professor of medicine and pathology at the State University of New York at Stony Brook and director of the allergy/immunology training program at the Nassau University Medical Center/North Shore University Hospital in East Meadow and Manhasset, New York.

Calcium. Corticosteroids, especially the oral variety, can increase your risk of osteoporosis. So if you use these drugs, it's essential that you get enough calcium. The Daily Value is 1,000 milligrams a day. For postmenopausal women and other adults at risk for osteoporosis, the recommended daily amount is 1,500 milligrams a day. Dairy products are the most concentrated source: One glass of fat-free milk contains 302 milligrams of calcium, while a serving of low-fat plain yogurt contains 415 milligrams. Good nondairy sources of calcium include tofu (135 milligrams in 3 ounces), freshly cooked broccoli (47 milligrams in ½ cup), collards (113 milligrams in ½ cup), turnip greens (100 milligrams in ½ cup), and sardines with bones (325 milligrams in 3 ounces).

Vitamin D. Vitamin D enhances calcium absorption, so you'll need to get the Daily Value of 400 IU, the amount contained in most multivitamins. Doses up to 1,000 IU have improved calcium absorption and bone metabolism, but don't take higher doses unless prescribed by a physician, says Dr. Frieri. Good natural sources include egg yolks, saltwater fish (herring, salmon, sardines), cow's liver, and vitamin D–fortified milk.

Note: Weight-bearing exercise—walking, hiking, stairclimbing, or jogging—is also an essential part of an osteoporosis-prevention program. Your goal should be to exercise at least four times a week. For walking, 45 to 60 minutes is recommended. If you've been inactive, consult your physician before beginning any exercise program.

smooth muscle. In an office setting, some doctors use intravenous magnesium to treat severe asthma attacks. Note that when taken orally, too much of it can cause diarrhea. Start with 300 milligrams a day, and work up to 350 milligrams a day. Reduce the dose if it gives you diarrhea, says Dr. Rountree. Chelated forms—such as magnesium glycinate and magnesium aspartate—seem to be better tolerated by many patients.

Pantothenic acid. This B vitamin is a natural anti-inflammatory. Take up to 2,000 milligrams a day for several months. Some people with asthma may need to take it for years, adds Dr. Rountree.

Vitamin B₆. This vitamin is a natural antihistamine. But easy does it: At daily doses of more than 200 milligrams, it can be toxic. Dr. Rountree recommends taking 50 to 100 milligrams daily for several months at a time. Among the side effects is neuropathy, a functional disturbance of the peripheral nervous system.

Note: Several different "antiasthma" formulas contain magnesium, pantothenic acid, and vitamin B₆.

In addition to these three supplements, Dr. Rountree also recommends taking up to 2,000 milligrams of vitamin C for as long as needed. It has shown promise for treating exercise-induced asthma. While studying 17 children with this condition, Japanese researchers found that 8 of them experienced fewer attacks and improved lung function after taking daily doses of 2,000 milligrams of vitamin C for 4 weeks.

• Dietary Supplements

"Before taking any of the following supplements, I recommend consulting with a physician first," says Dr. Rountree. "The decision regarding which supplements to use for an individual patient is quite complex, and I spend an extensive period of time with each patient deciding which supplements are appropriate."

Quercetin. This yellow bioflavonoid is found in apple skins. Take 400 to 3,000 milligrams of the supplement daily for as long as needed, says Dr. Rountree.

Proanthocyanidins. This technicolor bioflavonoid is the source of the blue in blueberries and the red in cranberries, and it is a potent antioxidant and anti-inflammatory. The most concentrated source, however, is in supplements. For asthma, Dr. Rountree recommends taking at least 100 to 300 milligrams a day for as long as needed.

Fish oil. "Everyone with chronic asthma should take a fish oil supplement, either as cod liver oil or an eicosapentaenoic acid (EPA) concentrate," Dr. Rountree says. Start with 1,000 milligrams a day of EPA and gradually work up to 2,000 to 2,500 milligrams.

Spirulina. Also known as blue-green algae, this supplement has been shown in animal studies to be a immunomodulator and natural antihistamine. Take 3 grams a day for as long as needed, says Dr. Rountree.

Caution: To avoid possible heavy-metal contamination, buy spirulina only from reputable sources. Check the label for a toll-free number for consumer questions or for an indication that it's been analyzed for heavy-metal content.

Borage seed oil/black currant seed oil. Both are potent anti-inflammatories because they're rich in gamma-linolenic acid (GLA). Take the equivalent of 300 milligrams of GLA every day for 6 months to a year, says Dr. Rountree.

N-acetylcysteine (NAC). This mucolytic agent breaks up phlegm, making it ideal for people with "wet" coughs. It also prevents recurrent infections. Take 500 milligrams two or three times a day for as long as needed, says Dr. Rountree.

Reishi mushroom concentrate. This natural antihistamine and immune system booster can prevent flare-ups in people with chronic asthma. Capsules generally contain 500 milligrams of extract. Take two to four capsules a day for as long as needed.

Perilla seed oil. When Japanese researchers fed 26 asthma patients 10 to 20 grams (about 1 tablespoon) a day of perilla seed oil (a derivative of an Asian mint plant), they found the patients' lung function significantly improved. Their hypothesis: Perilla seed oil works as a natural leukotriene modifier. Capsules that contain perilla oil are available at some health food stores.

• Herbs

Throughout most of the world, herbs are a mainstream treatment for asthma. Separate and distinct herbal regimens exist in China, Japan, India, and many other countries.

"Several of these herbs are very safe," says Marianne Frieri, M.D., Ph.D., professor of medicine and pathology at the State University of New York at Stony Brook and director of the allergy/immunology training program at the Nassau University Medical Center/North Shore University Hospital in East Meadow and Manhasset, New York. Just like prescription drugs, however, herbal remedies carry their own sets of risks and benefits.

For example, in Japan, the herbal medicine Saiboku-to is often used as an effective steroid-sparing agent. Problem is, it can increase the risk of drug-induced inflammation of the lungs. It has been linked to numerous cases of serious and destructive lung disease.

Since there's little quality control, herbs can be contaminated with many bioactive substances. They also can trigger the very thing you want to prevent: asthma.

One example is echinacea, an herb widely used by people with allergies to boost immunity. Research shows that it can cause a variety of allergic reactions, including asthma and anaphylaxis. (For more information about herbs that cause allergic reactions, see Food Allergies and Intolerances on page 278.)

Here are some herbs that are commonly used to treat asthma in the United States, says Dr. Rountree. These herbs are typically taken individually, except for boswellia and curcumin, which are usually found in combination. Before using any of the herbs below for self-care, however, Dr. Rountree recommends consulting first with an herbalist or naturopathic physician trained in the use of these herbs.

Garlic. In laboratory studies, garlic increases production of anti-inflammatory chemicals. In clinical practice, however, it seems to get mixed reports as an anti-in-

Licorice Root Is "Lung Candy"— If You Use It Correctly

Of all the herbs used to treat asthma, licorice root is one of the most effective and best-studied. "It's awesome stuff," says Robert Rountree, M.D., a holistic physician in Boulder, Colorado, and coauthor of *Immunotics.*

But it's also risky stuff. Since it can cause salt retention, don't use it for more than 2 weeks if you're prone to high blood pressure. It also lowers blood levels of potassium, which can cause an irregular heartbeat.

When used properly, however, this herb serves as a potent anti-inflammatory and can soothe irritated mucous membranes. It also can be used to help reduce your reliance on oral and inhaled corticosteroids.

No longer found in most "licorice" candy—most of which is flavored with anise— licorice root contains the sugarlike substance glycyrrhizin, which is 50 times sweeter than sugar. So-called deglycyrrhizinated licorice root has fewer side effects, but it has no anti-inflammatory properties. If you're not using any form of corticosteroids, take 1,000 to 2,000 milligrams a day of the powdered herb for no more than 2 to 3 weeks at a time, says Dr. Rountree.

Even if you're not prone to hypertension, you should have your blood pressure monitored regularly if you take licorice for more than a few weeks.

If you're using oral prednisone (Deltasone), which is similar to corticosteroids, be careful. "If you start taking licorice, you can get into trouble because of the additive effect," Dr. Rountree says. If you use inhaled corticosteroids, you'll also get an increased steroidal effect from licorice, which is undesirable.

In his practice, Dr. Rountree has successfully used licorice root to wean patients off oral and inhaled corticosteroids. By using a little of both licorice root and the corticosteroids, he's found that he can get the same anti-inflammatory effect with a lower risk of side effects. "In essence, this is true integrative medicine," Dr. Rountree says.

Try this approach only under the approval and guidance of a knowledgeable doctor or other medical professional.

flammatory. Take up to three 500- to 600-milligram capsules a day for as long as needed, says Dr. Rountree.

Coleus. Distantly related to the coleus houseplant, this traditional Ayurvedic herb contains forskolin, a natural bronchodilator. In Europe, researchers have demonstrated good results from coleus-containing metered-dose inhalers. Since these products are not available in the United States, you have to get this herb in capsules. Take 50 milligrams two or three times a day, says Dr. Rountree. It has few side effects, but you'll need to take it for a week or two for the beneficial effects to become noticeable.

Note: This herb may enhance the effects of medications for asthma or high blood pressure, so do not use it unless under medical supervision.

Ginkgo. This widely used herb blocks platelet-activating factor, one of the main triggers of bronchospasm. But reports are mixed on its efficacy as an asthma remedy. Take 60 milligrams three times daily of an extract standardized to 24 percent ginkgo flavone glycosides and 6 percent terpenes. You'll need to take it for a month before the full benefits are noticeable.

Curcumin, from turmeric. Turmeric is a well-known spice, a staple in Indian cuisine, and its compound curcumin is a natural anti-inflammatory. Take 500 milligrams twice a day. The results should be noticeable within a couple of weeks.

Boswellia. This traditional Ayurvedic herb has long been used to treat inflammation because it inhibits the formation of inflammatory chemicals. Take 1,000 milligrams daily. The results should be noticeable within a couple of weeks.

Note: Curcumin works best when combined with boswellia. Some supplements contain both. Dr. Rountree often tells his asthma patients to take this combination along with a magnesium, pantothenic acid, and vitamin B_6 combination.

Caffeine. If you're on the road without your quick-relief inhaler, drinking two to three cups of strong coffee can help open you up. But you probably won't notice the effects for at least 30 minutes. If you are sensitive to caffeine, however, it's probably best not to try this approach, says Dr. Rountree.

Ginger. This herb is sometimes helpful for asthma. Take one 500-milligram capsule three times a day. The results should be noticeable within a couple of weeks.

Astragalus. Although technically not an antiasthma remedy, this Ayurvedic, immune-boosting herb is renowned for its ability to prevent respiratory infections, a common asthma trigger. Take two 250-milligram capsules daily. It can be taken throughout the cold and flu season for several months at a time, adds Dr. Rountree.

Traditional Chinese Medicine (TCM) remedies. Researchers from the Mount Sinai School of Medicine in New York City and the Johns Hopkins University School of Hygiene and Public Health in Baltimore studied the effects of two TCM formulas—

Ding-Chuan-Tang (DCT) and Jia Wei San Zi Tang (Modified Three Seeds Decoction, or MTSD)—on mice with asthma. Both formulas proved to have various anti-inflammatory actions, including suppressing the production of IgE antibodies, MTSD more so than DCT.

Note: TCM remedies should be used under the supervision of an oriental medicine doctor (OMD) in concert with your regular physician. It is important to stress that the quality control of TCM remedies is not rigorous, and some TCM remedies have been found to be contaminated with

Help Your Lungs by Helping Your Sinuses

"Treatment of any respiratory problem should be directed at both the upper and lower airways," says William Storms, M.D., clinical professor at the University of Colorado Health Sciences Center in Denver and a practicing allergist in Colorado Springs. "We shouldn't treat just one while ignoring the other." Since 80 percent of people with asthma also have allergic rhinitis (hay fever), most doctors recommend treating both.

By effectively treating your upper airways, you should be able to decrease the amount of treatment you need for your lower airways.

Here are some natural hay fever remedies that can indirectly improve your asthma.

Allergy sinus solution (Sinusol). This nose spray contains menthol, eucalyptus oil, birch oil, and spearmint oil. It works as a nonsteroidal anti-inflammatory, decongestant, and antifungal, and can be used every 2 to 3 hours as needed to wash allergens out of your sinuses.

Saline irrigation. By snuffling salt water up your schnozz, you can reduce the sinus drainage that worsens your asthma. If you want to go the deluxe route, you can buy an irrigator that attaches to a Waterpik or an Indian neti pot. (For information on ordering these products, see the Resource Guide on page 497.) The simplest method is to dissolve 1/4 teaspoon of salt in a cup of warm water and squirt the solution into one nostril at a time with a spray bottle or rubber-bulb syringe. Spit the water out through your mouth.

Homeopathy. You can try "desensitizing" yourself with homeopathic remedies containing extremely weak dilutions of allergens. Some combination remedies contain up to 15 different pollens. Others contain a mixture of molds. Take three to five pellets two or three times daily for 2 months. "This is working right at the cellular level. You get the immune system to not recognize these substances as harmful," says Mark Stengler, N.D., a naturopathic and homeopathic physician in La Jolla, California.

For more detailed advice about allergic rhinitis, see Hay Fever on page 307.

heavy metals and synthetic steroids.

Lobelia. Also known as Indian tobacco, this natural decongestant also has a long history as an asthma-attack remedy—a sometimes dangerous one. Lobelia poisoning, which is usually a consequence of using the herb to get high, can result in rapid heartbeat, coma, and death. Because of this, lobelia should be used only under the supervision of a qualified herbalist.

To treat an asthma attack with lobelia, Dr. Weil recommends mixing three parts tincture of lobelia with one part tincture of capsicum (red pepper or cayenne pepper). Take 20 drops of the mixture in water. Repeat every 30 minutes for a total of three or four doses.

Note: Because of lobelia's possible dangerous side effects, you should never use it without first consulting your doctor. It is not a "self-help" herb.

• Mind-Body Interventions

From the demands of our jobs to the demands of our families, our lives seem to be filled with greater and greater amounts of stress. And although most people are aware that stress can affect their general health, few realize that stress can actually affect asthma symptoms as well.

"Stress has an effect on the allergic response," says Gailen D. Marshall Jr., M.D., Ph.D., director of the division of allergy and clinical immunology at the University of Texas–Houston Medical School. "In chronically stressed individuals, there's an increase in IgE that could result in increased cell responsiveness."

To make matters worse, asthma itself is stressful. So are many of the many asthma medications. "We have patients who don't want to take albuterol because it makes their hearts race," Dr. Marshall says.

Here are some natural stress busters that can help relieve asthma.

Acupuncture. Several studies show that even a single acupuncture treatment can significantly improve short-term lung function. But other studies are either inconclusive, poorly designed, or dismissive. In clinical settings, however, a few doctors see dramatic improvements. "I've seen people come in with bad asthma, get one acupuncture treatment, and basically pop right out of it," Dr. Rountree says.

Behavioral change. In one study, 13 participants completed a 7-week behavioral-change program that included interactive education, social support, relaxation training, and humor therapy. Among the changes they incorporated into their daily routines were drinking 10 glasses of water, exercising for 30 minutes, and practicing relaxation for 30 minutes. Among the benefits they experienced: less chest tightness and fatigue, more energy, and better asthma control.

Biofeedback. Ordinary biofeedback for relaxation produces only a modest improvement in lung function. Biofeedback for respiratory sinus arrhythmia, a pattern of heart fluctuations, produces much more significant results, however. It may be especially useful for people with emotionally triggered asthma.

Breathing exercises. Many different breathing exercises have been recommended for asthma. But perhaps the most promising one is the Buteyko technique developed in the former Soviet Union. Through live or video instruction, patients are taught to control the hyperventilation associated with asthma, says Susan Neves, a Buteyko practitioner in Indianapolis. At least two double-blind studies show that the technique can significantly reduce the need for asthma medications. More information is on the Web at www.buteyko-usa.com.

Guided imagery. One controlled study showed that 47 percent of asthma patients who used guided imagery were able to decrease or discontinue their medications. Similar improvements were seen in only 18 percent of the control group.

Hypnosis. Many studies suggest that hypnosis, including self-hypnosis, can be an ef-

fective treatment, especially for children with asthma. One controlled study showed that patients who received 6 months of hypnosis treatment reduced bronchodilator usage from an average of 89 times a month to 22 times a month. The best response was among people under age 30 who had had asthma for less than 20 years. Another catch: Hypnosis works best in the 5 to 10 percent of the population that is highly responsive to hypnotic suggestion.

Journaling. Writing about stressful life experiences is not only an emotional release, it might help you breathe easier, too. One controlled study showed significant improvements in lung function after 4 months in asthma patients who wrote about the single most stressful event that occurred in their lives. Patients who wrote about an emotionally neutral topic didn't improve.

Massage. One small study showed improved lung function in children who re-

Breathe to Relieve Asthma

To help the next time you feel your asthma beginning to act up, practice this diaphragmatic breathing exercise, says Robert Rountree, M.D., a holistic physician in Boulder, Colorado, and coauthor of *Immunotics*. First, find a comfortable position and rest your left hand, palm down, over your navel. Place your right hand over your heart.

While inhaling, imagine that you're filling a pouch that is between your hands. For the first 2 weeks, limit inhalation to 3 seconds, then gradually increase to 4 or 5 seconds. Exhale slowly while silently reciting this affirmation: "My breath is calm, deep, and quiet."

Practice this exercise up to 15 times daily, especially when your asthma is acting up.

ceived 20-minute massages from their parents every night for 1 month. Other research, at the University of California, Davis, suggests that massage produces no measurable benefits. But that doesn't mean that massage is useless. Researchers speculate that massage therapy's team approach might make patients feel more empowered and encourage them to become more compliant with their medications.

Nebulizer therapy. Although nebulizers are used to dispense drugs, they also allow you some quiet time while taking the medicine. This "quiet time" is helpful to many asthma patients. "I've often felt that a major part of nebulizer therapy effectiveness is that it makes patients sit still and relax for 10 to 15 minutes," Dr. Marshall says.

Stress reduction. Since stress makes asthma worse, research shows that stress reduction can make it better. Here's some specific advice for people with asthma.

1. Take notice of the things, events, and people that add stress to your life and work to reduce their impact.

2. Learn and use constructive ways to reduce anger, anxiety, and fear.

3. If you can, take yourself away from stressful situations.

4. Reduce noise and clutter in your work area and at home.

5. Exercise to let off steam.

6. Get help. Friends, family, organizations, support groups, and therapy can make it easier to handle emotional issues.

7. Be sure to take time each and every day to enjoy the good things in your life.

For more information on stress reduction, see Allergy-Free Stress Busters on page 173.

Guided Imagery Exercise

Through guided imagery, patients are taught to visualize their relationship to their asthma and imagine themselves breaking free of it. The following exercise is from Fran Greenfield, M.A., coauthor with Kathryn Shafer of *Asthma Free in 21 Days*.

Close your eyes and breathe out three times, exhaling through your mouth and inhaling through your nose. See before you the image of your difficulty, disease, or symptom. See the chains that bind you together. Know that this difficulty has created a life of its own. See and feel how you are a slave to this life of darkness.

Breathe out one more time. Find a way to unlock or to break these chains and release yourself from bondage. Do this now—and as the chains fall away, take your first steps in the direction of freedom and truth.

What happens? How do you feel?

Now breathe out and open your eyes.

Asthma
ACTION PLAN

Because asthma is such a variable disease, you need to work with your doctor to devise a treatment plan that is tailored to your individual needs. The tips below provide general strategies for managing asthma symptoms. Discuss them with your doctor to see which might best be incorporated into your individualized treatment plan.

indicates a natural remedy

- Take charge of your environment by reducing or eliminating any known allergy triggers, such as dust mites, mold, and tobacco smoke. In addition, check your local weather forecast, pollen count, and smog index, and stay indoors as much as possible when conditions outside are likely to cause asthma attacks.
- Work with your doctor to learn how to use a peak-flow meter, and use it regularly to monitor your asthma symptoms more effectively.
- Asthma medications can significantly improve your quality of life. Work with your doctor to find the medications and dosages that best manage your symptoms. These may include inhaled corticosteroids or nonsteroidal drugs such as cromolyn or nedocromil.
- Consider the benefits of inhalation devices such as metered-dose inhalers. Discuss your options with your health care professional.
- If you develop asthma symptoms from vigorous exercise, your doctor may prescribe medications such as beta$_2$-agonists, cromolyn or nedocromil, or leukotriene modifiers. Because each of these medications needs to be taken within a certain time period before beginning exercise and because they prevent symptoms for anywhere from 1 to 24 hours, it is important that you play an active role in helping your doctor choose the medication that best fits your lifestyle.
- Consider immunotherapy, also known as allergy shots, if your doctor believes you are a good candidate for it.
- Make sure that you're eating a diet rich in antioxidants and vitamin E, which some studies have suggested could reduce asthma symptoms. In ad-

dition, make fish a regular part of your diet, since the omega-3 fatty acids it contains have been shown to improve lung function. The fish with the highest levels of these acids are the darker, richer-fleshed varieties such as salmon, mackerel, and bluefish.

- Drink at least eight glasses of water a day, since dehydration may trigger or worsen asthma symptoms.

- Limit your intake of foods that contain trans fats, since they have been associated with increased asthma rates. Avoid foods that list "partially hydrogenated oil" on the nutrition label.

- In addition to prescription medication, Dr. Rountree recommends taking the following three supplements: 300 to 350 milligrams of magnesium (taken daily), up to 2,000 milligrams of pantothenic acid (taken once a day for several months), and 50 to 100 milligrams of vitamin B_6 (taken daily for several months). There are numerous other dietary supplements that may also lessen your symptoms; check with your doctor before trying them.

- If you're interested in using herbs as part of your asthma action plan, discuss your options with your doctor, herbalist, or naturopathic physician.

- Managing your stress levels can help you to manage your asthma symptoms. Explore stress-busting activities such as biofeedback, journaling, and guided imagery. Some people who have tried these techniques have been able to reduce the amounts of asthma medications they were taking.

Drug
ALLERGIES

WHEN PENICILLIN WAS first manufactured in the 1940s, it was hailed as a miracle drug, capable of eliminating many common diseases and vanquishing infections. It was the first of a new class of potent drugs called antibiotics that would change the way we live. So, what drugs are most likely to cause allergic reactions?

Antibiotics. It is precisely because penicillin is so commonly used to treat infections that it is linked to drug allergies. The reason? The more frequently your body is exposed to a drug, the more likely your immune system will become activated against it and be ready to cause an allergic reaction the next time it's used. When you do take the drug again, antibodies summoned by your immune system mistake it for a harmful substance and launch an attack.

Penicillin is an example of a true allergic reaction in that it is IgE-mediated. IgE is short for immunoglobulin E, an antibody that is present in very low levels in most people but found in large quantities in people with allergies and certain infections. It is believed to be the primary antibody responsible for classic allergic reactions. The most common drug allergy symptoms are hives, skin rash, stuffy nose, wheezing, dizziness, and swelling of body parts. There are medications that your doctor can prescribe to help relieve these symptoms. Most will go away when you stop using the drug.

If you experience hives, a skin rash, wheezing, vomiting, or swelling of body parts after taking a drug, you should consult your physician immediately, says Mark Dykewicz, M.D., associate professor of internal medicine and director of the training program in allergy and immunology at St. Louis University School of Medicine. In addition, be aware that blisters are a serious complication of a drug rash. Their appearance can be a sign that you're developing

Stevens-Johnson syndrome, which can be fatal if not treated; therefore, you should seek medical assistance immediately, cautions Dr. Dykewicz.

When you experience any of the side effects above, your physician will usually take you off the medicine that was prescribed. Usually, another drug can be safely substituted.

The most drastic drug reaction is anaphylaxis (a severe allergic reaction that involves the entire body), which can be fatal if not treated immediately. The first symptom is usually itchiness, especially on the soles of the feet and the palms of the hands. There can also be swelling in the face or other parts of the body. The bronchial muscle (which is the muscle in the airway that leads to the lungs) constricts, making it difficult to breathe.

Symptoms associated with anaphylaxis can be fast and progressive, and they most often occur within 1 hour after the drug is taken. In 5 to 20 percent of cases, a recurrence of the reaction may transpire up to several hours later. If medical attention is not sought immediately, the blood vessels dilate, blood pressure drops, and the person goes into shock. Since the brain and nervous system are deprived of oxygen, they can't narrow the blood vessels again, and the person will die unless he gets immediate medical treatment. Patients experiencing anaphylaxis are given a shot of epinephrine (a drug similar to the natural adrenaline in our bodies), which constricts blood vessels and opens up the bronchial tubes. If you experience any of the symptoms mentioned, seek medical assistance right away. (For more information, see Anaphylaxis on page 211.)

One other note: A family history of allergy to penicillin or any other drug does not mean that your children will have an increased chance of a reaction. "Contrary to popular belief, the vast majority of drug allergies are not inherited," says I. Leonard Bernstein, M.D., clinical professor of medicine and environmental health at the University of Cincinnati College of Medicine in Ohio. In addition, according to the American Academy of Allergy, Asthma, and Immunology, 70 percent of people who are allergic to penicillin lose their allergy over a 5- to 10-year period.

Before you can understand what the medical profession calls true drug allergies, you should understand how they differ from side effects, dose-response differences, intolerance, and idiosyncratic reactions.

Nonallergic Drug Reactions

All drugs have side effects. Drug side effects are not the result of medical errors and are not drug allergies. They are the result of taking the drug properly and at normal doses, without any complicating factors such as interactions with other drugs. By the time the FDA approves a drug, the main side effects of the drug are usually known. If you look at any magazine ad for a prescription drug, a summary of the main side effects will be listed in the "balance statement," which the FDA requires pharmaceutical companies to put in their ads. For example, the ad for the heartburn drug Prevacid says, "Prevacid has a low occurrence of side effects, such as diarrhea (3.6 percent), abdominal pain (1.8 percent), and nausea (1.4 percent)."

Sometimes a reaction to a drug is not a side effect but a dosage-related response. We are all different. Just as some people can tolerate more liquor than others, people's tolerance for drugs differs as well. For example, three people can take the same dosage of Benadryl and have different reactions, claims Dr. Dykewicz. One person may experience relief from their allergy symptoms and have no side effects. Another person may get relief but become drowsy and may fall asleep. The third person may experience dizziness. (That's why you see the warning about not operating heavy equipment or machinery in many advertisements for drugs.)

Adverse reactions can include intolerance or idiosyncratic reactions to certain drugs. Neither of these reactions depends on having taken the drug previously. Intolerance means that even at the normal dose for the drug, the person taking it shows undesirable effects, as though he had overdosed. An idiosyncratic reaction occurs when an individual has an abnormal susceptibility to a drug that causes him to act in an unusual or unpredictable way. For example, fewer than 1 percent of people who take Motrin (ibuprofen) have reported hallucinations, bleeding episodes, and arrhythmias (abnormal heartbeats).

True Drug Allergies

Drug allergies are generally divided into four types, ranging from the potentially life-threatening, such as anaphylactic reactions, to the merely irritating, such as allergic contact dermatitis.

• Type I are the anaphylactic reactions discussed earlier. Again, these are true medical emergencies that require immediate treatment.

• Type II reactions cause cell destruction. They can result in a decrease in red blood cells (anemia), a potentially fatal blood disorder of the white blood cells that increases the risk of infections (granulocytopenia), and a decrease in the number of blood platelets (thrombocytopenia). Type II allergies are rare and are usually reactions to medications. If you suspect you are having a reaction, see your doctor, who can make a final determination.

• Type III reactions occur when a drug combines with antibodies and causes serum sickness reactions, which can include fever, skin lesions, hepatitis, kidney problems, and even arthritis. Unlike anaphylaxis, which has a sudden onset, serum sickness usually occurs 1 to 4 weeks after drug use. If you experience any of these symptoms, seek medical assistance.

• Type IV reactions are delayed reactions as well, but they don't take as long to develop as serum sickness, and they're not as dangerous. The classic Type IV reaction is allergic contact dermatitis, a rash from touching something to which you are allergic, such as an antibiotic cream. It usually takes 1 to 3 days to occur. If you develop a rash after using a cream or ointment, seek medical assistance.

The Usual Suspects

What drugs besides penicillin and other antibiotics cause the most allergies? Most

A Matter of Life and Death

Pop a pill and feel better, right?

In November 1999, the Institute of Medicine (IOM) of the National Academies issued a report that shook up the medical profession, the public, Congress, and then-President Clinton. The IOM reported that between 44,000 and 98,000 Americans die in U.S. hospitals each year because of medical errors.

According to the report, even at the lowest estimate, that would still mean that more Americans died of medical errors than from motor vehicle accidents, breast cancer, or AIDS.

Of this large number of deaths due to medical error, the IOM report found that about 7,000 were caused by medication errors either in hospitals or at other health care facilities, such as outpatient clinics, day-surgery clinics, retail pharmacies, and nursing homes. This exceeds the number of deaths that result from workplace injuries, which get much more attention in the news.

It is important to remember that a medication error is not always caused by a drug allergy (and that not all drug allergies are associated with medical errors). For example, if a patient who doesn't have a history of allergic reactions to drugs suffers an allergic reaction to an antibiotic, this patient has suffered an adverse drug event, not a medical error.

Many drugs don't interact well with other drugs and should never be given at the same time. For example, many people used the drug Seldane to treat allergies before it was taken off the market by the FDA. When taken with other drugs such as the antibiotic erythromycin, Seldane caused potentially fatal heart-rhythm disturbances in some people. Unfortunately, some dangerous reactions are simply not known until the drug is on the market and people take it with other drugs.

people are surprised to learn that aspirin and other classes of pain relievers are the next biggest culprits. Unlike allergies to penicillin, those to aspirin and other pain relievers usually are not based on antibody response, so doctors cannot test for them.

The drugs that commonly cause allergic-type reactions are:

Angiotensin-converting enzyme (ACE) inhibitors. These drugs, such as lisinopril (Prinivil) and benazepril (Lotrel), are used to treat high blood pressure and heart failure. They produce coughing in 10 to 25 percent of patients within 1 to 12 months after therapy.

Aspirin and related anti-inflammatory drugs. Between 8 and 19 percent of adult patients with asthma and 30 to 40 percent of adult patients with nasal polyps and sinusitis develop reactions from aspirin and related drugs such as ibuprofen. These reactions may include rhinitis, angioedema, or even anaphylaxis.

Cytokines. These are drugs, such as interferon, that are used in the treatment of viral hepatitis and cancers. Cytokines, which are proteins normally produced by body cells, can cause low blood pressure, capillary leakage syndrome (the cells that hold the blood vessel walls together become detached, causing the leakage), and flulike symptoms.

Insulin. As a protein, insulin tends to activate the immune system. So it is no surprise that reactions ranging from anaphylaxis to allergic contact dermatitis have

been reported. Human insulin causes fewer allergic reactions than insulin derived from pork. Humulin and Novolin are the most commonly prescribed types of human insulin.

Since insulin is injected into the body, about half of people with diabetes get skin rashes as a result. Usually, these reactions are minimal and clear up over time. It is common, however, for patients with diabetes to develop antibodies to insulin after several weeks. Since insulin is vital, the treating physicians must find the right insulin preparations for their patients. Fortunately, several types of insulin are becoming available that may be tolerated by those who have become allergic to one type of insulin. Allergy skin testing can also help select insulin that is more likely to be tolerated.

In addition, patients with diabetes who have taken NPH (neutral protein hagedorn) insulin, which is a commonly used long-acting insulin, are 40 times more likely to have an increased risk for anaphylaxis after heart surgery. This happens because protamine (a drug given to restore normal clotting after heart surgery) is contained in NPH insulin, and the continued exposure to this causes the body to become sensitized to it.

Radiographic contrast media. An x-ray dye, this is injected through an IV during lab tests such as CAT scans. If a person has had a reaction, another agent can usually be found that is safe to use.

Drug Allergy
ACTION PLAN

If you're taking a drug for the first time, how do you know if you're allergic to it? While you can never be 100 percent certain, simply being informed about drug allergies is an important first step, says Dr. Bernstein. Most medical students get very little training in drug allergies, and most physicians—and even some allergists—are not informed about all the issues, he cautions.

Further, drug allergies often are not taken seriously, believes Dr. Dykewicz. "Even though this is very rare, over-the-counter drugs such as Advil and Motrin can cause reactions such as meningitis and liver damage. Drug reactions should be taken seriously, and both the public and physicians need to be better educated about them," he says.

In addition to being an informed health consumer, you can take some other practical measures to decrease your chances of experiencing a drug allergy.

🌿 *indicates a natural remedy*

- Always tell your physician about every drug you're taking. Don't forget to mention any herbal medicines or vitamin supplements you use, since they can have interactions with prescription drugs. (Some can cause allergic reactions by themselves, too.) If you've had a reaction to a drug before, it is essential to tell your doctor, since you could also be allergic to drugs that are chemically related to it. So that you don't forget to mention any medications, you might simply put all the drugs you take—including alternative ones—in a bag and take them along with you to your doctor.

- Consider skin tests, which can be useful in determining if you are allergic to certain drugs. If you're being tested for Type I allergy, a small amount of the suspected substance is placed on your skin and pricked, or injected under your skin, and read after 20 to 30 minutes. If you're being tested for a Type IV reaction, the drug is applied on top of your skin with a patch that is kept in place for 2 to 3 days before it is removed and the skin is examined. Redness or swelling is the sign of a positive reaction, meaning you are allergic to that substance.

The most successful of these tests is for penicillin. By testing for allergic antibodies and substances formed after penicillin is given, doctors can determine if you're allergic to the drug. Sometimes it's not the penicillin but rather the natural substance formed after the drug is taken that causes a reaction. This test is considered more than 98 percent reliable for predicting Type I reactions such as anaphylaxis. It cannot predict other types of drug reactions, however, such as measles-like rashes. Skin tests with other antibiotics, such as Ceclor, can also be done, but they're not as reliable. Other drugs for which allergic reaction tests can be done include insulin and tetanus shots. Unfortunately, not every drug can be tested yet with such accuracy.

- Obviously, avoiding the drug that is causing an allergic reaction is the safest way to go, but this is not always an option. Whenever possible, take the drugs orally rather than intravenously to lessen the chance of a severe reaction, advises Dr. Dykewicz.

- If you had a previous reaction to radiographic contrast media (x-ray dye) and you need to have a similar test, request one of the newer agents that have less chance of causing an allergic reaction and ask your doctor for premedication that will reduce or eliminate a reaction, he suggests.

- Wear a MedicAlert necklace or bracelet with a personalized tag that is engraved with medical information about your specific condition or allergies. This personalized alert allows for prompt recognition of your allergy, disease, chronic condition, or other health problems in an emergency. This is one of the first things that medical and paramedical personnel look for in patients who cannot talk or who are unconscious.

By the
numbers

10

Percentage of the population that has allergies to penicillin, sulfa drugs, and other antibiotics

Dust Mites, Roaches, and Other Insect ALLERGIES

POET T. S. ELIOT must have known a great deal about allergies, judging from this ominous line from his poem "The Waste Land":

"I will show you fear in a handful of dust."

Indeed, if you swept up a fistful of dust in your home and examined it under a microscope, you'd probably see some ingredients that are fearsome. Not to mention downright gross.

You would likely find dust mites and bits of roaches as well as droppings of their waste materials. Just 1 gram of dust—the weight of a paper clip—may contain several hundred dust mites.

Researchers from the National Institute of Environmental Health Services in Research Triangle Park, North Carolina, and the U.S. Department of Housing and Urban Development in Washington, D.C., found plenty of that kind of stuff when they examined the dust from 831 households around the United States. Their results indicate that about 43

million homes in the country have enough dust mite allergen to potentially cause allergies, and 13 million have enough dust mite allergen in the bedding to possibly trigger asthma symptoms in sensitive asthmatics. Plus, the researchers estimate, about 6 million households have detectable levels of cockroach allergen in the bedding.

"Those numbers, perhaps, were a surprise. We would not have predicted that the problem was as widespread as it is," says Darryl Zeldin, M.D., a lung doctor and the principal investigator on the study.

"This is not just a problem of the poor or people with bad housekeeping habits," Dr. Zeldin adds. The study included free-standing houses, multi-unit dwellings, homes of the affluent, and homes of the poor, all in different regions and climates throughout the country.

"These days, mite is perhaps the most common allergy we see in people," says

Hobert Pence, M.D., associate clinical professor of medicine at the University of Louisville. Other sources agree that mites are generally the greatest risk factor for asthma in temperate and humid regions, though in some spots that honor goes to the cockroach.

Virtually any bug that you encounter in great enough numbers—including cute little lady beetles—may cause you trouble, however. Let's take a closer look.

But not *too* close. We don't want to start sneezing.

Mighty Mites and Roaches: Tiny but Powerful

Sure, humans can be hard to count, but if the census bureau ever wants a real challenge, they should try to get a head count of all the mites in our homes. At least they could spend most of their time searching specific areas.

To find these microscopic mites, you need to hunt in places with soft, squishy, porous surfaces that offer moisture for them to drink, food to eat, and places to hide. Unfortunately, many of our homes offer these sorts of places in abundance.

Wall-to-wall carpeting is a veritable continent for mites to explore and conquer. When the vacuum roars overhead, they cling deep within the fibers with their sticky feet and blissfully ignore the noise. They'll also hide in your couch, hitch a ride in your clothes, and thrive in your children's stuffed animals.

These tiny relatives of the spider live for a month, and during that time an egg-laying female can bring 30 new mite babies into the world. Mites spend their days munching on skin cells that constantly shower off your body and come to rest on your sheets, carpeting, and other surfaces in your house. The droppings that mites produce break down into a fine powder that clings to surrounding surfaces.

To get water, mites soak up moisture through their coating. They thrive in areas of 75 to 80 percent humidity, but as the humidity falls below 40 to 50 percent, they die off. That's why at high altitudes and other dry climates, their numbers are scarce.

In the United States, mite allergen levels are highest in August and September and lowest in November and December.

A roach will encroach in your home for the same reasons as mites—food and water—says Larry Williams, M.D., associate professor of pediatrics at the Duke University Medical Center in Durham, North Carolina, and admittedly one of few physicians who study these nasty critters. "Roaches just sort of randomly forage, trying to avoid getting into open areas. They like to be up against the walls and under things if possible."

The kitchen and bathroom are the two biggest places for roaches to hang out, notes Dr. Williams. It makes sense, then, that these two rooms often have the highest amounts of cockroach allergen. While keeping your home immaculately clean will give roaches less to eat, even a bit of moisture on wood in your home will grow enough microorganisms for them to eat, drink, and thrive, he says.

While scurrying about, roaches leave trails of allergy-triggering saliva, waste products, and shed body parts, all of which can become airborne. When the bugs die, their bodies decay into even more allergens.

As these little souvenirs that the mites and roaches leave behind float through the

Lady Beetles: Cute but Not Harmless

The lady beetle holds something of a rare position in the insect world—it's a bug that people tend to find cute. Button-shaped and whimsically colored, it doesn't bite like a mosquito or scurry malevolently like a roach. So when a man with a history of allergies entered the office of Hobert Pence, M.D., complaining that lady beetles were causing his asthma symptoms, the doctor was a bit skeptical.

Dr. Pence, associate clinical professor of medicine at the University of Louisville, started his patient on medications and tried with no luck to find a mention of lady beetle allergy in the medical journals. About this time, he attended an allergy conference in which other doctors presented papers on—surprise!—lady beetle allergy.

Dr. Pence had his patient bring in a few of the thousands of lady beetles infesting his home, then extracted proteins from them and tested them on the man. Bingo—his body reacted to them. The doctor found the allergy-triggering proteins both inside the bugs' bodies and in a yellowish fluid they secrete.

If a lady beetle lands on your jacket, that's no cause for panic. But if you regularly find yourself in clouds of them, you may be at risk of becoming sensitized to them. The bugs tend to enter homes in hordes during the winter, Dr. Pence says, much like they did in his patient's case. The man noticed his symptoms the most during the winter, and they went away in the summer.

If you're noticing lady beetles in your home, take care to seal up any entry points in your home to keep them outside. And use caution if you're among the growing number of gardeners buying masses of lady beetles to eat harmful bugs in the garden. Dr. Pence thinks we'll see more and more allergy problems from the bugs as they become more popular for pest control.

Finally, if you are regularly exposed to other sorts of bugs and are having symptoms of asthma or allergies, report this situation to your doctor, since the bugs may be contributing to your problem.

air, rest on your pillow, and zip up your nose as you inhale, they may be giving you asthma or allergies—or making them worse.

Allergens Plus Genetics Can Equal Trouble

To become allergic to bugs, you need two things: proteins from these bugs in your environment and a genetic background that predisposes you to become allergic to them, Dr. Zeldin says.

Let's say that, hypothetically speaking, Abel and Mabel live in a mite- and roach-infested home. If Abel's genes are so inclined, he's more likely to come down with asthma or hay fever (also known as rhinitis). But if Mabel isn't genetically set up to become allergic, she'll probably be fine despite the bugs. If they had chosen a different home, free of roaches and with minimal levels of dust mites, they'd likely both be free from allergy and asthma caused by these bugs.

As the bugs shed proteins throughout the house, they get knocked aloft into the air currents when Abel and Mabel walk on the carpet, lie down on the bed, and run the vacuum. As Abel breathes in the proteins that the bugs shed, his body's immune system sensitizes him, making antibodies that detect these specific proteins—and remember, his genes dictate that this will happen.

As he keeps breathing in these proteins, his body sends cells to his lungs, releasing chemicals that leave his lungs inflamed and in the throes of asthma, Dr. Zeldin says. These allergens can also trigger allergic rhinitis, which can flare up along with asthma or on its own, and may also contribute to atopic (allergic) dermatitis, or eczema.

This leads us to some important questions that scientists are still trying to answer: How much allergen is enough to give you asthma or allergies? And once you have these conditions, how much allergen is enough to make them flare up?

Researchers have some assumptions about how high an allergen level needs to be to lead to trouble, but the definitive numbers are elusive, in part because the studies that look at groups of people and measure their exposures to allergens are extremely hard to do. If you're genetically prone to these allergies, however, just remember this: You don't need much exposure to bug allergens to have a reaction.

"The more allergen the person is exposed to, the greater the chance he will become sensitive if he has the genetic makeup," Dr. Zeldin says. "Furthermore, the more allergen that one is exposed to, the more severe the symptoms in general."

Another complication in dealing with these allergens is that it's tough to measure them in a home with constantly changing real-world conditions. Thus, it's difficult to know for certain just how much we have in our homes and how much remains after we take steps to clear it out.

Prioritizing Is Key to Limiting Mites

We've long known that taking people with mite allergies out of their normal environ-ments and putting them into mite-free en-vironments—like hospital rooms or high-el-evation locations—will improve symptoms for many of them, points out Euan Tovey, Ph.D., a mite researcher with the University

Get Out the Vacuum to Test for Allergens

If your curiosity won't let you rest until you know just how many mites, cockroaches, and other allergens are in your home's dust, technology can provide an answer.

All you need to do is vacuum up a sample of the dust and send it off to a testing lab. Technicians will then use intricate processes to refine the sample and determine its contents. They'll then report back to you with what they find.

One lab that offers this service is the Dermatology, Allergy, and Clinical Immunology Reference Laboratory at the Johns Hopkins University in Baltimore. The lab can be reached at (800) 344-3224 or (410) 550-2029. It will screen dust for allergens from dust mites and cockroaches as well as from cats, dogs, and mice, says director Robert Hamilton, Ph.D.

The lab sends clients a disposable, socklike filter to tuck into their vacuum cleaner's suction hose and use to gather dust and debris from specific spots around the home. Clients then drop the filter into a sealable plastic bag and mail it back to the laboratory, Dr. Hamilton says. There, the dust is run through a sieve, and aller-genic proteins are extracted and analyzed. Clients are then told how high the protein levels are in the dust and how these levels may be affecting their health. The lab also gives clients advice on ways they may want to remedy the problem.

Though the tests aren't terribly expensive—about $25 for each allergen analysis—the lab urges people to be evaluated by an allergist to determine whether the aller-gens are even a health problem before they order a test on their dust. "(Some) people think that this is a panacea and they'll find something magic about their house if they do this testing. And yet if they're not allergic to dust mites, cats, dogs, or cock-roaches, it's meaningless," Dr. Hamilton cautions.

If you're tempted to use one of the at-home allergen-testing kits that some allergy-product catalogs carry, be aware that they might not give a detailed answer to how much of the allergen is present. Plus, the fact that several experts weren't even aware that they exist casts doubt on the usefulness of these kits.

of Sydney in Australia. A murkier issue is how to do the inverse—bring down the levels of mites and their allergens in the home so that they're low enough to reduce allergy symptoms.

Since much about measuring the levels of allergens and knowing how much is bad for us remains a mystery, it's hard to judge for certain which tactics work around the home and which don't. "Right now, folks are just flying blind," Dr. Williams says. "In the clinic, you see people doing things that are unhelpful—all the way from people who don't believe the allergens have anything to do with their health problems and don't do any intervention to improve their situations, to people who think everything that ever happens to them is related to allergens in the house, and they do much more than they ever should do."

Researchers are still trying to determine which methods of bringing down mite and cockroach allergen work well enough to warrant your time and expense. Because mites are so widespread, keeping up with them is a steady pursuit.

Some improvements you can make are relatively cheap and easy but still probably effective, like reducing the allergens in your bedding. Some are expensive and effective, like ripping out your carpeting. Others are relatively cheap but ineffective, like sprinkling mite-killing chemicals on your carpet. Dr. Tovey has reviewed the research and offers the following list of recommendations for limiting mites in your home.

Definitely useful: Experts say that the best place to begin your war on mites is your bedroom, particularly your bed, because that's where you spend a large chunk of your life. Dr. Tovey recommends encasing your mattress, box spring, pillows, and, if possible, blankets and duvets in special impermeable covers, which keep the critters and the allergens they shed from invading the bedding. Some of these covers are made of tightly woven material that lets air and moisture pass in and out, making them more comfortable than the vinyl-type materials of earlier days.

It's also crucial to wash your sheets, pillowcases, and unprotected blankets regularly—every week to 10 days or so—to wash out the allergens. Washing them in water hotter than 130°F will kill the living mites, but Dr. Tovey says that it's most important to just make sure you wash out their droppings and other allergens. As far as detergents go, one will work as well as the next at washing away allergens.

Finally, wipe down the encasings with a damp cloth or clean them according to the manufacturer's directions each time you wash the rest of the bedding.

Probably useful: Remove carpets and replace them with smooth flooring that can be cleaned with a damp mop. This removes a huge reservoir of mite and other allergens, but it's also an expensive choice.

In addition, wipe shiny, hard surfaces in your home weekly with a damp cloth or paper towel. This simple act removes a lot of dust and allergens. It's cheap, too, though it requires a good deal of elbow grease.

Possibly useful: Air filters may take some dust mite allergens out of the air, but these allergens are so heavy that they're usually resting on a surface and only briefly stay aloft when they're disturbed. As a result, a faraway filter is unlikely to grab them. Research has shown, however, that when used along with bedding encasings, free-standing HEPA (high-efficiency particulate air) filters can help reduce symptoms of mite allergy better than the encasings alone.

Unfortunately, vacuuming doesn't make a dent in the population of live mites—their sticky feet keep them in place. But it does lift out dust and other allergens, which is helpful. Just be sure to use a vacuum with a HEPA filter or double-lined bags to minimize the dust that spews out of the machine, and wear a dust mask for extra protection.

Probably not useful: Acaricides, which are mite-killing chemicals applied to the carpet or upholstered furniture, haven't been proven to be helpful enough to warrant using them.

Ridding Your Residence of Roaches

In a sense, knowing whether roaches are making your allergies and asthma worse is simple. After all, unlike microscopic dust mites, roaches are visible to the naked eye.

"If the patients never see cockroaches in their homes, they can be relatively sure that they are not a part of their problem," says Dr. Williams. "Folks who see cockroaches every day in their household and have asthma probably have somewhere around a 50 to 60 percent chance of having allergy to cockroaches, and that is probably one of the things that keeps their asthma going."

And like that battery-powered rabbit in the TV commercials, roach allergens keep going and going. Studies have shown that with exterminating and thorough cleaning, you can bring down the levels of roach allergen in the kitchen by about 90 percent after 6 months. But even after running roaches away and cleaning up, some roach allergens will persist in your home for months or even years.

The best way to cope with roaches in your home is to ensure that they don't come inside in the first place. The way to do that is to take away their entry points by sealing cracks in your home, deprive them of drinks by keeping your humidity low and making sure your home stays dry, and shut off their sources of food by sealing food containers tightly and keeping the home free of crumbs.

If roaches do make an appearance in your home, the best way to tackle them is with gels and baits instead of sprays, which can be irritating to people with asthma, says Dr. Williams. (For more details on types of roach killers, check the Roach Allergy Action Plan on page 277.) Take extra care to regularly clean your home afterward—that's what will bring down the remaining roach allergens.

Dust Mite Allergy
ACTION PLAN

Before making expensive or time-consuming modifications around your residence, make sure that you or the person with allergies is actually allergic to the triggers you're trying to reduce. Obviously, if the allergens aren't triggering the problems, getting rid of them won't help the symptoms.

An allergist can test you, diagnose your allergy triggers, and recommend how vigorously you should try to reduce them.

If you and your allergist do determine that dust mites are the cause of your symptoms, here are the best strategies for reducing their impact in your home.

🌿 *indicates a natural remedy*

🌿 Because about a third of our lives takes place in the bedroom—which often contains the most dust mites—give that room special attention when you start working to bring down allergens. Slip your mattress, box spring, pillows, and comforter into allergen-proof encasings. Be sure to choose a style that allows moisture to pass through so they won't grow hot and sweaty as you sleep. Woven styles tend to be more comfortable than crinkly plastic styles.

🌿 Wash your sheets and pillowcases every week to 10 days in hot water. Wipe down the protective encasings or wash them according to the manufacturer's directions.

🌿 Keep the humidity in your home at 50 percent or lower, using an air conditioner or a dehumidifier if necessary. Pick up a humidity gauge, also known as a hygrometer, at your local hardware store to help you track the level in your home.

🌿 Repair any water leaks or other sources of moisture around the home.

🌿 Remove carpeting, especially in the bedroom, and replace it with a hard, shiny surface like wood. (This is an expensive proposition, so check with your doctor to see if your situation warrants this.) If you must have carpeting, select a type with a low pile or use scatter rugs that you can wash in hot water each week.

🌿 Replace upholstered furniture with wood, leather, or plastic pieces that you can wipe clean of dust.

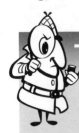

THE HIDDEN CONNECTION

Think Twice Before Ordering That Escargot

From the "Someone Should Warn the French" files: Research has found that people who are allergic to dust mites should think twice before eating snails. Scientists have identified a cross-reaction between these two organisms. Fortunately, in most cases, the symptoms are only mild, but scientists warn that asthma or even anaphylaxis could occur.

If you're a person who enjoys munching on a snail or two—personally, we can think of a better snack, but don't let us stop you—and you're allergic to dust mites, you might consider getting tested for sensitivity to snails and other invertebrate animals.

- Use curtains or shades instead of venetian blinds and thick drapes. Regularly wash them if they're washable.
- Clean your home thoroughly on a regular basis. Vacuum each week, ideally with a vacuum equipped with a HEPA filter or special double-lined bags.
- Dust all the hard surfaces in your home with a damp cloth each week.
- Don't keep a lot of dust-collecting knickknacks around, like books, figurines, and stuffed animals, especially in the bedroom. Instead, keep these items in enclosed bookcases or cabinets.
- Use HEPA filters, available from your hardware store, on your air-conditioning and furnace system. Change or clean them regularly, according to the manufacturer's directions.
- Consider a freestanding HEPA filter in the bedroom. Remember, though, that this is a measure that will be helpful only if you've also taken care of the other recommendations like putting encasements on the bed, lowering the humidity, and removing carpeting.
- Place a filter made of a piece of cheesecloth under the faceplate of the bedroom vent to catch dust blowing out. Change it regularly.
- Wash teddy bears and other stuffed animals regularly in hot water.
- Consider getting immunotherapy shots to make you less sensitive to mites.

Roach Allergy
ACTION PLAN

The best way to deal with roaches is to ensure that they don't come into your home in the first place. If they've already set up house, though, there are still a number of practical things you can do to limit their allergens and encourage them to move on.

indicates a natural remedy

- Seal any crevices and cracks in the perimeter of your home that give roaches an entryway.
- Keep your home free of food sources. Store your food in sealed containers, use trash and recycling containers with lids and empty them regularly, clean up food crumbs and spills, and don't leave dirty dishes in the sink.
- Mop the kitchen floor and wipe down the countertops each week.
- Ensure that your home is free of sources of moisture. Fix leaky pipes, use exhaust fans in your bathroom and kitchen, and make sure that rainwater drains far away from your home.
- To kill roaches, set out bait stations containing the ingredients fipronil or hydramethylnon. Fipronil will kill roaches quickly; hydramethylnon does it more slowly but gives the roach time to get back to its nest and spread the poison for other roaches to eat it.

  Be sure to set the stations in spots where roaches will likely encounter them—in corners and along the angle where the floor meets the wall under sinks, dishwashers, stoves, and refrigerators. You also may find that coating roach thoroughfares with a thin layer of boric acid will cut down on their numbers. Boric acid is low in toxicity to people and pets. Just be sure to keep this white powder away from surfaces where you prepare food.

- Talk to your doctor about immunotherapy shots to make you less sensitive to roaches.
- For more ideas, see The Allergy-Free Home on page 73.

Food Allergies and
INTOLERANCES

IT MIGHT BE COMFORTING to think that the primary culprits in food allergy are manmade chemicals like herbicides and pesticides sprayed on food crops, antibiotics and hormones fed to food animals, and preservatives and flavor enhancers added to processed foods.

But that wouldn't be the truth.

Although such substances can cause adverse reactions, they're typically *not* what sets off food allergies. The usual triggers are as natural as food itself: proteins. Examples include caseins and whey in cow's milk, ovomucoid in egg whites, and tropomycin in shellfish.

Although food allergy appears to be an increasingly common problem, it's nothing new. Two thousand years ago, the ancient Roman philosopher/poet Lucretius wrote, "What is food to some may be bitter poison to others." He wasn't speaking metaphorically. He was simply lamenting the fact that some people can stuff themselves silly on food and drink that makes other people seriously ill.

If you have a food allergy, you probably lament it, too. Being allergic to a favorite food is a cruel twist of fate. With other kinds of allergies, at least there's some consolation in knowing that the offending substances aren't essential to survival. The last we heard, there were no recommended daily allowances for pollen, mold, and dust mites. Food allergy, on the other hand, can make getting essential nutrients problematic.

Further, food allergy can affect any part of the gastrointestinal tract, from the mouth to the anus. Since allergenic food molecules can travel anywhere in the body, they also can cause hives, eczema, and other rashes, as well as allergic rhinitis (hay fever) and asthma.

Environmental-medicine doctors and alternative practitioners believe that the allergic response is intensified by leaky-gut syndrome, a controversial theory, which holds that the Western diet, antibiotics, and other stressors make the gut more "porous." This enables toxins to leak out into the bloodstream and surrounding tissue, triggering an allergic response in many different parts of the body.

In severe cases, food allergy can cause anaphylactic shock. In fact, it's the leading cause of anaphylaxis outside of a hospital setting, accounting for an estimated 30,000 emergency room visits and 100 to 200 deaths each year.

Fortunately, food allergy is manageable. With conventional strategies, you can avoid the foods that cause allergies and sensitivities, enjoy great-tasting alternatives, and still get all the nutrients you need to keep your-

The Promise of Probiotics

When Finnish researcher Erika Isolauri, M.D., Ph.D., treated children with severe eczema, she discovered a seemingly paradoxical effect: The children's eczema cleared up after they received probiotic supplements, which contain bacteria that are believed to be beneficial to human health.

Why would treating the gut affect a skin condition? Dr. Isolauri suggests it's because probiotics restore the gut's natural bacterial balance, reverse leaky-gut syndrome, and reduce allergic inflammation. The children's eczema improved because the supplements treated its real cause: an underlying food allergy.

Such research has sparked interest in the use of probiotics as a treatment for food and other allergies. "Everybody with allergies should probably take acidophilus," says Robert Rountree, M.D., a holistic physician in Boulder, Colorado. Unlike some practitioners, he believes that probiotics supplements are the best sources of beneficial bugs. His recommendation: Take daily supplements containing the equivalent of 10 to 20 billion live organisms.

Other practitioners argue that natural sources of probiotics are just as effective. Mark Stengler, N.D., a naturopathic and homeopathic physician in La Jolla, California, recommends eating a diet rich in low-fat plain yogurt, cottage cheese, kefir, miso, and sauerkraut. In addition, you can support the growth of acidophilus, lactobacillus, and bifidobacteria by eating foods that contain an indigestible carbohydrate called FOS. Among the best sources of FOS are bananas, garlic, honey, chicory, wheat, onions, soybeans, tomatoes, and, especially, Jerusalem artichoke.

self hale and hearty. And with alternative strategies, you can even strengthen your gastrointestinal tract, improve your digestion, and decrease or eliminate your sensitivity to certain foods.

We'll show you how to do all of this in this chapter. First, though, let's clear up some misconceptions about food allergy.

Understanding Food Allergies

Many people think that food allergy is as widespread as the common cold. In truth, though, food allergies are much rarer than commonly believed. The reason lies in the definition of an allergy.

According to conventional medicine, a true food allergy is an immediate reaction mediated by the so-called allergy antibody, immunoglobin E (IgE). A classic example of this is the hives that people get shortly after eating shrimp.

Does that mean that people who don't have true food allergies are experiencing no ill effects? Not at all. It simply means that foods are making them sick in ways that don't involve IgE. They might have a food intolerance, which could produce milder reactions such as stomach cramps and diarrhea. A prime example is lactose intolerance, which results from an insufficient amount of an enzyme called lactase. Another possibility is that they experienced an epidosde of food poisoning or toxicity.

This is a mild-to-severe reaction caused by foods contaminated with bacteria or chemicals.

Why is the distinction so important? Well, if you're allergic to milk, for example, a few drops could kill you. If you're intolerant to milk, the worst you can expect is gas, diarrhea, and social embarrassment.

A Food Allergy Attack on a Plate

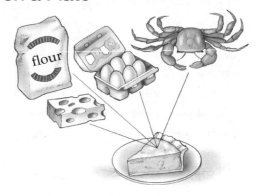

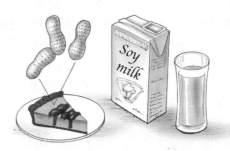

You've heard the expression "a heart attack on a plate." Now meet a "food allergy attack on a plate." The dinner above—seafood quiche, soy milk, and peanut butter pie—contains the culprits responsible for the vast majority of true food allergies: dairy products, wheat, peanuts/tree nuts, fish/shellfish, egg, and soy.

Immediate and Delayed Reactions

People who experience adverse reactions to foods can be divided into two camps: those who develop reactions within 2 hours of eating a suspect food and those who develop reactions more than 2 hours and up to several days later.

Immediate reactions are instantly recognizable. Soon after ingesting even a small amount of a problem food, you can experience any of the following symptoms.
- Tingling of the lips, palate, tongue, or throat
- Hoarseness
- Nausea, vomiting, cramping, or diarrhea
- Hives, eczema, itching, and flushing
- Chest tightness, wheezing, and shortness of breath
- Nasal congestion, runny nose, and sneezing
- Decreased blood pressure
- Loss of consciousness

Conventional doctors believe that immediate reactions are the most dangerous because they include anaphylaxis, which seriously affects the respiratory and cardiovascular systems and can be fatal. "Anaphylaxis is rapid, generalized, and often unanticipated," says John James, M.D., a specialist in allergy, asthma, and clinical immunology at Colorado Allergy and Asthma Centers, P.C., in Fort Collins. "The most worrisome symptoms involve the respiratory system. Throat tightening, hoarseness,

wheezing, and coughing are all red flags that the reaction is involving the respiratory system."

Immediate reactions are relatively easy to diagnose. If you undergo skin or blood tests, you'll probably test positive for specific IgE antibodies to eggs, peanuts, cow's milk, soy, tree nuts, shellfish, fish, or wheat. Although you can be allergic to practically any food, these eight foods account for approximately 90 percent of true allergic reactions to foods.

Delayed reactions are more common, but in these circumstances the cause-and-effect relationship is more difficult to identify. Up to 72 hours after eating a relatively large amount of a problem food, you can experience any of the above-mentioned symptoms as well as eczema, abdominal pain, and headaches.

If you undergo skin or blood tests, you'll probably test negative for specific IgE antibodies to the most common allergenic foods. In most cases, a well-designed oral food challenge can establish that you do indeed experience adverse reactions to a particular food or foods. The specifics of this food challenge must be worked out between you and your doctor. Conventional doctors acknowledge that some delayed non-IgE food reactions are serious. Celiac disease, for instance, is caused by a sensitivity to the gluten found in wheat, oat, rye, and barley. Its symptoms include abdominal distention and gas, oral ulcers, and an increased risk of cancer.

THE HIDDEN CONNECTION

Aspirin and Foods

If you're sensitive to aspirin, also known as acetylsalicylic acid, you should be aware that certain foods contain high amounts of natural salicylates and could potentially cause an allergic reaction. These include almonds, apples, apricots, blackberries, boysenberries, cherries, cucumbers, currants, dewberries, gooseberries, grapes/raisins, nectarines, oranges, peaches, pickles, plums, prunes, raspberries, strawberries, and tomatoes.

In general, though, conventional doctors believe that immediate food allergies are most deserving of immediate attention. They're also skeptical of claims that delayed food allergies are the hidden causes of scores of serious conditions.

"It's pretty much, you eat the food, you have a reaction," says Jay Portnoy, M.D., chief of allergy, asthma, and immunology at Children's Mercy Hospitals and Clinics in Kansas City, Missouri. "The hidden food allergies you read about, they pretty much don't exist."

All too often, say conventional doctors, the real problem is a "masquerader" of food allergy, such as food intolerance, hiatal hernia, gastrointestinal reflux disease, inflammatory bowel disease, pyloric stenosis, pancreatic insufficiency, gallbladder or peptic ulcer diseases, irritable bowel syndrome, and bacterial, viral, and parasitic infections.

"The public's perception of food allergy is slanted," says Barbara Magera, M.D., an allergist and medical director of Asthma, Allergy, and Immunology Clinic for Adults and Children, L.L.C., in Charleston, South Carolina. "That's because it's safe to blame symptoms on food allergy. In about 25 percent of adults complaining of food allergy, there's no evidence of IgE-mediated disease."

Environmental-medicine doctors and alternative practitioners respond that conventional doctors are too focused on IgE. In their view, delayed allergies may be due to a reaction to another antibody, IgG. In addition, the adverse food reaction may not involve a true food allergy but may be due to other causes like food intolerance or gastrointestinal problems. For example, if someone has an ulcer, he may not be able to eat spicy foods or more than a breadplate–size portion of food.

Although both sides agree that food allergy is strongly associated with asthma, allergic rhinitis, and eczema, environmental-medicine doctors and alternative practitioners believe that food reactions—especially the delayed variety—are associated with more than 100 other conditions. Among them are rheumatoid arthritis, attention deficit hyperactivity disorder, depression, fatigue, insulin-dependent diabetes, irritable bowel syndrome, migraine, and recurrent infections.

"Almost always, it's a reasonable assumption that any kind of chronic illness potentially has a food allergy component," says Robert Rountree, M.D., a holistic physician in Boulder, Colorado, and coauthor of *Immunotics*, a book that provides natural remedies for balancing and strengthening the immune system. "The reason it's a safe assumption is that if you're wrong, there's no harm done in having looked for it. There's no downside in just looking for food allergy." If a food is eliminated and the condition improves, everyone is a winner.

Who Has Food Allergies?

Although food allergy can strike anyone at any age, it's most prevalent in those who are least equipped to cope with it: infants and young children. According to conventional doctors, as many as 10 percent of American youngsters have true, IgE-mediated food allergies, most often to milk, eggs, wheat, soybean products, and peanuts. About 25 percent of them also have an intolerance to orange juice and other fruit juices.

In many cases, food allergy is a step in the "atopic march" that progresses into eczema (atopic dermatitis), allergic rhinitis, and asthma.

When Should You See the Doctor?

You absolutely must be evaluated by a doctor if you've ever experienced even a single episode of food-induced anaphylaxis. You also should see a doctor if you've experienced the following symptoms of a "true" food allergy within 2 hours of eating a suspect food.

- Gastrointestinal symptoms: itching or tingling of the lips, palate, tongue or throat; swelling of the lips or tongue; hoarseness and sensation of tightness in throat; loss of voice; nausea/vomiting; colic or abdominal cramps; diarrhea
- Skin symptoms: hives or angioedema (swelling of the tissues beneath the skin), atopic dermatitis, flushing, itching
- Respiratory symptoms: nasal congestion, itching, sneezing; chest tightness, wheezing, shortness of breath
- Eye symptoms: itching, tearing

Here are some risk factors for developing food allergy.

Heredity. If both of your parents had some kind of allergy, you have a 40 to 60 percent chance of developing allergies, including food allergy. If one parent is allergic, you have a 20 to 40 percent chance of becoming allergic.

Other allergies. Children and adults who already have eczema, allergic rhinitis, or asthma are more likely to develop food allergies. About 35 percent of children with eczema are allergic to one or more foods.

Passive tobacco exposure. A German study of 342 children shows that food allergies are more than twice as common among children of smokers than among children of nonsmokers. Interestingly, prenatal and early exposure to smoke did not increase the risk of allergies to such inhalants as pollen, mold, and animal dander.

Bacterial infection. Researchers have found that infection by CagA-positive *Helicobacter pylori*—the same bacterium that causes ulcer—may increase the risk of food allergy.

Fortunately, most children outgrow their allergies to eggs, milk, wheat, and soybean products by age 10. Unfortunately, they rarely outgrow allergies to peanuts, tree nuts, fish, and shellfish. Together, these four foods account for 90 percent of the food allergy seen in older children and adults. Since they're strongly associated with hives, angioedema (swelling of the tissues beneath the skin), and anaphylaxis, the standard conventional treatment is to permanently exclude them from the diet.

While conventional doctors believe that only 2.5 percent of American adults actually have true IgE-mediated food allergies, environmental-medicine doctors and alternative practitioners believe that such statistics grossly underestimate the extent of the problem. In their view, at least 25 percent of Americans have some kind of food allergy or sensitivity.

Environmental-medicine doctors and alternative practitioners agree that most food allergy begins in childhood, although adult-onset food allergies also occur. But they're more likely to believe that such allergies frequently go unrecognized until adulthood, and they're often likely to pin the blame on a single food: cow's milk.

In their view, a typical scenario unfolds like this: A mother who is allergic to cow's milk passes her allergy to her unborn baby. After birth, the baby does just fine on breast milk as long as the mother does not consume cow's milk. After being switched to cow's milk, however, the baby may develop repeated ear infections, some so serious that drainage tubes must be surgically implanted in the baby's eardrums.

Since the doctor believes that the problem is of bacterial instead of bovine origin, the baby receives repeated courses of antibiotics through childhood. Not only does this not treat the underlying milk allergy, it increases the risk of developing other allergies as well. In fact, many researchers—both conventional and alternative—believe that early antibiotics actually prevent the development of a normal immune system. Their suspicion is based on the "hygiene hypothesis," which holds that allergies are on the rise because our immune systems aren't properly stimulated by infectious organisms in early childhood.

In this scenario, it is not until many years after the fact that it dawns on anyone, including the patient, that the problem began with the introduction of cow's milk. "The patient didn't realize what was going on," says Charles Hinshaw, M.D., an environmental-medicine doctor in Wichita, Kansas, and past president of the American Academy of Environmental Medicine. "They just thought they had all these infections. But they got the infections because of food allergy."

When people develop food allergies in adulthood, an entirely different dynamic comes into play. Both conventional and alternative practitioners agree that the probable cause is years of exposure to a small number of staple foods.

"Constant exposure to large amounts of any one food may lead to sensitization," says Robert Nathan, M.D., associate clinical professor of medicine at the University of Colorado Health Sciences Center in Denver and an allergy practitioner in Colorado Springs. That helps explain why fish allergy is common in Scandinavia and rice allergy is common in Japan.

According to conventional doctors, adults who have allergic rhinitis are prime candidates for developing food allergies. In their view, the usual suspects are peanuts, tree nuts, fish, and shellfish, and the usual symptoms are IgE-mediated.

In contrast, environmental-medicine doctors and alternative practitioners believe that in some cases it's the food allergy that *causes* symptoms similar to rhinitis. "A lot of people think they have environmental reactions when they actually have food sensitivities," says Mark Stengler, N.D., a naturopathic and homeopathic physician in La Jolla, California.

Since environmental-medicine doctors and alternative practitioners don't restrict themselves to investigating IgE-mediated allergies, their list of suspect foods also includes corn, sugar, chocolate, citrus, or any food that you simply "must" have. "The food to which you are most reactive is the food you eat the most and crave the most," explains Allan Lieberman, M.D., an environmental-medicine doctor in North Charleston, South Carolina.

Unlike most conventional doctors, environmental-medicine doctors and alternative practitioners believe that many chronic conditions are associated with food allergy. As an example, Dr. Hinshaw recalls a young tennis instructor whose marriage was on the rocks because of her arthritis.

"She was raised on a farm where she ate beef and corn once or twice a day all year long," Dr. Hinshaw says. Tests revealed that she was allergic to both of these staple foods. When she eliminated them from her diet, her arthritis symptoms disappeared, and her marriage stabilized.

No one knows why some adults suddenly become sensitive to favorite foods while other people can safely eat such foods every day for decades. For now, the best explanation appears to be bad luck. "My patients ask me, 'Why did I develop a food allergy in my fifties? What did I do wrong?'" says Dr. Magera. "The answer is your immune system is just changing. That's the nature of the game."

Oral Allergy Syndrome

If you have a food allergy, you may have noticed that your symptoms are worse during certain times of the year. That's because food allergy symptoms often intensify when trees, grasses, or weeds are pollinating. In some cases, people *only* experience food allergy symptoms when pollen counts are high.

This strange phenomenon is oral allergy syndrome, a little-known condition named after its most notorious symptom: an intense itching and swelling of the lips, tongue, throat, and roof of the mouth. This syndrome almost exclusively affects people with allergic rhinitis. Researchers believe that certain foods cross-react with certain pollens because they share similar proteins.

Although the condition isn't usually life-threatening, it can cause such serious symptoms as generalized hives, severe asthma,

vomiting, diarrhea, and anaphylactic shock.

Unlike most food allergies, oral allergy syndrome isn't triggered by eating foods such as fish, shellfish, eggs, milk, soy, and wheat. Instead, the usual culprits are fresh fruits, vegetables, and nuts.

The good news is that the condition can be prevented. While cooking has no effect on other food allergies, heat usually destroys the protein responsible for oral allergy syndrome.

Conventional doctors believe that the following pollen/food combinations are responsible for most cases of oral allergy syndrome.

• Birch pollen: kiwifruit, apples, pears, plums, prunes, peaches, nectarines, apricots, cherries, celery, carrots, parsnips, parsley, dill, anise, cumin, coriander, caraway, fennel, potatoes, tomatoes, green peppers, lentils, peas, beans, peanuts, hazelnuts, walnuts, almonds, sunflower seeds

• Grass pollen: watermelon, melon, tomatoes, oranges, kiwifruit

• Mugwort pollen: apples, kiwifruit, watermelon, melon, celery, carrots

• Ragweed pollen: bananas, watermelon, cantaloupe, honeydew, zucchini, cucumbers

Natural-rubber latex proteins also can cross-react with certain foods to produce an allergy syndrome. Among them are bananas, kiwifruit, avocado, and chestnuts. (For more information about the latex/food allergy connection, see Latex Allergy on page 327.)

Environmental-medicine doctors often diagnose a similar condition called con-

THE HIDDEN CONNECTION

Pollens and Food

Environmental-medicine doctors believe that a condition called concomitant food allergy can cause increased allergic reactions to specific foods during pollen seasons. They warn their patients about the following cross-reactions:
- Tree pollen: eggs, beef
- Grass pollen: legumes
- Weed pollen (especially ragweed): dairy products, melons, banana, mint
  Environmental-medicine doctors typically advise their patients that when pollen counts are high for a specific type of pollen, avoid eating the foods that cross-react with it.

comitant food allergy. This food sensitivity is intensified by reactions occurring simultaneously between a food and a pollen—but the list of suspect foods is somewhat longer. (See "The Hidden Connection: Pollens and Food.")

Food-Dependent Exercise-Induced Allergy

For most people, food and exercise are two of life's essentials. For some unfortunate souls, however, food and exercise can be a dangerous combination that causes hives, wheezing, and anaphylactic shock.

Athletic women are especially vulnerable to this curious condition, which goes by the unwieldy name of food-dependent exercise-induced allergy. Researchers first identified the condition in 1974. They were struck by the fact that some athletes experienced allergic symptoms when they engaged in vigorous exercise after eating certain foods. Paradoxically, the same athletes experienced no symptoms if they didn't exercise after eating those foods. Today, researchers suspect that the rise in body temperature during exercise somehow triggers the release of histamine and other noxious chemicals.

The reaction usually starts 3 to 4 hours after eating a suspect food, but it can occur up to 24 hours later. One minute, you might be jogging along a city street. The next minute, you develop large hives, tingling and itchy skin, swelling, and faintness.

If you're really unlucky, you might develop the labored breathing and vascular (blood vessel) collapse characteristic of anaphylactic shock. Should you suffer such an attack, you will need an immediate injection of epinephrine. That's why people with

THE HIDDEN CONNECTION

Exercise and Food

For people who have food-dependent exercise-induced allergy, working out after eating certain foods can lead to reactions such as hives, itchy skin, and faintness. In extreme cases, it can even lead to anaphylaxis. Foods associated with this condition include celery, apples, peaches, cabbage, parsnips, shellfish, chicken, and wheat. Spices such as anise, caraway, coriander, cumin, thyme, and sage have also been implicated in the condition.

this condition are advised to avoid problem foods, wait at least 4 hours after eating any food before exercising, and always carry an epinephrine injector. (For more information, see Anaphylaxis on page 211.)

How Are Food Allergies Diagnosed?

Diagnosing a food allergy—especially a delayed food allergy—is a tricky procedure. Since no single skin or blood test has proved reliable in all situations, a combination of steps is usually necessary to make a definitive diagnosis. These steps—and the tests used—may vary depending on what type of doctor you visit.

• Conventional Diagnostic Procedures

One of the first things a conventional doctor will probably do is take a detailed medical history. Some of the things the doctor will

be looking for include symptoms that don't respond to usual therapy, dramatic improvement or worsening of symptoms following a significant change in diet, extreme cravings and dislikes of certain foods, a personal or family history of allergic disorders and food sensitivity, and evidence of oral allergy syndrome or food-dependent exercise-induced allergy, says Marianne Frieri, M.D., Ph.D., professor of medicine and pathology at the State University of New York at Stony Brook and director of the allergy/immunology training program at the Nassau University Medical Center/North Shore University Hospital in East Meadow and Manhasset, New York.

You can play an active role in this process by keeping a food diary for 2 weeks. It should include a detailed record of the foods you eat, listing dates, times, and any symptoms that occurred afterward.

After taking your medical history and examining your food diary, your doctor will conduct tests to measure your sensitivity to specific food allergens. Such tests include skin-prick tests—during which food extracts are scratched into the skin to see if they cause swelling and redness—or blood tests to measure IgE sensitization. If you don't have a strong history of food allergy, the predictive value of a skin-prick test is poor. But if you do, its predictive value is very good. Although blood tests such as a radioallergosorbent test (RAST) and an enzyme-linked immunosorbent assay (ELISA) have become more reliable in recent years, in most cases they still don't provide definitive results.

The final type of test your doctor might use is known as a food or additive challenge. According to Dr. Frieri, this is the *only* definitive diagnostic test for food allergy. Suspect foods are eliminated from your diet for 10 to 14 days, then reintroduced one at a time in gradually increasing portions until you either develop symptoms or can tolerate a normal serving. An "open challenge" test, during which one or two foods are tested daily, can be conducted in a doctor's office or under the supervision of a dietitian. But the gold standard—a double-blind, placebo-controlled food challenge in which neither you nor the doctor knows what you're ingesting—can be performed only in an office setting. The biggest drawback of food challenges is that they're costly and time-consuming. For obvious reasons, they're never performed with foods that are likely to cause anaphylaxis or other severe reactions.

• Environmental and Alternative Diagnostic Procedures

Since conventional laboratory tests for food allergy are unreliable, environmental-medicine doctors and alternative caregivers have developed their own diagnostic procedures. Here are some of their preferred tests.

Provocation/neutralization. During the provocation phase, an extract of the suspect food is administered by injection or sublingual drops. The doctor determines how much allergen is required to produce such symptoms as coughing, throat clearing, watery eyes, rapid pulse, and behavioral changes. During the neutralization phase, the doctor determines how much allergen is required to relieve the symptoms. Only doctors trained in environmental medicine perform this provocation test.

IgG blood tests. Many environmental and alternative practitioners believe that delayed food allergies are mediated by IgG antibodies, so they often send patients' blood samples to laboratories that test for IgG. Since such tests are not standardized, however, they are at best rough guides to identifying problem foods.

Fascinating **fact!**

Medical literature is rife with instances of unusual food reactions. One of the most bizarre cases, however, involved a 66-year-old woman who complained that she got a strawberry-shaped rash on her left buttock whenever she ate strawberries. To verify her complaint, her doctor subjected her to an oral challenge. Sure enough, within 48 hours after eating strawberries, a suspiciously shaped rash appeared just where she said it would.

Electro-dermal testing. The patient holds the suspect food in one hand and a low-voltage wire in the other. A machine measures changes in electrical conductivity. If the reading is low, it's a sign that the patient has an allergy or sensitivity to the food.

Since insurance typically doesn't cover the cost of such tests, patients usually pay for them out of pocket. Mainstream allergy associations oppose their use, citing a lack of credible evidence in their favor. Environmental-medicine doctors, however, note what they believe to be credible evidence. So the debate on insurance coverage for certain tests is ongoing, and we may see changes in the future, says Dr. Hinshaw.

How Are Food Allergies Treated?

Once you've been diagnosed with an allergy to a food or food additive, the only sure way to stay allergy-free is to banish these bad actors from the stage.

Especially if they've ever caused an anaphylactic reaction, it is vital that you systematically and permanently remove from your diet any foods to which you are allergic. "A person can avoid peanuts for 20 years, and then somebody at the next table starts munching on peanuts, and the person keels over," Dr. Rountree says. "It takes only one or two molecules of it to cause a reaction."

In theory, avoidance sounds simple. In practice, however, it can be maddeningly difficult. Not only must you avoid eating the offending foods at home, but you must also find ways to avoid them when eating at restaurants, school cafeterias, picnics, and get-togethers with family and friends.

Fortunately, most people with food allergies are allergic to fewer than four foods. But even if you're allergic to only one or two foods, it can be extremely difficult to

Don't Make This Mistake

If you have an allergy or a sensitivity to a food you love, friends may have told you that you can eat all you want of it as long as you first premedicate yourself with Benadryl or some other over-the-counter antihistamine.

Bad idea.

"Benadryl decreases skin symptoms, but it doesn't do anything for anaphylaxis," says Barbara Magera, M.D., an allergist and medical director of Asthma, Allergy, and Immunology Clinic for Adults and Children, L.L.C., in Charleston, South Carolina. "We're trying to educate patients and doctors—even emergency room doctors—that the first drug of choice for anaphylaxis is not an antihistamine, but injectable epinephrine."

excise them since they're often hidden in processed and restaurant foods.

In addition to avoidance strategies, conventional, environmental-medicine, and alternative practitioners use various modified diets and other techniques to help their patients with food allergies. Let's discuss each school's approach to treatment, beginning with conventional medicine.

• Conventional Treatments

Because conventional doctors realize how difficult it is to not accidentally ingest certain food allergens, they don't just send you out the door with vague instructions to "avoid" certain foods. Their first priority is to give you an unusual kind of "prescription" known as the therapeutic elimination diet.

Often working with a registered dietitian, the doctor will provide detailed instructions on eliminating suspect foods from your diet. Most likely, you will *not* be asked to avoid entire food families. (*Note:* This is not the same as the elimination diets recommended by environmental-medicine doctors and alternative practitioners, which do ask you to avoid entire food families.)

"The key is education and awareness," says Anne Muñoz-Furlong, founder and president of the Food Allergy and Anaphylaxis Network in Fairfax, Virginia. "Know where the traps are. Build on your success and learn from your mistakes, and little by little, you become an expert. It'll take time, but someday you'll ask yourself, 'When did I become so comfortable with this?'"

Although drug interventions are important in treating other allergies, they're controversial in treating food allergy. About the only strategy endorsed by all conventional doctors is using injectable epinephrine to treat anaphylactic and anaphylactoid reactions. Still, since the process of eliminating certain foods is tricky and accidental ingestion can occur, the following drugs are sometimes used to prevent or treat food allergies. In general, however, they do not prevent serious anaphylactic reactions.

Oral antihistamines. First- and second-generation antihistamines can help relieve mild-to-moderate skin or gastrointestinal reactions. In Europe, the antihistamine ketotifen (Apo-Ketotifen) is widely used to prevent IgE-mediated food allergies. It is not commercially available in the United States.

Aspirin and other NSAIDs . These are particularly useful in treating nonallergic, gastrointestinal symptoms.

Oral cromolyn (Gastrocrom). Although not all conventional doctors agree on its efficacy, some argue that it can prevent allergic reactions if taken 15 minutes before meals and snacks.

Other drugs. Some doctors prescribe corticosteroids and leukotriene inhibitors such as zafirlukast (Accolate) to modify food allergy symptoms.

Immunotherapy, a cornerstone of conventional treatment in which the patient is given minute amounts of the allergen in an attempt to "desensitize" him, has not been proven effective for food allergy. In fact, it can be dan-

(continued on page 294)

Food Allergens Run in "Families"

If you're allergic or sensitive to a particular food, you might also experience adverse reactions to other foods in the same family, because they share similar proteins. For example, if you're allergic to cantaloupe, you might also be allergic to pumpkin.

Here are some "families" in which cross-reactions are common. If you are allergic to any item in the family, be especially cautious about consuming other foods in that family.

Cereal Grains
- Bamboo, barley, corn, hominy, malt (germinated grain), millet, oat, popcorn, rice, rye, sorghum, sugarcane, wheat (bran, germ, gliadin, globulin, glutenin, leucosin, proteose, whole)

Dairy Products (cow and goat)
- Butter, buttermilk, casein, cheese, ice cream, lactalbumin, milk (condensed, evaporated, homogenized, powdered, raw, skim), select infant formulas, sour cream, whipped cream, yogurt

Eggs
- Ovomucoid, ovovitellin, white, whole, yolk

Fish and Shellfish
- Fish: anchovies, black bass, bonito, bullhead, carp, catfish, cod, crappie, croaker, drum, eel, flounder, grayling, grouper, haddock, hake, halibut, herring, mackerel, mullet, muskellunge, perch, pickerel, pike, pollack, pompano, porgy, redfish, red snapper, rockfish, salmon, sardines, scrod, sea trout, shad, smelt, sole, sprat, sturgeon (caviar), sunfish, swordfish, trout, tuna, weakfish, white bass, whitefish
- Crustaceans: crab, crayfish, lobster, prawn, shrimp
- Mollusks: abalones, clams, cockles, mussels, octopus, oysters, quahogs, scallops, snails (escargot), squid

Fruit
- Apple family: apple cider vinegar, apples, cider, crabapples, pears, quince, quince seed
- Banana family: bananas, plantains

- Citrus family: citron, grapefruit, kumquats, lemons, limes, oranges, tangelos, tangerines
- Gourd (melon) family: cantaloupe (muskmelon), casaba (winter muskmelon), Chinese watermelon, citron melon, cucumbers, gherkins, honeydew melon, Persian melon, pumpkin, summer squash, watermelon, winter squash
- Grape family: champagne, grapes, grape wine, raisins, wine vinegar
- Heath family: black huckleberries, blueberries, cranberries, wintergreen
- Mulberry family: breadfruit, breadnut, fig, hop
- Olive family: jasmine, olives
- Palm family: cabbage palm, coconut, dates
- Papaya family: papain, papaya
- Plum family: almonds, apricots, cherries, peaches, nectarines, plums, prunes
- Saxifrage family: currants, gooseberries

Fungi

- Mushrooms, truffles, yeast (baker's, brewer's, distiller's, Fleischmann's yeast, lactose-fermenting, lager beer)

Herbs and Spices

- Ginger family: cardamom, East Indian arrowroot, ginger, turmeric
- Laurel family: avocado, bay leaf, cinnamon, sassafras
- Mint family: balm, basil, catnip, horehound, Japanese artichoke, lavender, marjoram, mint, oregano, peppermint, rosemary, sage, savory, spearmint, thyme
- Myrtle family: allspice, clove, guava, myrtle, pimento
- Nutmeg family: mace, nutmeg

Legumes

- Acacia, alfalfa, black-eyed peas (cowpeas), broad beans (fava beans), carbo beans (St. John's bread), chickpeas (garbanzo), common beans (kidney, navy, pinto, string), Jack beans, lentils, licorice, lima beans, mesquite, peas, peanuts, soybeans, tamarind, tragacanth

Meats

- Poultry: chicken, Cornish hen, duck, goose, grouse, guinea hen, partridge, pheasant, pigeon, quail, squab, turkey

(continued)

Food Allergens Run in "Families" (cont.)

Meats (cont.)

- Red meats: cow (beef, calf, steer, veal), gelatin, goat, ox, pig (bacon, boar, ham, hog, pork, sausage, scrapple, sow, swine), sheep (lamb, mutton), sweetbreads

Nuts

- Beech family: beechnuts, chestnuts, chinquapin
- Birch family: filberts, hazelnuts, wintergreen
- Cashew family: cashews, mangoes, pistachios
- Cola nut family: chocolate (cocoa), cola (kola) nuts
- Pine family: juniper, pine nuts (pignoli)
- Walnut family: black walnuts, butternuts, English walnuts, hickory nuts, pecans

Vegetables

- Buckwheat family: buckwheat, rhubarb, sorrel
- Goosefoot family: beets, lamb's-quarters, spinach, Swiss chard
- Lily family: aloe, asparagus, chives, garlic, leek, onions, sarsaparilla, shallots
- Mallow family: cottonseed, marshmallow, okra
- Morning glory family: sweet potatoes, yams
- Mustard family: broccoli, brussels sprouts, cabbage, cauliflower, collards, garden cress, horseradish, kale, kohlrabi, mustard, radishes, rutabagas, turnips, watercress
- Nightshade family: bell peppers, cayenne pepper, chiles (paprika, red pepper), eggplant, ground cherries, melon, pears, potatoes (white), strawberry tomatoes, tobacco, tomatoes, tree tomatoes
- Parsley family: anise, caraway, carrots, celeriac, celery, coriander, dill, fennel, parsley, parsnips
- Sunflower family: absinthe (sagebrush, wormwood), artichoke, chamomile, chicory, dandelion, endive, escarole, Jerusalem artichoke, lettuce, oyster plant (salsify), safflower, sunflower seeds, tansy, tarragon

gerous. At least one death has resulted from experimental trials to "desensitize" patients to problem foods. Still, researchers hope to develop safe and effective immunotherapies for food allergy within 10 years.

Meanwhile, you might want to consider trying traditional immunotherapy, especially if you're allergic to pollen, mold, and other inhalants, says Dr. Frieri. Such immunotherapy may indirectly help relieve food allergies, she adds, especially the oral allergy syndrome related to inhalant allergy.

• Environmental-Medicine Treatments

Since environmental-medicine doctors use tests that usually diagnose multiple food allergies, they're more likely than conventional doctors to prescribe an extremely stringent elimination diet.

Environmental-medicine doctors also often insist that patients stay on an elimination diet indefinitely. One such diet instructs patients to avoid all dairy products, wheat, corn, eggs, citrus fruits, refined sugars, and artificial colors, flavors, preservatives, and sweeteners. Allowable foods include soy milk, oats, millet, barley, buckwheat, rice, amaranth, quinoa, legumes, all vegetables except corn, and all fruits except citrus.

"If you put people on a really good diet, you can decrease their food allergies because it reduces the total load on their immune systems," says Steven Bock, M.D., cofounder and codirector of the Rhinebeck Health Center in Rhinebeck, New York, and the Center for Progressive Medicine in Albany.

The problem is that some patients find an elimination diet so difficult to follow that they give up. Other patients adhere to the diet so zealously that they become malnourished. In extreme cases, patients misinterpret signs of starvation as symptoms of food allergy, which prompts them to eliminate even more foods from their diets.

"If you're ever asked to go on an elimination diet, it takes an incredible amount of motivation, and it's not designed for chronic

Battle Food Reactions with Baking Soda

Among environmental-medicine doctors and alternative practitioners, one of the most potent weapons in the war against food allergy reactions is ordinary baking soda.

"Allergic reactions are basically associated with intracellular acidosis," says Charles Hinshaw, M.D., an environmental-medicine doctor in Wichita, Kansas, and past president of the American Academy of Environmental Medicine. "The acid-base balance in the cell is slightly skewed toward the acid side."

To prevent or relieve a food reaction, you can use plain baking soda (sodium bicarbonate) or Alka-Seltzer Gold, which contains sodium bicarbonate and potassium bicarbonate. Follow the manufacturers' recommendations for heartburn relief on the side of either box. Both products contain an alkali that's quickly absorbed by the stomach, so you should get a response in 10 to 15 minutes.

Note: This remedy should be used only to treat mild-to-moderate reactions. For more serious reactions, such as anaphylaxis, follow the Anaphylaxis Action Plan on page 217.

use," says Dr. Magera. "I've actually seen some patients who go on eating only lamb, water, rice, and chicken, and they are obviously not getting enough nutrition in their diets. Not only are you what you eat, you are what you don't eat."

Recognizing the risks inherent in strin-gent elimination diets, many environmental-medicine doctors offer a somewhat easier-to-follow prescription, known as the rotary diversified diet.

Patients on this diet are instructed to not eat any food, in any amount or form, more often than once every 4 days. Obviously, this

Dr. Rountree's Natural Food-Allergy Protocol

When he treats anyone with allergies—including food allergies—Robert Rountree, M.D., a holistic physician in Boulder, Colorado, and coauthor of *Immunotics*, a book that provides natural remedies for balancing and strengthening the immune system, recommends the following regimen of vitamins, minerals, and nutrients. But, depending on the severity of your allergy, he suggests that you consult a nutritionist, chiropractor, or naturopath before taking supplements.

- Tocopherol (vitamin E) complex: 200 to 400 IU
- Selenium: 200 micrograms
- Zinc: 20 to 40 milligrams
- Vitamin C: 2,000 milligrams
- Quercetin: 500 to 3,000 milligrams
- Proanthocyanidin (grape seed extract): 50 to 150 milligrams
- EPA (eicosapentaenoic acid from fish oil): 500 to 3,000 milligrams
- GLA (gamma-linolenic acid, from borage or black currant seed oil): 300 milligrams

"Quercetin is by far my favorite supplement for all allergies," Dr. Rountree says. "It's also good for leaky-gut syndrome. You're treating the gut and also getting an anti-inflammatory effect that keeps the mast cells from exploding."

Other supplements Dr. Rountree recommends for food allergy include betaine hydrochloride, glutamine, and nettle. "Some people have reported freeze-dried nettle as being very helpful for food allergies," he notes. He recommends nettle mostly for respiratory symptoms like sneezing, runny nose, or wheezing. "Nettle is sometimes helpful for hives as well," Dr. Rountree adds. Take two 300-milligram capsules immediately after the onset of allergic symptoms and continue every few hours until symptoms improve.

requires some planning. Environmental-medicine doctors believe that by not eating any one food too often, patients can become less likely to react to certain foods. They also believe that this diet can help prevent food allergy in patients who haven't developed food sensitivities.

Here are some other treatments.

Optimal-dose immunotherapy. Unlike conventional doctors, environmental doctors believe that by using provocation/neutralization testing, food allergies can be safely diagnosed and treated simultaneously. Injections of food extracts are

For hard-to-diagnose food allergies, Dr. Rountree recommends a 3-day fast (liquid cleansing), either under a doctor's supervision or on your own. Obviously, any kind of fast should be undertaken only if your overall health is good. Don't fast if you have insulin-dependent diabetes, hypoglycemia, or a seizure disorder or are in a generally weakened condition, says Dr. Rountree. Following are two types of fasts Dr. Rountree recommends; note that a traditional water fast can be too hard on your system.

UltraClear fast. This brand-name product is essentially a rice protein with extra nutrients for liver support and is available through licensed health care practitioners.

Juice fast. During this type of fast, you drink a wide variety of organic fruit and vegetable juices, supplemented with a small amount of watery cream of rice cereal. "If you feel fabulous after a fast, then you know your problems are caused by something you're eating," Dr. Rountree says. "Then you can go on a modified elimination diet, where you take out the most obvious offenders like wheat, dairy, corn, soy, eggs, and citrus."

Once you've identified foods that cause immediate immunoglobulin E (IgE)–mediated allergies, your only recourse is to avoid them. But if your problem foods are responsible for delayed immunoglobulin G (IgG)–mediated reactions that aren't too severe, it's possible to reintroduce them into your diet with a strategy called oral tolerance.

"You might start out once a week with ⅛ teaspoon of milk," Dr. Rountree says. "You use a tiny amount about once a week, then go to once every 3 days or so, until your body can handle a fairly large amount." He cautions, however, that this can take many months or even a year.

typically given at least once a week.

Enzyme-potentiated desensitization. Used to desensitize patients to a broad range of foods, this procedure involves the injection of extremely small amounts of food extracts, which have been mixed with the enzyme beta-glucuronide to increase, or "potentiate," the effect.

Intravenous sodium bicarbonate. Environmental-medicine doctors base this treatment on the premise that the blood becomes too acidic during allergic reactions. By injecting patients with an alkaline solution of sodium bicarbonate, they can often neutralize even a strong reaction in 2 to 10 minutes.

Mainstream allergists consider most environmental-medicine treatments to be experimental and unproven.

• Alternative Treatments

Alternative practitioners treat food allergies much the same as they treat other allergies. Modalities include vitamin, mineral, and herbal supplementation; homeopathy; elimination and rotary diets; chiropractic manipulation; and acupuncture.

The following dietary supplements are used by Dr. Stengler to strengthen the gut, improve digestion, and prevent adverse reactions to food. Check with your caregiver before trying dietary supplements to treat food allergies.

Digestive herbs. Gingerroot, dandelion root, and gentian root—sometimes called "king of the bitters"—stimulate stomach-acid enzyme production and retrain the di-

gestive system to work more efficiently. These bitter herbs are best taken 5 to 15 minutes before each meal. Recommended dosages for each are one 300-milligram capsule or 30 drops of extract.

Note: Such herbs can cause allergic reactions. People with stomach ulcers should avoid gentian root.

Microbial enzymes. Derived from fungi, these contain a full spectrum of digestive enzymes. "I typically recommend microbial enzymes over other enzymes because of their potency, purity, and stability," Dr. Stengler says. Take as directed on the container, usually one to two capsules with meals.

Plant enzymes. The two best-known examples are bromelain from pineapple and papain from papaya. Both can be taken with meals to help with the digestion of protein. When taken on an empty stomach, bromelain has a natural anti-inflammatory effect. Take as directed on the container.

Animal enzymes. Pancreatic enzymes are derived from pig or sheep pancreas. Bile enzymes and salts are derived from ox gallbladder. Take as directed on the container.

Note: Although they appear to have therapeutic benefits, animal enzymes are of questionable purity. Even the enteric-coated varieties are vulnerable to stomach acids.

Homeopathy. According to Dr. Stengler, homeopathy can desensitize patients to certain foods. Remedies include a grain mix, which contains wheat, barley, and rye, as well as a dairy mix. They're usually given in low potency such as 3X or 6X. Patients are instructed to take 5 to 15 drops of the solution one or two times daily, usually for at least 1 month and sometimes for several months. "Homeopathic drops (for patients who are sensitive to particular foods) and microbial enzymes are usually where I start," says Dr. Stengler. The other treatments may follow.

Dietary Supplements Can Cause Allergies, Too

If you take herbs for allergies or any other condition, you should know that many of them have been documented as causing allergic reactions. "Herbal medications need careful evaluation for potential adverse events, especially in individuals with allergic rhinitis, asthma, and atopic dermatitis," says Marianne Frieri, M.D., Ph.D., professor of medicine and pathology at the State University of New York at Stony Brook and director of the allergy/immunology training program at the Nassau University Medical Center/North Shore University Hospital in East Meadow and Manhasset, New York.

Dr. Frieri has seen four patients who developed hives after taking ginseng and glucosamine, one who wound up in the emergency room after taking bee pollen, and one who developed an autoimmune disease after taking kava-kava.

Another patient developed symptoms from drinking tea made from chamomile. "She came to me with the worst case of angioedema (swelling of the tissues beneath the skin) and urticaria (hives) that I've ever seen," Dr. Frieri says.

She also cites research showing that bioflavonoids—substances that get high marks from alternative allergy practitioners—can cause anemia and kidney damage.

Here are some other medicinal plants frequently associated with allergic reactions.

• Angelica	• Elecampane	• Meadowsweet
• Aniseed	• Euphorbia	• Motherwort
• Apricot	• Feverfew	• Parsley
• Arnica	• Fucus	• Pilewort
• Artichoke	• Gravel root	• Plantain
• Asofoetida	• Guaiacum	• Pulsatilla
• Boneset	• Holy thistle	• Rosemary
• Cassia	• Hops	• Royal jelly
• Celery	• Hydrangea	• Tansy
• Cinnamon	• Hydrocotyle	• Vitex
• Cowslip	• Juniper	• Wild carrot
• Dandelion	• Lady's slipper	• Yarrow

Food Allergy ACTION PLAN

Successfully coping with a food allergy requires you to be alert everywhere—the supermarket, restaurants, picnics, and parties. By being a savvy consumer, you'll be on your way to avoiding even hidden sources of food allergens.

Deciphering Food Labels

• Read every line. It doesn't matter if you've purchased a product 500 times. Manufacturers often change ingredients. Unless you read the fine print, you might not notice that, say, a milk derivative has become part of the lineup. (Several major food industry groups have voluntary guidelines to identify allergy-provoking ingredients on the labels of processed foods. The industry groups strongly encourage their members to follow these guidelines.) You must know your triggers and be familiar with all their other names. For example, casein and whey indicate the presence of cow's milk. In addition, pay attention to the following other potentially troublesome areas.

The "2 percent rule." The FDA requires companies to list ingredients on the package in rank order. But when they get to the very small quantities—2 percent or less—the ingredients don't have to be listed. They can be lumped. That's where you're going to see flavorings and spices, which can include almost any food that commonly causes allergies.

"May contain." This generally indicates that the food was processed with equipment that processed other foods, such as peanuts. Some manufacturers use an alternative label: "May contain the occasional nut."

"Nondairy" foods. Because of a loophole, foods that contain the milk derivatives casein or caseinates can legally be advertised as nondairy.

Kosher labels. A "D" on the label means the product contains dairy. "DE" means it was processed on dairy equipment. If you're allergic to milk, either symbol is a sign to stay away.

Food additives. Regulations now require manufacturers to list food colorings such as yellow dye no. 5 (tartrazine) as well as the sources of protein and hydrolysates. Therefore, a statement that once read "protein hydrolysates" must now read "wheat hydrolysates, soy hydrolysates," and so on.

- When in doubt, don't buy it. Avoid buying foods that don't have an ingredient listing. Also beware of foods with foreign-language ingredient statements. Labeling laws in other countries aren't as strict as they are in the United States.
- Call a toll-free number. If you see "natural flavors," "artificial flavors," or "spices" on a label, call the company and ask specifically if that means milk, eggs, peanuts, or whatever you're trying to avoid.

Smart Shopping

- Beware the bulk-food bins. If you've ever seen how people spill food from bin to bin, you know why it's a good idea to stay away.
- Choose wisely at the deli. Avoid buying deli meats if you're allergic to milk. The same machine is often used to slice both cheese and meat products.
- If you're allergic to nuts, shun the baked goods aisle. Muffins and other baked goods often contain nuts or other ingredients that you may not suspect. An "almond-coated" doughnut, for instance, can actually be coated with sliced peanuts.

Home Food Preparation

- Organize your pantry. Use separate shelves to store allergenic and nonallergenic foods.
- Use different pots and pans. When cooking allergenic and nonallergenic meals, use separate pots, pans, and utensils to prevent cross-contact. If you must use the same pots and pans, wash them thoroughly with soap and water. The same goes for kitchen cabinets, counters, and chopping boards. Wiping or rinsing will not remove allergenic proteins.
- Use separate grills. Avoid barbecuing allergenic and nonallergenic foods on the same grill.
- Know your cooking oils. Highly processed oils are considered safe because they don't contain allergenic proteins. The ones to watch out for are the gourmet oils labeled as cold-pressed, extruded, or expelled. In addition, be sure not to use the same cooking oil for allergenic and nonallergenic meals.
- Stock your freezer. Cook several allergy-free meals at a time and keep at least one spare meal in the freezer.

• Plan ahead for "mistakes." Even the most careful cook can accidentally cross-contaminate meals. Get a written emergency plan from your doctor. Make sure everyone knows where medications and doctors' phone numbers are kept. Hold a practice drill.

Eating Out

• Call ahead. To find a restaurant that will work with you, call the manager and explain the seriousness of your food allergy. Ask about the ingredients the restaurant uses in its meals. Ensure that the allergy is noted on the reservation.

• Be specific. Don't simply ask the waiter or waitress, "Does this have milk in it?" Show a card that lists all the different names for milk products and ask, "Does this contain any of these products?" Also, be aware of what common menu terms indicate about the ingredients in a dish. For example, "souffle" usually means eggs. "Hollandaise" means egg and butter. "Au gratin" means cheese. "Seviche" or "carpaccio" means raw fish. "Bisque" means cream. "Deviled" means mayonnaise, which means that eggs were used.

• Order simple meals. When ordering from a menu, choose simply prepared foods such as baked potatoes, steamed vegetables, or broiled meat.

• Avoid the plethora of peanuts. Chefs have used peanuts and peanut products in everything from brown gravy, piecrusts, chili, and spaghetti sauce to egg rolls, brownies, and cheesecake. Even pesto sauce sometimes includes peanuts instead of pine nuts because peanuts are cheaper.

• Steer clear of fried foods. Since many restaurants fry a variety of foods in the same oil, your "nonallergenic" meal can contain residues of many allergenic proteins.

• Think twice about Asian restaurants. If you have a peanut, nut, or fish allergy, Asian restaurants are high-risk because woks are typically wiped clean instead of washed clean after they're used to prepare a meal.

• Keep the lid on covered dishes. You never know what's in a pot pie or other covered dish until you bite into it.

• Beware of wheat imitations. Chefs sometimes use wheat flour to prepare imitation chicken or beef pieces in vegetarian dishes. In particular, steer clear if the menu mentions seitan, which is a key ingredient in the popular Chinese vegetarian dish Buddha's Delight. Seitan is made from the protein in wheat.

- Put a buffer between you and buffet desserts. These are notorious for containing hidden nuts.

- Inquire about your fast food. If the restaurant fries both potatoes and cheese sticks, and they use a common fryer, your french fries may be contaminated with dairy.

- Attend a safe party, picnic, or sleep-over. Alert the host or hostess that you or a family member has food allergies. Offer to bring an allergy-free dish or dessert.

Identify Hidden Sources of Trouble

Knowledge is the key to managing your food allergies. Check out the following categories of common food allergens and the unlikely places they're found. Keep this information handy the next time you go grocery shopping.

Dairy

- Shirk suspect foods. Cow's milk is not only found in obvious sources like fresh, powdered, and evaporated milk; buttermilk; cheese and cream cheese; yogurt; ice cream; pudding; butter; and sour cream and imitation sour cream. It's also in some breads and pastries (except "kosher parve" or similar breads); margarine (except margarine made with soybean oil); flavorings (caramel, Bavarian cream, coconut cream, brown sugar); milk chocolate and other candies; cream sauces and soups; sherbet; puddings; pastas; some luncheon meats, hot dogs, and sausages; high-protein flour; nondairy milk substitutes containing caseinate; baking mixes; pies with cream filling or made with butter; granola; salad dressings; and many "nondairy" products.

  Note: Manufacturers add caseinates (a milk derivative) to canned tuna so it won't look like cat food.

- Learn the aliases. Some of them are casein, caseinates (ammonium, calcium, magnesium, potassium, sodium); whey (sweet, delactosed, protein concentrate); lactalbumin and lactalbumin phosphate; lactose and lactulose; rennet casein; hydrolysates (casein, milk protein, protein, whey, whey protein). Look for the names on food labels and avoid those foods.

- Become familiar with milk substitutes. Water, soy milk, rice milk, fruit juices, and 100 percent soy margarine can substitute for milk in most recipes. If you're worried about not getting enough calcium in your diet, drink calcium-fortified soy milk and eat calcium-rich foods such as spinach, salmon canned with bones, bok choy, napa cabbage, sesame seeds, collard greens, kale, turnip greens, dandelion greens, mustard greens, and broccoli.
- Realize how little is needed to cause a reaction. If you're severely allergic to milk, you can have a reaction even if a few drops are spilled on your skin.

Eggs

- Unearth uncommon hiding places. Egg white (the most allergenic part) can be found in "lemon" drinks, cocktail mixes, processed meats, wine, and coffee. It's also used as a foaming agent in root beer.
- Don't be fooled by a name. All of the following translate into "egg," so steer clear of products that list them as ingredients: albumin, ovomucin, ovomucoid, livetin, ovovitellin, and vitellin.
- Use caution with flu vaccines. If you're allergic to eggs, you may have been told to forgo getting a flu vaccine since it contains small amounts of egg protein. Research shows, however, that you may be able to safely receive an influenza vaccine in a two-dose protocol if the vaccine contains less than 1.2 micrograms of egg protein per milliliter. Ask your doctor about this option.

Food Additives

- Know which additives to subtract from your diet. Of the hundreds of additives found in food, only a handful have been linked to adverse reactions. Most of these reactions were not associated with allergies. The potentially harmful additives include the following:

  Aspartame. Commonly known as Nutrasweet, this artificial sweetener can cause swelling of the eyelids, lips, hands, or feet.

  Benzoates. These preservatives are used in the processing of bananas, cake, cereal, chocolate, dressings, fats, licorice, margarine, mayonnaise, powdered milk, oils, powdered potatoes, and dry yeast.

  BHA/BHT. Butylated hydroxyanisole (BHA) and butylated hydroxytoluene (BHT) are antioxidants usually added to foods containing fats and oils, most often cereal and other grain products. BHT is found in ready-made foods, bread, milk, fats, oils, margarine, mayonnaise, soft drinks, and instant drinks.

Carmine. A red dye derived from the dried bodies of certain insects, carmine has been associated with allergic reactions and is found in many foods and cosmetics.

MSG. Monosodium glutamate, a flavor enhancer, is often used in processing peanuts, dried tomatoes, soups, oriental foods, and soy sauce. It's commonly found in processed foods and Chinese cooking. Many Chinese restaurants will honor requests to eliminate MSG from a meal.

Nitrates and nitrites. These preservatives and flavor enhancers are most often found in spinach, beets, radishes, lettuce, and packaged meats such as sausage, bacon, lunchmeats, and hot dogs.

Sulfites. These preservatives include sulfur dioxide, sodium or potassium sulfite, bisulfite, and metabisulfite. They're most often found in dried fruits and vegetables; gelatin products; pickles; sausage; wine, wine coolers, and cider; vinegar; some fruit juices; cider; molasses; cookies and crackers; shellfish; beer; citrus drinks; prepared potatoes and potato chips; mushrooms; and guacamole. In 1986, customer complaints prompted the FDA to ban the use of sulfites in restaurant salad bars.

Yellow dye no. 5. The Food, Drug, and Cosmetic Act of 1938 approved a number of dyes used in foods and beverages. They are identified on labels by color and number. FD&C yellow no. 5—or tartrazine—has been associated with asthma. Although it's less commonly used now than in the past, it can be found in flavored drinks, candies, sherbet, pudding, frosting, dry cereals, and some medicines. Beware of any food product or medicine colored yellow or green.

Fish and Shellfish

- Beware of surimi. If you're allergic to fish, it's not enough to avoid fish fillets and chowders. You also need to watch out for surimi. Used to make imitation crab legs, crabmeat, and lobster products, surimi is reconstituted fish muscle. It's also sometimes used in pizza toppings and meatless hot dogs.

- Don't get glued. If you're extremely allergic to fish, you can react to the fish extracts used in some glues.

- Know that a whiff can be enough. Some people can develop asthma symptoms just from the odor of cooking fish.

Peanuts and Tree Nuts

- Know where nuts might lurk. Peanuts are found in M&M's, spaghetti sauces, and many precooked foods that don't list them on the label. Minced, ground, and otherwise camouflaged nuts are often among the ingredients in "plain" chocolate, barbecue sauce, chili, ice cream, and baked goods.
- Watch who you kiss. If you're severely allergic to peanuts, you can have a reaction simply by kissing someone who's recently eaten a peanut product.

Soy

- Become acquainted with the many products containing soy. Soy isn't found only in such obvious sources as soy milk, soybean noodles and pasta, soy sauce, soy cheese, and tofu. It's also found in breads, cakes, crackers, candy, cereals, hydrolyzed vegetable protein, ice cream, lecithin, miso, nondairy frozen desserts, margarine, infant formulas, processed meats and sausages, salad dressings, sauces, shortening (including Crisco), soups, soy protein isolates, soy fiber (okara, soy bran, soy isolate fiber), textured soy protein, soy nuts, soy nut butter, tempeh, and yuba (also called dried bean curd, bean curd sheets, and bean curd skin).

Wheat

- Be wise to wheat. Not only is wheat found in breads, buns, and pastas, it's also found in breaded foods; gravies thickened with flour; soups and sauces; candies, cookies, and other baked goods; beer, malted milk, and soft drinks such as Coca-Cola; breakfast food and cereals; canned baked beans; chili; and meat products such as hamburgers, meat loaf, hot dogs, and sausage.
- Watch out for "wheat" words. Avoid products that list wheat bran, gum, cornstarch, gluten, food starch, enriched flour, or vegetable starch/gum on the label.
- Investigate wheat substitutes. Try using other grains such as quinoa, amaranth, and millet.

Hay FEVER

THE NEXT TIME you have hay fever, with its accompanying itchy nose, watery eyes, and sneezing fits, don't think of it as "hay fever."

Think of it as Rodney Dangerfield.

Hay fever is an outdated term from the days when more people lived around farms. We now know it has nothing to do with hay and doesn't involve having a fever. These days, it affects up to 40 million Americans, making it the fifth most common chronic illness in the country.

Since it has become such a widespread problem and we know so much more about it, from now on in the chapter we'll use its official name, "allergic rhinitis," which means an inflammation in the nose caused by allergies.

So how does Rodney Dangerfield enter the picture? William Berger, M.D., compares the condition to the bumbling comedian because neither gets any respect.

"At first look, it appears that it's no big deal—just a runny nose. But as you really investigate and start to understand this disease, you realize that it actually causes more problems than almost any other disease," says Dr. Berger, clinical professor in the department of pediatrics and department of allergy and immunology at the University of California, Irvine, and author of *Allergies and Asthma for Dummies*.

The Cause of More Than Just Sniffling

Thinking of your nose as just a lump on the front of your face is like seeing the front porch but overlooking the whole house behind it.

Your nose—that is, the empty space behind your nostrils—is connected to your sinuses, ears, mouth, and lungs. When the symptoms of rhinitis strike, these related body parts can be affected, too.

Allergic rhinitis can lead to sinusitis, an infection in the sinuses that can make life truly miserable. It can also contribute to ear infections, which can lead to muffled hearing and learning difficulties in children. Because the nose and lungs are part of the same pathway, allergic rhinitis is frequently seen in patients with asthma.

And here's a real surprise: The condition, which most often develops before the age of 20 and frequently between ages 5 and 15, can cause crooked teeth and changes in the shape of the face, too. Since congestion in the nose often leads people to breathe through their mouths when they're asleep, they tend to thrust their tongues forward into their teeth. "I'd say that the majority of my teenagers with allergic rhinitis are wearing braces," Dr. Berger says.

If the thought of all those maladies isn't enough to make you view that lowly stopped-up nose in a new light, simply consider the way it can drag down your everyday life. "There have been studies that have shown that allergic rhinitis actually causes greater quality-of-life issues than heart disease, in terms of the patient's daily activities being affected," Dr. Berger says. In a study of people with allergic rhinitis conducted by the Children's Hospital of

Allergic Rhinitis May Cause Itching at the Table

Normally an apple, banana, or melon leaves behind just a fruity taste on the tongue. But for some people with allergic rhinitis, a mouthful of one of these foods can feel like a mouthful of itching powder.

This condition, known as oral allergy syndrome, is often found in people with seasonal allergic rhinitis. After eating fresh fruits and vegetables, the person's lips, tongue, palate, and throat will start to itch, due to a cross-reaction between some pollens and foods.

Melons and bananas cross-react with ragweed pollen. Apples, carrots, hazelnuts, potatoes, and almonds cross-react with birch pollen. Celery, apples, and kiwifruit cross-react with mugwort pollen. And bananas, kiwifruit, avocado, and chestnuts cross-react with latex.

While oral allergy syndrome is more of a minor annoyance than a health threat, you should seek medical help if your throat starts closing or you break out in hives and feel itchy all over your body after eating a food. This is a life-threatening reaction not to be confused with oral allergy syndrome. (For more information, see Food Allergies and Intolerances on page 278.)

Pittsburgh, 42 percent said that the condition had recently caused them to have difficulty sleeping. Twenty-eight percent said that they had been unable to do routine activities, and 14 percent had been unable to perform their normal workload. In another study, at the Hennepin County Medical Center in Minneapolis, symptoms such as increased irritability, fatigue, and increased sadness occurred in 81 percent of the allergic patients studied.

Still, the public isn't especially worked up over allergic rhinitis. You certainly won't find celebrities rallying to call attention to it (and let's not even think about what color the commemorative ribbon would be). And doctors stay busy enough dealing with life-threatening conditions like heart disease and diabetes. In fact, that same Children's Hospital survey showed that nearly two-thirds of people with allergies had never heard from their doctors about the other conditions that can be connected to allergic rhinitis. Allergies just don't get respect—except from the pharmaceutical industry.

Pharmaceutical companies have long provided a whole arsenal of drugs to combat the symptoms of allergic rhinitis. Antihistamines have long been a mainstay in treating the condition, but the older, over-the-counter versions are infamous for making the user sleepy. Newer prescription nonsedating versions, like loratadine (Claritin) and fexofenadine (Allegra), burst onto the scene with a flurry of advertisements that were as hard to ignore as a sneezing fit in church.

Doctors have grown enthusiastic about using inhaled steroid nasal sprays to fight allergic rhinitis symptoms, and supermarket customers have shelves full of over-the-counter decongestants to try as well.

While your medication choices for treating this problem are legion, so are your natural treatment options. The first step experts recommend is as natural as they come: Learn to avoid your allergy triggers. In addition to avoidance, conventional and alternative doctors alike have embraced the notion of washing symptoms away with salt water. Plus, supplements like quercetin and nettle may give you even more ways to control your allergic rhinitis.

Before we consider how to fix it, though, let's talk about what's causing the problem.

What's Going On in There?

While you may associate your nose most often with your ability to smell, it serves many other valuable functions. As you breathe in through your nose, it quickly warms and humidifies the air, making it more comfortable before it hits your lungs. The mucus-producing lining also protects you from germs, dust, and other bits of debris that get sucked into your nose.

Your nasal passages, and the sinuses connected to them, are lined with microscopic hairs called cilia. These hairs beat back and forth in waves, propelling a blanket of mucus over them. Imagine a crowd in a football stadium passing along a banner overhead, person to person, and you get the picture of how cilia work.

As you breathe in unwanted particles, the sticky mucus captures and carries them as it is passed along to the back of your throat, where you swallow it, and then your stomach disintegrates it all. You produce

Rhinitis Comes in Many Styles

About half the people with rhinitis have types that aren't brought on by allergies or that are a combination of allergic and nonallergic rhinitis, according to William Berger, M.D., clinical professor in the department of pediatrics and department of allergy and immunology at the University of California, Irvine, and author of *Allergies and Asthma for Dummies*. Here's a quick look at some of the common types and triggers of nonallergic rhinitis.

Infectious. The same symptoms of allergic rhinitis—sneezing, burning in the nose and throat, and runny nose—are often caused by the common cold virus.

When you have a normal cold uncomplicated by other problems like a bacterial infection, expect your symptoms to go away in 4 to 10 days. If you have asthma, take care to manage extra airway problems, which often crop up during a cold.

The rest of what you should do falls closely to Mom's traditional advice: Get plenty of rest and drink lots of hot fluids.

Vasomotor. This type typically crops up during middle age and is the most likely cause when a person older than 50 suddenly starts having symptoms of rhinitis. The main problem with vasomotor rhinitis tends to be nasal congestion and postnasal drip, but unlike in allergic rhinitis, there usually aren't sneezing fits or eye trouble.

Symptoms are usually worse in cold weather and dry climates—skiing is a common trigger—and the lining of the nose becomes very sensitive to irritants like smoke, smog, perfumes, cooking spices, aspirin, and alcoholic drinks. Allergy skin tests will generally come up negative.

The first thing you should do to handle vasomotor rhinitis is to avoid the irritants that you know trigger the symptoms. You might also find that rinsing your nasal passages regularly with saline is helpful. Also, if your main complaint is congestion, a decongestant medication may help, and if a runny nose is giving

about a quart of mucus and fluid each day for this process.

Among the airborne specks you inhale are allergens, particles with the potential for triggering allergic rhinitis and asthma. When they land on the moist mucous membrane in your nasal passage, they can quickly dissolve and spark an allergic reaction if, of

you fits, the prescription drug ipratropium (Atrovent) may dry you up.

Pregnancy. Hormonal changes during pregnancy can cause new cases of rhinitis. They typically crop up in the second month and last until childbirth, then rapidly subside. In addition, an existing vasomotor rhinitis or allergic rhinitis may grow worse.

Work with your doctor to discover which type you have, and use medications cautiously. Oral decongestants are not recommended during the first trimester, as they can cause birth defects. You may find that washing your nose with salt water or spraying with cromolyn—regarded as safe during pregnancy—can help control your symptoms.

Medication. The severe congestion that can result from using too many nasal decongestant drops or too much spray is a type of rhinitis called rhinitis medicamentosa. To avoid this problem, do not use these types of drugs for more than 3 or 4 days at a time.

Medicines to bring down high blood pressure, particularly the ones known as alpha-blockers, can also induce nasal congestion, says Russell Settipane, M.D., assistant clinical professor of medicine at Brown University in Providence, Rhode Island. These can cause a stuffy nose by dilating the blood vessels in the area.

Nonallergic rhinitis with eosinophilia syndrome. Also called NARES, this form of rhinitis brings congestion and sneezing, generally without a link to allergen exposure, and gets its name from eosinophils, a type of cell connected to allergy. But tests looking for allergies when you have this condition won't make any useful findings.

The condition is often found along with nasal polyps, which are growths in the nasal area. The standard treatment is nasal steroid sprays or sometimes short courses of systemic steroids. These can reduce rhinitis symptoms and shrink polyps.

course, you react to that particular allergen.

Allergic rhinitis comes in two styles, which are labeled according to when and how long you have the symptoms.

Seasonal allergic rhinitis. This type is usually caused by grass, tree, and weed pollen as well as mold. The problems usually crop up when the pollen and mold counts rise in your area, and they dwindle after the first frost. Symptoms due to pollen are usually worse in the morning and clear up toward evening.

Perennial allergic rhinitis. Usually triggered by allergens like dust mites and pet dander, perennial allergic rhinitis strikes year-round. If dust mites are the cause of your problems, the symptoms will likely be worse at night. You may also have some problems year-round with more severe symptoms during pollen season.

As we've discussed elsewhere in this book,

Take a Shot at Allergic Rhinitis

In general, experts recommend that you first try to solve your allergic rhinitis by avoiding the allergens that trouble you. If that doesn't work, then you should step up to treating it with drugs and other remedies. If that's not effective, experts recommend that you start immunotherapy, or allergy shots.

While immunotherapy can be an effective way to make your body react less explosively to allergens, it's relegated to the third option because it's not much fun to do. "Shots may represent an inconvenience to many people because they must be given in the doctor's office," says Jonathan Corren, M.D., associate clinical professor of medicine at UCLA and director of the Allergy Research Foundation in Los Angeles. "Initially, a new patient may be making these doctor's visits once or twice a week. Also, the patient must wait 30 minutes following the shot in case there's an allergic reaction, which happens in about 1 out of every 200 shots. This happens mostly in the buildup section of the therapy, where the doctor is increasing the amount gradually until a maintenance dose is reached."

In immunotherapy, the doctor injects you once or twice a week with very dilute amounts of the allergen that gives you grief. The doses increase until, after 6 to 9 months of therapy, you can tolerate enough that you only need a shot every 4 weeks to maintain your desensitized status. Treatment usually takes 3 to 5 years.

You may want to consider immunotherapy if medicines for your rhinitis aren't working for you, are too expensive, or cause side effects, or if you just have to take too many of them, says Dr. Corren.

if you have allergies, sensors in your mast cells and other cells cause them to burst open in a cascade of inflammatory chemicals when particular allergens touch them.

When this process erupts in your nose during allergic rhinitis, these chemicals—such as histamine, leukotrienes, and prostaglandin—cause the sneezing fits, runny nose, congestion, and itching in your nose, eyes, ears, and palate.

Other symptoms include stuffy ears, a scratchy throat, coughing, and postnasal drip. Sometimes allergic rhinitis will lead to a horizontal crease across your nose as a result of the "allergic salute," or rubbing the nose upward. And your eyelids may grow swollen from fluid accumulation, and you may develop dark circles under your eyes from rubbing them, which are known as allergic shiners.

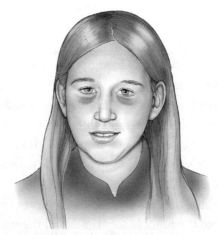

Mouth breathing and "allergic shiners," a darkening of the skin under the eyes, often occur in people with allergic rhinitis.

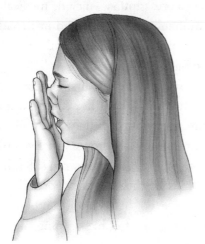

Repeated nose wriggling, wiping, and pushing are common responses to the nasal itching associated with allergic rhinitis, especially in children. Allergists call the upward rubbing of the nose the allergic salute.

Often people trying to cope with these symptoms, which can interrupt their restful sleep, will grow irritable and fatigued and will have trouble concentrating during the day.

Of course, as we mentioned, allergic rhinitis can be like a train engine as it pulls loads of other conditions along behind it. Here's how they happen.

• Your sinuses—small, air-filled cavities in your face and forehead—are connected to your nasal passage by tiny openings. When the mucous lining swells during an allergic reaction, these openings can be pinched shut, trapping air and mucus in the sinuses and forming a breeding ground for bacteria. (You can read more about this in Sinusitis on page 381.)

• Similarly, the opening of the eustachian tube, a thin tunnel connecting the back of the nose to the middle ear, can also be pinched shut by the swelling during rhinitis, setting up the ear for an infection. This is most common in children and is discussed in greater detail in Symptom Solver: Ear Problems on page 434.

• Allergic rhinitis also predisposes you to polyps, which are fluid-filled outgrowths that hang like grapes from the mucous lining in your sinuses and nose. These need to be treated medically or surgically.

• Because the lining of the airways from the nose to the lungs is very similar all the way down, the chaos in the upper end can easily affect the lungs as asthma. In fact, about 40 percent of patients with allergic rhinitis develop asthma, and virtually everyone with allergic asthma has rhinitis.

If you've had allergic rhinitis for a long time, you have a greater chance of developing asthma than someone who doesn't, says Jonathan Corren, M.D., associate clinical professor of medicine at UCLA and director of the Allergy Research Foundation in Los Angeles. If you have both, treating the rhinitis can lessen your asthma symptoms—and leaving one untreated will just allow it to worsen the other, he says. You and your physician should try to tackle both the problems at once. (For more information on this condition, see Asthma on page 222.)

Obviously, allergic rhinitis can open the door to enough ailments to keep several specialists busy full time. But taking care of all the symptoms of just plain allergic rhinitis, with no other complications, can be a chore in itself. Symptoms that range from runny nose and congestion to sneezing and watery eyes may require a well-orchestrated approach.

Let's take a look at prescription and over-the-counter drug treatments, followed by your natural options.

The Drug Approach

Because an awful lot of activity is going on in your nose during allergic rhinitis—with many different symptoms cropping up as a result—drug treatment can follow several different approaches. Here's a rundown of the more common choices.

Antihistamines. These are the most commonly prescribed drugs for allergic rhinitis. They've been around long enough that they've become divided into two different types: first and second generation.

The first-generation drugs—which don't require a prescription—include medications like diphenhydramine, found in Benadryl, and chlorpheniramine, found in Chlor-Trimeton.

A drawback to these first-generation antihistamines is that they tend to make people sleepy, though they don't all cause the same amount of drowsiness. Even when taken the night before, they can still muddle your thinking the next day. (For small children, however, the sedation can be helpful if they're having trouble sleeping, although antihistamines should not be given to children under 12 without the advice of a physician.)

The second-generation drugs, such as

Allegra and Claritin, which were developed more recently, have a less sedating effect. As a result, these tend to be the preferred type of antihistamine. They're far more expensive, however, and require a doctor's prescription.

As you may recall, when the allergic process takes hold of your nasal area, histamine is released from special cells. This chemical causes the runny nose, itching, and sneezing. But the histamine has to connect with receptors in your eyes, nose, and throat to trigger these effects.

When You Need to Be Alert

Newer, or second-generation, antihistamines have a much-touted advantage over the older brands: They are less likely to make you sleepy.

Two recent studies examining the sedating effects of both old and new antihistamines turned up some surprising information and some guidance on how to use these drugs safely.

The first study, done at the University of Iowa, compared the effects of the drug in Allegra (a second-generation antihistamine), the drug in Benadryl (an older antihistamine), and alcohol on driving.

The participants who'd taken the newer antihistamine drove no differently in a driving simulator than the ones who'd taken a placebo, or a neutral product with no effect. On the other hand, the people who took a dose of diphenhydramine (Benadryl) drove more poorly than the ones with a blood-alcohol level of 0.1 percent.

Based on these results, use caution if you're taking a first-generation antihistamine. Whether drivers felt drowsy or not didn't predict how well they'd drive, which means that you shouldn't rely on your sense of alertness to decide whether or not to drive after taking the antihistamine.

The second study, conducted in Great Britain, followed the effects of four second-generation antihistamines—fexofenadine (found in Allegra), loratadine (Claritin), cetirizine (Zyrtec), and acrivastine (Semprex-D). It found that the risk of sedation was low for all drugs, with no increased risk of accident or injury with any of them.

The drug in Zyrtec, however, was 3.5 times more likely to result in sedation than Claritin, and Semprex-D was 2.8 times more likely. There was no significant difference between Claritin and Allegra.

The authors of the study suggest that if you have a job in which any chance of sedation is unacceptable—flying a plane, for example—Claritin and Allegra are the better choices.

When you take an antihistamine for allergic rhinitis, it blocks those receptors so the histamine can't squeeze in. It's like filling a lock with cement so the key won't fit. As a result, antihistamines work much better when you take them *before* you're exposed to an allergen, rather than waiting until the process has already begun. They're useful for sneezing, itching, runny nose, and itchy eyes, but not especially helpful for congestion.

While most antihistamines are taken in pill form, doctors can also prescribe an antihistamine-type drug called azelastine (Astelin) that you can spray up your nose. While this works faster because you're putting the medication directly where it's needed, it also can cause sedation and often leaves a very bitter taste in the mouth.

Not all doctors are enthusiastic about antihistamines. For example, Terence Davidson, M.D., an otolaryngologist and professor of surgery at the University of California, San Diego, opposes them on the grounds that they make the mucus in the nasal region thicker and impair the tiny hairlike cilia that keep it healthy.

In addition, Harold Nelson, M.D., senior staff physician at National Jewish Medical and Research Center in Denver, says that he rarely uses them because he finds nasal corticosteroid sprays to be cheaper and more effective.

Nasal corticosteroids. Nasal corticosteroids, such as beclomethasone (Beclovent), are commonly regarded as the most effective type of drug for treating allergic rhinitis, even though antihistamines are more popular.

Maybe that's the case because antihistamines have a longer history in the American consciousness, or because we prefer pills over sprays, or even because the pharmaceutical companies advertise them more, Dr. Nelson speculates. But it could be that the populace just doesn't like the sound of "steroids."

"Whenever you use the word *steroid* for the first time, it means you're going to have to spend 5 to 10 minutes talking about steroids," Dr. Nelson says. "In the primary care realm, that may be a major factor, because doctors don't have the time to talk to the people. It's much easier to write a prescription where there'll be no 'Oh, steroids' comments, because then they won't have to sit down to explain them."

What some doctors may not explain is that these aren't the kind of steroids commonly associated with muscular bodybuilders and athletes. Nor do they affect you like the systemic corticosteroids that you take orally, which have side effects including weight gain, weakened bones and skin, and high blood pressure.

Nasal corticosteroids are drugs sprayed into the nose that reduce inflammation in the mucous membranes and make the area less reactive. They're useful for sneezing, runny nose, coughing, and itching on the roof of the mouth. And unlike antihistamines, these will substantially clear up your congestion.

These drugs generally affect only your nasal area, though there has been some concern that they can cause children to grow more slowly, Dr. Nelson says. This doesn't appear to be a serious issue, however.

"If there is any slowing, it's very transient in the first couple of months and is not continuous and cumulative, so that you don't take the slowing of growth the first 3 months and multiply it by 12 years and say,

'The kid's going to be 6 inches shorter!' That doesn't happen," Dr. Nelson assures.

Plus, most of the studies looking at this possible side effect have used the drug beclomethasone, which is more easily absorbed into the body through the digestive tract (after it heads down the back of the nose and the throat) than other nasal corticosteroids like budesonide (Pulmicort), mometasone (Nasonex), or fluticasone

Which Medication Is Best for My Symptoms?

The following chart neatly summarizes which medications are most helpful for treating certain symptoms of allergic rhinitis. Use it when you consult with your doctor about your treatment options.

Medication	Sneezing	Itching	Congestion	Runny Nose	Eye Symptoms
Oral antihistamines (Claritin, Allegra)	++	++	+/−	++	++
Nasal antihistamines (Astelin)	+	+	+/−	+	−
Intranasal corticosteroids (Beclovent)	++	++	++	++	+
Oral decongestants (Semprex-D)	−	−	+	−	−
Intranasal decongestants (Beclovent)	−	−	++	−	−
Intranasal mast cell stabilizers (NasalCrom)	+	+	+	+	−

− = Provides no benefit
+/− = Provides little or minimal benefit
+ = Provides modest benefit
++ = Provides substantial benefit

What to Do When You Can't Smell

During an attack of allergic rhinitis, an innocent bystander that might get taken out is your sense of smell. Here's how it happens.

Your nostrils lead into an open chamber, and high in the roof of this chamber is an area of nerve endings that serve as smell receptors. When you inhale molecules from an odor-producing object, they touch those nerve endings and send a message to your brain, which registers it as a particular smell.

When anything prevents those molecules from touching those receptors, you could be left with the inability to smell, known as anosmia (pronounced uh-NOZZ-me-uh), or a partial loss of smell, known as hyposmia (high-POZZ-me-uh).

Allergic rhinitis can inflame your nasal passages and block off the smell receptors, says Alfredo A. Jalowayski, Ph.D., a respiratory physiologist with the Nasal Dysfunction Clinic at the University of California, San Diego. A more likely scenario to hamper your smell, though, is when an allergic inflammation in your nose allows an infection to take hold of your nasal passages or sinuses, he says.

It's important to see a doctor when you've lost your sense of smell to figure out what's causing it, as some viral infections can cause permanent damage to the smell receptors themselves, Dr. Jalowayski says. Other causes of anosmia or hyposmia include head injury and polyps, which are growths in the sinuses often associated with rhinitis.

If your congestion impairs the normal draining of the sinus area between your eyes, the area might become infected and even more inflamed than is usual with allergic rhinitis. This may prevent the flow of vapors to your olfactory, or smelling, receptors, so your doctor might prescribe a steroid such as prednisone (Sterapred)—which brings down inflammation—for a week or so, says William S. Cain, Ph.D., professor of surgery in the division of otolaryngology, head and neck surgery, at the University of California, San Diego. If your sense of smell comes back, it's a good sign that the problem is fixable with antibiotics. To keep your nasal passages and sinuses clear over the long term, you may need decongestants, antihistamines, antibiotics, nasal steroids, cromolyn, or other remedies.

You shouldn't try to live with anosmia, as it can impair your quality of life in many ways, Dr. Cain says. Since much of a food's attraction is in the aroma it gives off, cooking and eating without smelling it isn't much fun. Food may even present a safety risk, as you're more likely to eat spoiled food if you can't smell it. Plus, you're at greater risk in the event of smoke or a gas leak in your home if you can't smell it.

(Flonase), says Dr. Nelson. This makes its effect on growth more likely than with the other drugs.

"Other than that, there's never been any at all convincing evidence that there's any systemic side effect from nasal steroids," Dr. Nelson says.

They can, however, cause stinging, burning, and bleeding in your nose. You can avoid this by aiming the spray bottle *away* from your septum, the stiff partition between your nostrils, rather than toward it.

If you use a spray regularly, be sure to use a dose just large enough to keep your symptoms at bay. For seasonal allergic rhinitis, you'll need to begin taking it when you start feeling symptoms or 2 weeks before the allergy season begins, and keep using it for a few weeks after the season ends.

Finally, some experts still warn that if you have kids on these drugs, you should track their growth and make sure they're using the minimum amount necessary to ward off symptoms.

Cromolyn. A nasal spray containing cromolyn can be very useful in keeping allergic rhinitis in check. It works by stabilizing your mast cells so they don't break open and unleash inflammatory chemicals when they encounter an allergen.

The drug is available over the counter in such medications as NasalCrom and is regarded as very safe, even for children over age 6 and pregnant women. It works for sneezing, itching, congestion, and runny nose.

Unfortunately, cromolyn works as a preventive therapy, *before* you're exposed to a troublesome allergen, not as a treatment for symptoms. Thus, it wouldn't help to take a few puffs of it when you're already sneezing from making ragweed bouquets. In addition, it works slowly, and the effect doesn't last long, so you'd typically need to spray it in your nose three or four times a day, starting up to a week before you need it to work, like when the pollen season begins.

Decongestants. These drugs shrink the blood vessels in your nose, cutting down on the amount of fluid that can leak out of them and cause congestion. Some decongestants are over-the-counter and some are by prescription. Some come as pills, some as sprays, and some are combined with antihistamines.

Decongestants don't help with sneezing, itching, or runny nose. And they do come with some harmful side effects. Oral forms can cause increased blood pressure, agitation, insomnia, and an irregular heartbeat.

Decongestant sprays work faster and have fewer effects throughout your body, but they have a whopper of a side effect. Using them too often can lead to *rhinitis medicamentosa*, a vicious cycle in which they make you even more congested and swollen. If you use these, do so no more than 3 or 4 days at a time.

Anticholinergic drugs. This type of drug calms the nerves that activate the mucus-secreting glands in your nose, which makes it effective for treating a runny nose. But be-

THE HIDDEN CONNECTION

Hay Fever's a Real Gas

A poll of 1,000 Londoners showed that the ones who used gas stoves instead of electric were 20 percent more likely to have allergic rhinitis. A by-product released when natural gas burns may cause irritation in some people, leading to rhinitis.

cause that's the only rhinitis symptom it will fix—and nasal corticosteroids and antihistamines handle runny nose as well as other problems—it's not commonly prescribed for allergic rhinitis, Dr. Nelson says. It's more often used for chronic rhinitis that isn't caused by allergies, he notes. The only type of anticholinergic drug available is ipratropium (Atrovent).

The Nondrug Approach

The very first step that experts recommend to rid your life of allergic rhinitis misery is completely natural: Avoid the allergens that set off your symptoms. This is little more than common sense. Nevertheless, a lot of people aren't getting this message. In that survey we mentioned at the beginning of the chapter, half the people said that their doctors never mentioned these sorts of changes. And of those who had heard the recommendations, less than 20 percent made them all.

By consulting an allergist, you can learn what type of allergen is at the root of your problem. Armed with that information, you may be able to avoid your triggers by taking steps such as the following:

• Keep your windows closed to keep out pollen.

• Bring down the moisture in your home to keep mold at bay.

• Encase your mattress and pillows in special covers to minimize dust mite allergens.

All of these tactics and more are discussed in detail throughout this book.

Unfortunately, totally avoiding allergens in the real world is sometimes about as likely as running through a storm and avoiding the raindrops. But staying away from allergens is just one of many natural options we can take to tackle allergic rhinitis. Read on for some additional remedies.

Nasal rinsing. Though this uses H_2O and NaCl, with a touch of $NaHCO_3$ if you'd like, it's still a natural, self-care option. These substances are easy to find: The first comes from the faucet and the second from the saltshaker (the third is plain old baking soda).

"Nasal hygiene" is the biggest priority in keeping clear of allergy misery, according to Robert Rountree, M.D., a holistic physician in Boulder, Colorado, and coauthor of *Immunotics*. "The biggest part of the

Choose Your Recipe for Saltwater Mixes

Not since Moses and his friends took off through the Red Sea have so many people gotten so up close and personal with salt water. But that's just what more and more doctors are recommending to their patients with nose and sinus conditions. Indeed, rinsing out your nasal passages with a saltwater solution is a simple, inexpensive way to get relief from your allergic rhinitis symptoms.

Not all saltwater mixtures are alike, however. Below are some of your options, both homemade and store-bought. Feel free to experiment and find the one you like best. To apply them, lean forward over a sink, start breathing through your mouth (to prevent the solution from coming out of your mouth and creating a very unpleasant choking sensation), and tilt your head to one side. Pour the mixture into the upper nostril.

Get into a pickle. This recipe is recommended by Diane G. Heatley, M.D., associate professor of pediatric otolaryngology at the University of Wisconsin in Madison.

Using measuring spoons for accuracy, mix 3 tablespoons of pickling and canning salt (it doesn't contain iodine) and 1 tablespoon of baking soda. You can make a stockpile of dry mix in this ratio and keep it in a sealed container.

When you need to use it, stir ½ teaspoon of this mixture into ½ cup of lukewarm tap water. If the water is too hot or cold, it will hurt your nose.

If ½ teaspoon of the mixture in water burns your nose, back off to ¼ teaspoon, but try to work up to the larger amount.

See sea salt. This option is recommended by Robert Rountree, M.D., a holistic physician in Boulder, Colorado, and coauthor of *Immunotics*.

Stir ¼ teaspoon of sea salt into 4 ounces of warm water. Add a pinch of baking soda—about ⅛ teaspoon.

Consider purchasing a mix. Both Dr. Heatley and Murray Grossan, M.D., an oto-laryngologist with Cedars-Sinai Medical Center in Los Angeles, sell their own pre-mixed packets of dry mixes that you dissolve in water as needed. Dr. Heatley's is called Sinucleanse, and Dr. Grossan's is called Breathe-Ease. (For information on ordering these products, see the Resource Guide on page 497.)

problem with allergic rhinitis is that you have mold, dust, pollen, animal dander, et cetera, landing on the mucous membranes. So if you just remove the offending agent, you can make a huge difference," he says.

The way to do that is to rinse them away with salt water—plenty of it, if needed. "You can do it all day long," Dr. Rountree says. "You can't go overboard. You can't overdo it."

Of course, we're not suggesting that you spend your days running through salt water like a mackerel, but during times of heavy pollen or mold, you may want to do it four or even six times a day.

The idea is very simple. You take salt water, mixed to about the same strength as the salty fluids that fill your body or a little stronger, and pour it into each nostril. (See "Choose Your Recipe for Saltwater Mixes" on page 321 for specific directions on making the saltwater solution.) It may emerge from the other nostril or from your mouth, since they're all linked. While this may be somewhat uncomfortable until you get used to it, it shouldn't be painful.

You have your choice of several different devices to get the water into your nose, like little genie lamplike devices called neti pots, squirting bulb syringes, and high-tech Waterpik machines with a special nose adapter. (For more information on the nasal washing technique, see "Give Your Nostrils a Jet-Powered Squirt" as well as the Sinusitis chapter on page

Give Your Nostrils a Jet-Powered Squirt

When all is working well deep within your nose, hordes of microscopic hairs called cilia are beating in unison at 16 waves per second to keep the area clean, says Murray Grossan, M.D., an otolaryngologist with Cedars-Sinai Medical Center in Los Angeles. But when they slow down, stop, or beat out of sync with each other, they sometimes need help to clear the gunk away and get them moving normally.

Dr. Grossan recommends a plug-shaped adapter that attaches to a standard Waterpik, which is a device used to clean teeth by squirting water on them. (In the interest of full disclosure, you should know that Dr. Grossan promotes his own line of these adapters.)

When you adjust the pressure on the Waterpik to the proper level (the stream from the adapter should be about an inch high) and stick the adapter into your nose, it works as a "pulsatile irrigator," not only washing the mucous membranes as recommended by many doctors but also spurting out salt water at 20 pulses per second, Dr. Grossan says. These little bursts of pressure dislodge mucus and help prompt the cilia to get back to waving at the speed they're supposed to move.

Be Careful with Store-Bought Sprays

Bottled saltwater sprays are a great way to hose your nose when you need to moisten or clean out your nasal passages. They're readily available in spray bottles from drugstores and supermarkets.

You should be aware, however, that to keep the contents fresh, manufacturers often add benzalkonium and other preservatives, says Diane G. Heatley, M.D., associate professor of pediatric otolaryngology at the University of Wisconsin in Madison. Unfortunately, the preservatives can be hard on the microscopic hairlike cilia, which move in unison to keep your nasal area clean. In fact, the stuff can keep them from moving.

A better bet is to buy a squirt bottle full of the stuff, empty the bottle, rinse it out, and refill it with your own saltwater mixture. Clean the bottle and replace the solution weekly.

381—the remedy is great for sinusitis, too.)

Quercetin. Dr. Rountree calls quercetin his number one favorite substance for treating allergic rhinitis. This flavonoid—found in buckwheat, citrus foods, and tea—keeps the mast cells stable so they don't unleash histamine and other inflammatory chemicals.

This works as a preventive measure, though, so it's not something to take after problems have kicked in.

Nettle. Capsules of this herb can help keep your symptoms under control when you can't avoid an allergen—say, if you're visiting a friend with a dog that triggers your allergies, Dr. Rountree says.

Also known as stinging nettle, this common plant gets its name from the bite it will give you if you brush by its stingers, which contain a burning chemical. Heating or drying the plant removes the sting; you can drink a daily cup of tea made from the plant or buy capsules of ground, dried herb.

Stress relief. Throughout history, many cultures have had special healing sites where people could go to seek relief from illness, says Murray Grossan, M.D., an otolaryngologist with Cedars-Sinai Medical Center in Los Angeles. Since these places typically offered a shelter from the hustle and bustle of daily life, the patient often benefited from the rest and stress reduction.

This can be even more important when you're dealing with the effects of allergic rhinitis, which can leave you irritable and fatigued. So make sure that you're getting plenty of sleep and relaxation when you're struggling with allergies.

Fatty acids. Dr. Rountree recommends oils high in gamma-linolenic acid (GLA), such as borage and black currant seed oil, to dampen inflammation in the body.

Antioxidants. Dr. Rountree believes that

people with allergies should be especially vigilant in getting their daily antioxidants to combat the effects of free radicals, those unstable molecules that course through your body, aiding in inflammation and damaging tissues.

Antioxidants include vitamins E and C, flavonoids, and proanthocyanidins from grape seed extract. Quercetin, which we mentioned earlier, is also an antioxidant.

To put more antioxidants in your diet, eat plenty of fruits and vegetables with deep, bright colors like green, yellow, orange, red, and blue, in addition to the supplements listed in the Action Plan.

Honey. Honey made by local bees has the potential to help some people with hay fever. "I think it's a very reasonable thing to use, but I wouldn't rely on it as my primary intervention," Dr. Rountree says.

Local honey could contain pollen from your area, which may be a trigger for your allergic rhinitis. The pollen in the honey might help make you less sensitive to the pollen in the air, sort of like immunotherapy.

Homeopathy. While homeopathy—which uses remedies that contain extremely diluted amounts of the active ingredient—may seem improbable to some, it might be useful in coping with allergic rhinitis.

A recent University of Glasgow study compared two groups of patients with allergic rhinitis. One group took a homeopathic dilution of the allergen that gave them the most trouble; the other group took a placebo (fake medication). At the end of the study, those who'd taken the homeopathic treatment could breathe better through their noses.

How Well Do You Smell?

If you think your sense of smell is out of whack, you can easily test it with a method devised by the University of California, San Diego, Nasal Dysfunction Clinic.

First, have a friend partially unwrap a small, disposable pad soaked in alcohol, known as an alcohol prep pad, which is available in drugstores, the first-aid section in supermarkets, or surgical supply stores. Then close your eyes and instruct your assistant to hold the pad under your nose at chest level. As you breathe normally, your friend should move the pad about ½-inch closer to your nose each time you exhale.

If you have a normal sense of smell, you should detect the odor when it's at least 8 inches from your nose. If you have hyposmia, or a hampered sense of smell, you'll detect the odor when it's 1 to 8 inches away. If you have anosmia, or a lack of smell, you won't smell it at all. If you suspect that you have a diminished or absent sense of smell, see your doctor, who can run tests to determine the extent of your problem.

Hay Fever
ACTION PLAN

There is no reason that you should suffer with the symptoms of hay fever (allergic rhinitis) when there are a host of treatment options available to you. Further, many of these are inexpensive things that you can do on your own.

🌿 indicates a natural remedy

- Consult with a doctor to learn which allergens are provoking your rhinitis—or if your rhinitis is even allergic in nature.
- 🌿 Take steps to avoid the allergens that cause you trouble. Take special precautions to make your bedroom an allergy-free zone. (For specific directions for doing this, see The Allergy-Free Home on page 73.)
- 🌿 Rinse out your nasal passages regularly to wash away allergens and keep the mucus in your nose moving. You can use a neti pot, a bulb syringe, a specially equipped Waterpik, or a refillable spray bottle to get the salt water into your nose.
- 🌿 Beware of saline sprays containing preservatives. A better option is to mix up your own solution from dry salt and other ingredients and refill a spray bottle as needed.
- 🌿 Monitor your stress levels. Practice stress-relieving exercises (see Allergy-Free Stress Busters on page 173), and get plenty of sleep each night.
- Talk to your doctor about your symptoms and medication options. These include nasal steroid sprays, antihistamines, cromolyn spray, and oral and nasal decongestants.
- If you take first-generation antihistamines, such as Benadryl, change your schedule to accommodate any possible sleepiness.
- If you spray decongestants into your nose, don't use them for more than 3 or 4 days at a time. They can cause even worse congestion if overused.
- If you use a nasal steroid spray, use the minimum amount necessary to ward off symptoms. Point it away from your septum, the wall between your nostrils.
- Consider using nasal cromolyn spray. This over-the-counter drug is regarded as safe for use over the long term to make your nose react less to allergens.
- 🌿 After trying avoidance techniques and pharmaceuticals, consider im-

munotherapy to make you less reactive to allergens. You may want to discuss it with an allergist if you're having to take too many remedies to keep symptoms in check or if they're causing side effects. It may involve 3 to 5 years of weekly shots, and you'll need to stay at the doctor's office for about a half-hour after each session to ensure that you won't have a bad reaction.

🌿 Nettle may be worth your while. For allergic rhinitis, the best form is freeze-dried extract of leaves. Dr. Rountree advises taking one or two 300-milligram capsules every 2 to 4 hours, as needed to control symptoms. Experts caution that you should take only one dose a day for the first few days to ensure that you're not allergic to the plant. (For information on ordering this product, see the Resource Guide on page 497.)

🌿 Try quercetin, a natural antioxidant, which stabilizes the mast cells that contribute the chemicals used in the allergic process. Dr. Rountree suggests that you take two 500-milligram capsules twice a day, for a total of 2,000 milligrams, at the first sign of your allergic symptoms or at the beginning of your typical allergic season. Continue taking this dose until your symptoms are resolved. If this dosage doesn't work, increase it to 2,500 or 3,000 milligrams a day, again divided into two doses.

🌿 Also take vitamin C, which acts as an antioxidant and cuts down on inflammation. Take 2,000 milligrams every day, divided into four doses of 500 milligrams each.

Other supplements suggested by Dr. Rountree to fight allergies are tocopherol, or vitamin E complex (200 to 400 IU daily), selenium (200 micrograms daily), zinc (20 to 40 milligrams daily), and proanthocyanidin as grape seed extract (50 to 150 milligrams daily). Take daily as a preventive measure. Ideally, he says, find a multiple vitamin that contains all of the above in a dosage as close as possible to his suggestions. If not, take them separately. Usually, the grape seed extract will have to be taken separately.

🌿 Get a daily dose of GLA, a useful fatty acid that helps control inflammation, by taking 300 milligrams of borage or black currant seed oil each day. It may take 6 months to a year before the full benefits become evident, says Dr. Rountree.

🌿 If you enjoy honey, try using honey made by bees in your area as a sweetener. Check with stores and farm stands for local honey. It may help desensitize you if you're allergic to pollen. Because it may contain dormant bacterial spores, honey can produce botulism, which poses little danger for adults but may be deadly for children less than a year old.

Latex
ALLERGY

INSIDE A NEW YORK CITY theater, Barbara Zucker-Pinchoff, M.D., and her family watched with delight as bungee-jumpers plunged from the rafters.

"It was like an old-time happening," Dr. Zucker-Pinchoff says. "Very cool."

But what happened next wasn't so cool.

"I could feel my nose and eyes starting to itch. I said, 'I'm not going to be able to stay here long. There's latex in here somewhere,'" she recalls.

Suddenly, a paper ceiling ripped open, releasing a barrage of balloons onto the surprised audience.

"I got out of there as fast as I could, but I was sick for 3 days," says Dr. Zucker-Pinchoff, a former anesthesiologist in New York City.

To many, the idea that something as innocent as balloons could trigger serious illness may seem hard to believe. Dr. Zucker-Pinchoff describes it this way: "How do you feel on the worst day of a crappy cold? How would you like it if you felt that way every single day you went to work?"

Latex allergy isn't just a glorified case of dishpan hands. It's a serious disease that causes disability and, in extreme cases, even death.

Most experts believe that latex gloves are the primary villain. Condoms are another leading culprit. Yet more than 40,000 everyday products contain latex, including some you'd never suspect, such as panty hose, poinsettia plants, and peaches. Even the little crumbs you get under your thumbnail when you buy a lottery scratch card contain latex.

Fortunately, not all latex products are equally allergenic. Only the most exquisitely sensitive patients react to products made of hard rubber, such as shoe soles. And some seemingly rubberized products contain no latex. These include electrical cords and most so-called latex paints.

"There are a lot of latex exposures out there, and many of them are unavoidable in a medical environment," Dr. Zucker-Pinchoff says. "For the vast majority of people with latex allergy, any exposure can be serious, and for people who are highly allergic to latex, this can lead to asthma attacks and anaphylactic shock, especially when they visit the doctor or dentist."

The First Step

Latex allergy is diagnosed by blood, skin, and patch tests. There's no cure and no immunotherapy to build resistance. "Unfortunately, the only treatment for latex allergy is avoidance," says Andrew Weil, M.D., director of the program in integrative medicine and clinical professor of medicine at the University of Arizona College of Medicine in Tucson.

Latex sensitization—which means that your immune system is producing detectable immunoglobulin E (IgE) antibodies to latex proteins but the reaction may not yet be strong enough to cause any symptoms—is the first step toward latex allergy.

Most people who are sensitized to latex don't know it, according to the National Health and Nutrition Examination Survey.

In the absence of symptoms, the only way to know for sure that you've been sensitized to latex is to get tested.

"If you're sensitized, it means you're walking on thin ice," says P. Brock Williams, Ph.D., clinical professor of medicine at the University of Missouri–Kansas City School of Medicine and research director for IBT (ImmunoBioTech) Reference Lab, which does testing for allergies and related immunologic diseases, also in Kansas City.

If you have a job that requires you to wear latex gloves, you've probably seen what happens to coworkers who fall through that ice. They may develop the dry, crusted lesions of irritant contact dermatitis, the weeping poison ivy–like rash of allergic contact dermatitis, and even immediate hypersensitivity reactions such as hives, allergic rhinitis (hay fever), asthma, and anaphylactic shock. In severe cases, they have to quit their jobs.

To keep this from happening to you, you have to stop the sensitization process. That means drastically limiting your latex exposure by wearing nonlatex gloves and asking your employer to establish latex-free working areas. Such approaches have worked at a number of hospitals.

Keep in mind, though, that you don't have to work with latex to become sensitized to it. Among those at increased risk are children with spina bifida and congenital urological abnormalities. Since such children undergo multiple surgeries at an early age, they're exposed to huge amounts of latex, so their sensitization rate is as high as 73 percent.

Other medical conditions associated with an increased risk of latex allergy include premature birth, multiple surgeries at any age (including C-sections), cerebral palsy, and a history of other allergies.

Gloves: The Worst Offender

Although latex gloves have been used for decades, today's gloves are more allergenic because of higher-volume manufacturing techniques that leave in more of the offending latex proteins, according to Bradley

The Organic Way to Avoid Latex Allergy?

Conventional wisdom blames the latex-allergy epidemic on the widespread use of powdered latex gloves. But P. Brock Williams, Ph.D., research director at IBT (ImmunoBioTech) Reference Lab in Kansas City, which does testing for allergies and related immunologic diseases, and clinical professor of medicine at the University of Missouri–Kansas City School of Medicine, is convinced that the real culprit is the ethylene gas that's commonly sprayed on fruits and vegetables to speed ripening.

The gas induces the same wound-repair proteins that have been identified as the most allergenic in natural rubber latex.

"Some of the foods we're eating have higher concentrations of these proteins. If you look at the foods that cross-react with latex—the banana, the kiwifruit, the stone fruits—they're all very high responders to ethylene gas," says Dr. Williams, who is a member of the latex committees at the American College of Allergy, Asthma, and Immunology and the American Academy of Allergy, Asthma, and Immunology.

Bananas release so much ethylene gas, in fact, that they can speed the ripening of other fruits just by being in close proximity to them. "People have known for a long time that if you want to ripen a piece of fruit like a pear, all you have to do is put it next to a banana," points out Dr. Williams.

Since studies have shown that food allergy can precede latex allergy, Dr. Williams suspects that people are first sensitized to latex by eating gas-treated food. His theory is that they only show symptoms after then being exposed to a high-latex environment, such as a hospital.

How do you avoid eating foods ripened with ethylene gas?

One way would be to buy organic produce from stores that get their produce from certified-organic farmers. But the best way might be to grow the food yourself. Besides, homegrown tomatoes taste better than those from the store, notes Dr. Williams.

Chipps, M.D., an allergist in Sacramento.

To meet the vastly increased demand for latex gloves that's been created by the AIDS epidemic, manufacturers have moved factories to a region of the world where rubber plantations are plentiful and labor is cheap: Southeast Asia. "Since the manufacturing is done in Third World countries, quality control is not as good," notes Dr. Chipps. "So you get a more highly allergenic glove."

Glove quality varies so much that Mayo Clinic researchers have found that some types release 3,000 times as many latex particles as others.

The Condom Conundrum

One of the other leading triggers of latex allergy is condoms. For those allergic to latex, so-called safer sex isn't safe at all.

"Symptoms can include contact dermatitis, hives, feeling faint, nausea, vomiting, abdominal cramps, runny eyes, breathing problems, and even anaphylactic shock," says Dr. Weil.

There's a good reason why condoms are often called rubbers. The overwhelming majority are indeed rubber products. But several brands of nonallergenic polyurethane condoms have made their way to drugstore shelves. These include the Reality Condom for women and the Durex Avanti Superthin Lubricated Nonlatex Condom and the Trojan Supra Microsheer Polyurethane Condom for men.

Thinner than latex condoms, the poly-

urethane varieties transmit more warmth and sensation. But they cost twice as much, are more likely to break, and may even be carcinogenic.

The priciest condoms of all—lambskin condoms, such as Trojan Naturalamb Natural Skin Lubricated Condoms—are made from loose-fitting animal membranes and transmit a high degree of sensitivity. While they offer protection against pregnancy, they're too porous to contain the microorganisms that cause sexually transmitted diseases, including AIDS. So they should be used only by mutually monogamous couples who are disease-free.

The ultimate answer to the condom conundrum could come from the French. At the Centre d'Allergologie at Hospital Trenon in Paris, researchers studied 14 women and 5 men who were allergic to latex and ranged in age from 21 to 60. Previously, all 19 had experienced genital rashes and swelling when exposed to natural rubber-latex condoms. Several patients had even experienced extra-genital hives, allergic rhinitis, and respiratory distress during or immediately after sexual intercourse.

For 6 weeks, the patients were instructed to use condoms that had been stripped of allergenic proteins by a special enzyme. Such "deproteinized" latex condoms are marketed in several European countries by Ansell France.

The result? "Nobody had a reaction to these condoms," says David A. Levy, M.D., an allergist at the hospital, who is one of the study's authors. They may be difficult to find in the United States. Ask your pharmacist if they can be ordered.

Toward a Latex-Free Future

Products made from dipped latex—gloves, condoms, and balloons—create the most havoc partly because they're often coated with cornstarch to make them less sticky. Cornstarch absorbs latex proteins, so when such products are used, a fine powder of latex protein particles is released into the air.

Although it typically takes months or years of exposure to such particles to develop a latex allergy, that's not always the case. Some people can develop allergic dermatitis after just one exposure.

Fortunately, there is hope. Thanks to the twin threats of lawsuits and federal regulation, latex manufacturers are adding extra steps to make their products less allergenic.

Hospitals, too, are switching to low-protein, powder-free latex gloves, with the ultimate goal of using only nonlatex gloves.

Among them is the University of

Does Your Job Put You at Risk?

Researchers for the National Health and Nutrition Examination Survey studied more than 5,000 American adults from 40 different occupations. They discovered that latex sensitization is widespread throughout the entire population. Here are their findings for some common jobs.

Occupation	Percentage with Latex Sensitization
Writers, entertainers, and athletes	29.1
Mechanics	28.3
Motor vehicle operators	25.5
Food handlers	22.6
Construction workers	20.5
Cooks	18.5
Health-care workers	18.0
Retail sales clerks	17.0
Teachers	16.9
Engineers and scientists	16.4
Secretaries	13.5
Waiters and waitresses	12.2
Sales representatives	10.8
Information clerks	6.5

Source: Third National Health and Nutrition Examination Survey (NHANES III)

Maryland Medical System in Baltimore. After screening 1,800 employees, researchers found 35 latex-allergic employees who were willing to use nonlatex gloves and have their blood tested at regular intervals. Within 18 months, their blood levels of latex allergen had decreased by an average of 30 percent. Those who adhered strictly to the use of only nonlatex gloves were more likely to have decreased levels.

"We even had three employees who went from a positive level to completely undetectable levels," notes researcher Mary Bollinger, D.O., allergy director and assistant professor of pediatrics at the University of Maryland Medical System Hospital for Children in Baltimore.

Such studies have fueled speculation that latex allergy could almost disappear over time, at least among health care workers.

Accept Substitutions

Latex is found in a mind-boggling number of products. Fortunately, acceptable alternatives are usually available. Check out the following suggested substitutions from the American Latex Allergy Association.

Instead of These Latex Products . . .	Use These Latex-Free Alternatives . . .
Automobile floor mats	Vinyl floor mats
Balloons	Mylar balloons
Balls (basketball, Koosh, rubber, tennis)	Vinyl or polyvinyl chloride (PVC) balls
Cosmetic applicators and sponges	Cotton balls or brushes
Crutches	Crutches covered with cloth
Food-storage bags with zip-lock feature	Plain plastic bags, waxed paper, plastic wrap
Garden hoses	Vinyl hoses
Gloves used for food handling	Synthetic or vinyl gloves
Gloves used for housekeeping	Heavy-duty nitrile gloves
Panty hose	Clothes tucked under panty hose waist band, panty hose made with Lycra spandex
Raincoats	Neoprene-coated nylon coats
Rubber bands	Plastic bands
Shoes (rubber boots, rubber thongs, shoes with arch pads or crepe soles, water shoes)	Rubber-free sport shoes or PVC waterproof boots
Socks	Cotton socks without elastic
Underwear with elastic	Underwear with elastic covered with cloth
Upholstery foam-rubber padding	Synthetic foam

Latex Allergy
ACTION PLAN

To reduce your risk of developing a latex allergy, you need to familiarize yourself with the places where latex proteins might lurk. If you already have a latex allergy, knowing the products and foods to avoid can go a long way in gaining control over this condition.

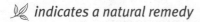 *indicates a natural remedy*

Prevention

Since there is such a wide variety of products made with latex, you're likely to come in contact with it nearly anywhere you go. Check out the following tips for the best ways to avoid or reduce your exposure.

At Work

The National Institute for Occupational Safety and Health (NIOSH) and the American Nurses Association offer the following advice on the proper use of latex gloves as well as a few cautions for your workplace.

- Use nonlatex gloves for activities that don't involve contact with infectious materials (such as food preparation and routine housekeeping).
- If you use latex gloves when handling infectious materials, use powder-free gloves with reduced protein content. Just be aware that so-called hypoallergenic gloves do not reduce the risk of latex allergy. They may, however, reduce reactions to chemical additives in the latex.
- When wearing gloves at work, use only those hand-care products that are not oil-based. Petroleum-based ointments can cause gloves to deteriorate.
- Remove gloves at least once each hour to air out and dry your hands.
- After removing latex gloves, wash your hands with a mild pH-balanced soap and dry them thoroughly.
- Outside of work, apply nonsensitizing moisturizers to restore your skin's protective barrier.
- For wet work, wear synthetic gloves or cotton liners with latex work gloves.
- Make sure that areas contaminated with latex dust are cleaned often.
- Request that ventilation filters and vacuum bags used in latex-contaminated areas be changed frequently.

At Home

Now that many Americans are assuming the role of home caregiver for sick relatives and friends, they're increasingly exposed to latex as they go through boxes of disposable gloves. This increased exposure can lead to hypersensitivity.

Most laypeople are not aware that they have a choice in gloves. There's no warning on the box about the sensitization risk, particularly for people with allergic diseases, such as asthma—the highest risk group. Here are your best bets.

- Look for nonlatex gloves at medical supply stores. Use synthetic gloves made of vinyl or nitrile for most home caregiving tasks that don't involve handling infectious materials.

- If there is a risk of disease from handling blood, urine, or feces, wear a powder-free latex glove over top of a cotton or vinyl glove for maximum protection.

Shrub May Solve Latex-Allergy Woes

The Brazilian rubber tree has long been the world's primary source of latex—and latex allergies. But people with allergies could get a break with the widespread cultivation of guayule, a shrub native to the American Southwest.

Pronounced "gwa-YOU-lee," the shrub produces a high-quality, hypoallergenic latex that's impervious to bacteria as well as the viruses that cause AIDS, hepatitis, and herpes.

"Guayule latex has a very low protein content, on the order of 0.05 percent, which is much lower than Brazilian rubber tree latex," says plant physiologist and lead scientist Katrina Cornish, Ph.D., of the U.S. Department of Agriculture (USDA) in Albany, California. "It is very unlikely that guayule-latex products will cause allergies."

Once a domestic source of rubber, guayule was rubbed out by foreign competition in 1929. But Dr. Cornish and other researchers are hopeful that modern strains will produce enough latex for a homegrown guayule industry to take root.

The San Diego-based Yulex Corporation, a bioagricultural company with ties to the USDA, is currently producing pilot guayule products and plans to market a complete line of guayule products soon, according to chief executive officer Jeff Martin.

At the Doctor's and Dentist's Offices

Here are some ways to minimize exposure to latex at your doctor's or dentist's offices, courtesy of ELASTIC (Education for Latex Allergy Support Team and Information Coalition).

- Find an office that uses nonlatex gloves or powder-free, low-protein gloves and nonlatex equipment.
- If that's not possible, choose a practice that has separate operatories—rooms that can be closed off and made latex-safe.
- Schedule your appointment for first thing in the morning. Other good times are the day the office opens after a vacation and the day after a cleaning crew has vacuumed all surfaces where latex dust can settle.

Preparing for an Emergency

If you're allergic to latex, the last thing you want to do is keep your condition a secret from the people who can save your life. This plan from ELASTIC will help ensure that your life won't be further endangered by latex exposure in the event of a medical emergency.

- Develop a written emergency plan with your physician that details the steps you need to take if serious symptoms develop. Include a list of the medications you'll need as well as critical telephone numbers.
- Learn to use emergency medications such as an epinephrine auto-injector. Always carry emergency medications with you.
- Share your emergency plan with family, friends, employers, and co-workers. Tell them where they can find your emergency medications.
- Wear a medical identification emblem, such as a MedicAlert bracelet.
- Place a "No Latex" reflective sticker or decal on your car to alert first responders in the event of an emergency.
- Carry a pair of nonlatex gloves for first responders to wear in case they need to administer first aid.
- Contact your local 911 dispatch office so personnel can "flag" your address for first responders.
- Share your latex-allergy status with others who might need to know, including your local emergency medical service, hospital and emergency room, and dentist and other health care providers.

THE HIDDEN CONNECTION

Latex and Food Allergies

You can't eat a rubber ball, and you can't bounce a banana. Yet, on a microscopic level, the two objects have much in common, especially proteins.

"Nature has a way of using proteins in different ways in different species," says P. Brock Williams, Ph.D., clinical professor of medicine at the University of Missouri–Kansas City School of Medicine and research director for IBT (ImmunoBioTech) Reference Lab, which does testing for allergies and related immunologic diseases, also in Kansas City.

The proteins shared by rubber balls and bananas are the same ones that cause contact dermatitis, hives, allergic rhinitis, and asthma in people who are allergic to latex. So if you're one of these people, you have a higher risk of being allergic to bananas and a host of other foods.

"About half of all the people who react to latex are also allergic to something else," says Andrew Weil, M.D., director of the program in integrative medicine and clinical professor of medicine at the University of Arizona College of Medicine in Tucson. "You'd know if you were sensitive to any of these foods by the itching in your mouth when you eat them."

If you are allergic to latex, says Bradley Chipps, M.D., an allergist in Sacramento, "you should have a blood or skin test to see if symptoms compatible to food allergy—swelling, itching, redness—are present."

Generally, people become allergic to latex before developing related food allergies. Sometimes, however, a food allergy precedes a latex allergy.

A Spanish study of 57 people—36 women and 21 men—with a clinical history of fruit allergy showed that 86 percent (mostly women) were sensitized to latex. More than 10 percent were found to have a clinical latex allergy.

"The repeated exposure of women to household gloves may be the reason," the researchers wrote. In other words, washing dishes with latex gloves might first make you allergic to the latexlike proteins in fruits, and only later allergic to the latex proteins themselves. Highly illogical, as Mr. Spock might say, but it's just another example of how unpredictable allergies can be.

The Spanish researchers concluded that all patients allergic to fruit should be screened for signs of latex allergy.

Buyer Beware

The following substances have been found to cross-react with latex allergy:

Common: almonds, apples, avocados, bananas, carrots, celery, chestnuts, hazelnuts, kiwifruit, melons, papaya, pears, raw potatoes, stone fruits (such as peaches, plums, and cherries), tomatoes

Less common: citrus fruits, coconuts, condurango bark, figs, mangoes, passion fruit, peanuts, peppers, pineapple, ugli fruits

Think Twice When Dining Out

Once you've identified the foods that cross-react with latex, you might think it's safe to eat in restaurants as long as you don't order, say, a guacamole burger, a side order of kiwifruit, and banana pudding.

Not necessarily.

Many food handlers wear latex gloves, including the powdered variety that shed latex protein particles like dogs shed dander.

In a laboratory study conducted at the Guthrie Institute in Sayre, Pennsylvania, researchers found that latex proteins can be transferred from powdered latex gloves to lettuce and sliced cheese.

"I've had reactions twice now from eating food that was prepared with powdered latex gloves," says Barbara Zucker-Pinchoff, M.D., a former anesthesiologist in New York City. "As they toss a salad with hands covered by powdered latex gloves, the moisture on the salad dissolves the protein, and it transfers beautifully to your dinner."

In another experiment, researchers from Massachusetts General Hospital and Beth Israel Deaconess Medical Center, both in Boston, concluded that a 46-year-old periodontist with latex allergy was experiencing the same symptoms after eating "safe" foods that had been in contact with a latex glove.

"The elimination of latex, which is already under way in the health care environment, should also be extended to the food-handling environment to protect consumers sensitized by other exposures," the researchers concluded.

Until that happens, people with latex allergy should probably avoid eating salads and other cold foods prepared in restaurants. They should also always carry an epinephrine auto-injector when they go out to eat, says Dr. Zucker-Pinchoff.

"In my personal experience, cooked foods are usually less of a problem because food handlers don't tend to stick their hands on them," Dr. Zucker-Pinchoff says.

Treatment

Appropriate treatment depends on the severity of the symptoms, but no treatment can take the place of avoidance.

Nonallergic Rashes

Not technically an allergy, irritant contact dermatitis results from repeated hand-washing and exposure to detergents, chemicals, endotoxins, or powders in gloves. In less enlightened times, it was called housewife's dermatitis because it was associated with rubber gloves used to wash pots and pans.

"Anyone who wears that type of glove for a long time is going to get a certain amount of skin irritation," says John Yunginger, M.D., an allergist at the Mayo Clinic in Rochester, Minnesota. "Moisture gets trapped inside the glove, and the skin macerates, or breaks down."

- Use a moisturizer or skin cream such as Vaseline Intensive Care Lotion several times a day, especially after bathing.
- Apply wet oatmeal to the rash once a day. Cover with a bandage and leave it in place for several hours.

Allergic Rashes

As its name implies, allergic dermatitis is a true allergy. It often is caused by chemicals added to latex or nonlatex gloves during the manufacturing process. This is a contact allergy that shows up as a skin rash—usually itching and redness—at the point of contact with the offending object.

- For immediate natural relief, use Oregon grape tincture or marshmallow leaf tincture, says herbalist Douglas Schar, Dip.Phyt. (diploma in phytotherapy), M.N.I.M.H. (member of the National Institute of Medical Herbalists), of London. These topical treatments help narrow blood vessels. Apply a few drops of one of these tinctures to the affected area with a cotton ball four times a day until the rash clears up. Noticeable improvements can take 2 to 3 months; lasting improvements, up to a year or more.
- For mild cases, use an over-the-counter topical steroid cream. But if you swell up like you've been bitten by a 10-pound mosquito and the itching is so bad that you want to scratch yourself with coarse sandpaper, you probably need a prescription steroid. Such creams are usually applied once or twice daily over 5 to 15 days. But don't overuse them without a doctor's supervision. Over long periods of time, they can cause thinning of the skin.

- For especially stubborn rashes, doctors may also prescribe oral steroids, antihistamines, phototherapy, or antibiotics.

Type I Allergic Reactions

The most serious but least common form of latex allergy, Type I allergic reactions produce a wide range of symptoms that can seriously affect the skin, eyes, nose, and lungs.

- For hives or hay fever–type symptoms, doctors often prescribe maximum doses of a nonsedating antihistamine such as fexofenadine (Allegra), as well as a sedating antihistamine such as hydroxyzine (Atarax) or doxepin (Sinequan).
- For occupational asthma, doctors often prescribe inhaled anti-inflammatories such as cromolyn (Gastrocrom) and nedocromil (Tilade).
- Most patients with Type I allergic reactions are instructed to carry an epinephrine self-injector (EpiPen Auto-Injector) at all times to help short-circuit life-threatening attacks of anaphylaxis. When patients are hospitalized because they've experienced a severe allergic reaction and the onset of anaphylactic shock, they're usually treated with epinephrine (Sensorcaine), diphenhydramine (also available as the nonprescription Benadryl), albuterol (Proventil), and supplemental oxygen.

When to Call the Doctor

Seek medical help if you experience any of the following symptoms within minutes of being exposed to latex: eye watering, nasal congestion, sneezing, or coughing.

Reactions such as hives, itching, or redness may also be a sign of latex allergy, and they should be checked. The most serious reaction—anaphylaxis—is identical to that caused by foods or insect bites. "You can have hives; swelling in your eyelids, lips, fingers, and toes; or trouble breathing," says Dr. Yunginger. "Some people get abdominal cramping or diarrhea or vomiting."

Anaphylaxis is a medical emergency. If you experience the symptoms described by Dr. Yunginger, immediately call 911, or the emergency number for your community, even if you've already used an epinephrine injector. Without further evaluation and treatment, you could die of anaphylactic shock.

Mold
ALLERGY

EVEN DURING Old Testament times, homeowners were struggling to rid their surroundings of mold.

Among guidance of a more spiritual nature, the Bible offers simple tips in the Book of Leviticus on how to tackle mold growing on clothing or walls. Solutions for the garment include cleaning it, cutting out the icky spot, or just destroying the whole thing. Similarly, advice for fixing the problem in the home ranges from tearing out the moldy wall material to demolishing the whole house.

Though we know much more nowadays about how mold can trigger allergies and cause other illnesses, some of the biblical advice regarding it remains true, says David Straus, Ph.D., professor of microbiology and immunology at Texas Tech University Health Sciences Center in Lubbock, Texas. The essence of that advice is still this: Don't give mold a chance to gain a foothold in your home. If it does, root it out quickly.

We have our work cut out for us. Probably about 1.5 million species of fungi exist in the world—a figure that includes mold, mildew, yeasts, and mushrooms—and about 75,000 have been identified, says Estelle Levetin, Ph.D., professor of biology and a mold expert at the University of Tulsa in Oklahoma.

While "fungus" conjures up an image as displeasing as "cockroach," some fungi are actually useful to us, like the *Penicillium* mold used to make the antibiotic penicillin and blue cheese. We like soy sauce, too, even though it gets its black color from mold—much as the tiles in your shower do.

On the other hand, about two dozen types of mold have been identified as significant allergens. These include *Alter-*

THE HIDDEN CONNECTION

Mold Lurks in Odd Places

Vincent Marinkovich, M.D., an allergist and clinical associate professor of pediatrics at Stanford University, gives his mold-sensitive patients a list of foods to avoid. Some are easy to spot, like fermented foods such as blue cheese, beer, and wine. Others are harder to monitor, like processed foods containing citric acid and fruit juices.

Processed foods? Juices? Where's the mold there?

The citric acid used to preserve many soft drinks and canned foods is produced in vats of *Aspergillus* mold, Dr. Marinkovich explains. The aspergillus isn't screened out very well, so along with the citric acid in the food comes an ample amount of mold.

Juicemakers use aspergillus when they process fruits to help break down the structure of the fruit so it yields more juice, notes Dr. Marinkovich.

Also on his list of foods for people with mold allergies to avoid are chocolate and soy sauce, which are also fermented with fungi, and bread, which contains an enzyme called amylase derived from aspergillus that bakers use to speed the production of the bread.

naria, *Cladosporium*, *Aspergillus*, and, ironically, *Penicillium*. These are such powerful allergy troublemakers because their chemical structure makes them especially allergenic and because they're in abundance, so you're more likely to encounter them.

When you breathe spores or other bits of fungi into your nose, they can give you the symptoms of allergic rhinitis (hay fever), such as a runny nose, congestion, and sneezing, by triggering the release of inflammatory chemicals in your nose. When they slip past your nose and into your lungs, they can give you symptoms of asthma. In fact, reactions for people who are sensitive to mold can be even more severe than the reactions experienced by people who are sensitive to pollen.

Other types of fungi can be harmful because they cause infections—like those that cause athlete's foot or the kind that when inhaled can cause histoplasmosis, a condition that affects the lungs and other internal organs. Still other molds are harmful because they generate toxins—like aflatoxin, which is produced by fungi often found on peanuts and is associated with liver cancer.

Outdoors, mold spores—the tiny grains by which mold reproduces—are found virtually everywhere in all climates, though levels drop when snow is on the ground. Indoors, spores drift in dust and scatter widely on most surfaces, with the exception of hostile environments like a steaming-hot autoclave that's just been used to sterilize medical equipment, Dr. Straus notes.

Given the sheer numbers of, as we used to say in elementary school, "the fungus among us," it would seem like an insurmountable task to keep them from growing in our homes or wafting into our noses. But don't despair. You can make your home unattractive to mold, take simple steps to protect yourself while you're in the great outdoors, and use medical assistance to help you cope when you experience an allergic reaction.

Thirsty and Bold Is What Describes Mold

If houseplants were as easy to grow as mold, our homes could look like well-stocked floral shops with a minimum of effort.

All mold really needs to thrive is something to eat and drink at the proper temperature. When it finds those, it can start growing to its full potential.

Mold travels by spores, tiny living particles containing genetic material that depart from an older mold colony to start new growths. "You might think of spores as little spaceships that these fungal colonies produce," Dr. Straus says.

These little spores waft into your home unannounced when you open a door or window, or they hitch a ride on your shoes and clothes. Once inside your home, they can drift on the air currents and fly through your air ducts. Indoors, these stray spores from outside aren't the major allergy

Mold Isn't Always a Creature of Darkness

The idea that mold and fungus will only thrive in darkness is a myth, says Elliott Horner, Ph.D., a mold expert and microbial laboratory director for Air Quality Sciences in Atlanta. What it needs is a location that supplies food and water at a suitable temperature.

It just happens that in your home, the moldy areas tend to be places you don't spend much time in, like the back of the closet, the crawl space under the house, or the closed-up room with the water heater. Hence, they're dark—but you're also less likely to keep them ventilated, clean, and dry like the places you inhabit, such as the living room.

problem—but they turn into it when they dig in and start multiplying, says Elliott Horner, Ph.D., a mold expert and microbial laboratory director for Air Quality Sciences in Atlanta.

Remember, all that mold needs are food, water, and the right temperature—which is the same temperature at which most of us keep our homes. These days, the food that mold likes to eat is in ample supply in virtually all modern buildings because we use it in construction.

The primary building ingredient on which mold likes to grow is cellulose. The reason we now use cellulose in building materials, like ceiling tiles, is that it's cheap, Dr. Straus notes.

In addition, many of us have carpeting in our homes, which stores moisture and holds shed skin cells and other gunk that mold will also eat.

Since the food supply mold needs tends to be widespread, the difference between a moldy home and a nonmoldy one is the presence of moisture. That's Dr. Horner's key philosophy, worth remembering in bold letters: **If you have a mold problem in your home, it's caused by moisture. If you don't have moisture in your home, you won't have a mold problem.**

Dampness in the home can flow from a number of sources, some obvious and others more sneaky. Moisture can condense on basement walls and concrete floors. If floors are carpeted—particularly a concrete basement floor—moisture can collect in the carpet fibers. Droplets can condense on a cold window and run down into the sill.

Pipes can drip and eaves can leak into walls. High humidity can saturate the air. Steam from boiling pots and hot showers can hang heavily. And on a *really* bad day, floodwater can pour into your home, soaking it to the core.

With water added to the food supply, the spores can start to grow. Typically, spores will produce tiny threadlike cells called hyphae, which grow into a tangled clump called a mycelium. Some molds will grow for quite a while before producing more spores, while others will start spitting them out almost immediately, Dr. Horner says.

When enough mold growth accumulates, you'll be able to see it or smell its distinctive stale, earthy smell.

If you've had a roof or pipe leak or other source of dampness in your home that was allowed to fester, and your family starts showing symptoms of allergic rhinitis or asthmalike wheezing, sneezing, and coughing or headache or mental confusion for unexplained reasons, mold might be the reason, Dr. Straus says. You'll need to clean or, more likely, remove the moldy material from your home.

A Wide World of Mold

Though we spend the vast majority of our time indoors, we run into mold spores whenever we step outside. In fact, you're likely to encounter a far greater variety of mold types outside than you will inside, Dr. Levetin says.

Outdoors, you'll find high concentrations of mold in places like decaying fallen leaves or deep in a grassy lawn. Other prime sites are compost piles and mulch out in the yard. You're likely to kick up a sizable amount of them when you go walking through the woods or mow your lawn.

"I've run an air sampler in my backyard when my husband's mowed, and the levels are almost uncountable, because the spores are one on top of the other. I'd say easily in the hundreds of thousands to millions (of spores per cubic meter of air)," says Dr. Levetin, whose area of expertise includes pollen and spore counting for her region. For comparison, a moderate day in her part of the country would have counts of about 20,000.

Pollen-counting stations will often also report the mold levels in the outdoor air. Check your local newspaper or tune in to your local television news broadcast for these counts. The levels tend to peak in the fall and run high until the ground is frozen or covered with snow in the winter, Dr. Levetin reports.

A Bleach-Free Option for Removing Mold

The recipe you'll typically find for a mold-killing brew is pretty simple: Mix 1 part bleach with 10 parts water, with a dash of detergent if you'd like, and use it to scrub off the fungus growing on a shower curtain, a wall, or other hard items.

This will kill most of the mold, but it isn't necessarily the best approach, says Elliott Horner, Ph.D., a mold expert and microbial laboratory director for Air Quality Sciences in Atlanta. The bleach probably won't kill all of the mold, leaving a bit waiting for the next damp period to grow again. Plus you'll be breathing in bleach fumes.

Here's another option: Mix a teaspoon of dishwashing liquid with a gallon of water, wet a sponge with the solution and scrub off the mold. You won't be killing the mold, but you'll be getting it off the target surface, which is the whole idea.

If you need something stronger to remove mold from the grout between shower tiles, for example, then fall back on the bleach solution or a mold-removing spray widely available at supermarkets and department stores.

Mold Allergy
ACTION PLAN

The first step in controlling mold allergy symptoms is to limit your exposure to mold. To do that, you need to clean up any areas in your home and yard where you know mold exists, and then make them as inhospitable to new mold growth as possible.

 indicates a natural remedy

Mold Prevention Indoors

- Pick up a humidity gauge, available for about $30 and up at hardware stores and allergy supply companies. Regularly monitor spots throughout your house to check the level of moisture in the air. Strive to keep the level between 40 and 60 percent.
- Use your home's heater or air conditioner to help keep the humidity low. You may need to run a dehumidifier in damp spots like the basement. If you use a dehumidifier, clean it according to manufacturer's instructions to keep it free of mold growth.
- Abstain from using a humidifier unless absolutely necessary. Raising the humidity encourages mold growth in the home, and humidifiers are prime locations themselves for mold growth. If you use one, clean it according to manufacturer's instructions and at least as often as recommended.
- Keep your home well-ventilated. This includes not only the rooms that you inhabit but also spare rooms, the attic, the basement, and any crawl spaces.
- Use your central air conditioner, if you have one, to cool your home instead of opening the windows.
- Use your exhaust fans when you run hot water in the bathroom or cook in the kitchen. Make sure these fans are vented to the outside. Your clothes dryer should be, too.
- Promptly fix any leaks, such as those from pipes or a hole in the roof. Thoroughly investigate to make sure that mold isn't growing on areas dampened by the leak.

- If you can, avoid having carpet in the bathroom, where it soaks up stray water, or on concrete basement floors. If you must have carpet on a basement floor, be extra cautious about keeping your humidity close to 40 percent.

  On account of the laws of nature, while the humidity level might be okay at shoulder height, it will increase close to cool surfaces, such as floors. At the carpet level, the humidity can make the fibers damp, turning the carpet into a rich harbor for mold.
- Household plants can scatter mold spores if overwatered, so keep them to a minimum in your home and out of your bedroom.
- If you store porous materials like clothing or newspapers in a damp area, check them regularly for mold growth or a moldy smell. Better yet, don't store them in a damp place.
- Regularly change or clean the filters on your air-conditioning and heating system according to the manufacturer's directions. Consider using HEPA (high-efficiency particulate air) filters on them to capture more spores.
- Have your air conditioner cleaned and serviced before cooling season. If your window air conditioner has a drip pan, keep it clean. The same goes for the drip pan under the refrigerator—they're both ideal spots for mold growth.
- Wipe down damp surfaces in the bathroom after a shower.
- Use allergen-proof encasings on your mattress, box springs, pillows, and covers.

Anti-Mold Gadgets May Be a Waste of Time

If the lure of a special ultraviolet light that kills mold tempts you to reach for your wallet, be cautious before you spend.

While ultraviolet light can be effective at killing bacteria floating in the air, such as the kind that causes tuberculosis, it's not so great at killing fungal spores, despite some advertising claims to the contrary, says Elliott Horner, Ph.D., a mold expert and microbial laboratory director for Air Quality Sciences in Atlanta.

Many of the molds that will grow in buildings are also used to floating around outside, where they're drenched with ultraviolet light from the sun, Dr. Horner points out.

• If your home is flooded, follow these steps.

If it's a sewage backup, any porous materials exposed to the mess should be removed.

If the water is from a potable water spill, a rain leak, or floodwater, any porous materials such as carpeting need to be cleaned and dried as quickly as possible. Within 24 hours is best, but you should still be okay as long as it's fixed within 72 hours. If not, the soggy material should be removed.

If the water rises several inches and gets the walls wet, remove the baseboards and cut an inch or two off the bottom of the drywall (you may need professional help for this) to allow the interior wall cavity to ventilate. Also remove outlet and light-switch cover plates to let more air circulate. When the walls are dry, replace the baseboards and covers.

Mold Treatment Indoors

🌿 If you see a moldy spot on a hard, nonporous surface—like shower tiles or curtains—scrub it clean. (See "A Bleach-Free Option for Removing Mold" on page 344 for more details.)

🌿 If you find mold on any porous item, throw it away. That includes items such as newspapers, books, and carpeting.

🌿 Use a HEPA filter in your bedroom to capture mold spores out of the air.

Preventing and Avoiding Mold Outdoors

• Avoid overwatering your lawn.
• If you must have mulch or compost material in your yard or garden, have a family member who doesn't have mold allergies work with it.
• Get someone else to mow the lawn, and stay inside during the mowing. If you must do the chore, wear a disposable dust mask that fits tightly against your face to filter out the mold.
• Similarly, if you can't get someone else to rake leaves, wear a mask while you do it.
• On warm, dry, windy days, minimize the time you spend outdoors. Mold counts will be high during these conditions.

Fascinating **fact!**

A puffball—the type of fungus that releases a hazy cloud when you stomp on it—can contain 7 *trillion* spores, or about 1,100 times more spores than there are people on the planet. On the other hand, a button mushroom—like the kind you can buy at the grocery store—has about 160 billion.

- Pay attention to mold reports from pollen- and mold-counting stations. Though they're not perfect, they can give you general guidelines on when you should stay indoors because mold levels are high.
- Minimize the time you spend out in the woods, particularly in autumn.

Medical Treatment for Mold Allergies

- If you suspect you have a mold allergy, check with an allergist, who can diagnose you by taking your history and running tests. He can suggest how active an approach you need to take to avoid mold.
- If you can't avoid going into a situation that will aggravate your mold allergies, pretreat yourself with the appropriate medications and remedies for allergy or asthma prescribed by your doctor, if any. (For more information, consult the Asthma and Hay Fever chapters.)
- Keep in mind that fungi can grow in your sinuses and lungs, leading to symptoms of sinusitis (marked by stuffy nose, fever, and facial pain) and bronchitis (marked by mucus-producing coughing). If it goes on long enough, you can develop flulike symptoms such as low-grade fevers, night sweats, headaches, fatigue, and achy muscles, says Vincent Marinkovich, M.D., an allergist and clinical associate professor of pediatrics at Stanford University. Your doctor may want to prescribe an antifungal medication, such as itraconazole (Sporanox), in these cases.
- Check with your doctor to see if you'd be a good candidate for immunotherapy to make you less sensitive to mold. Keep in mind, however, that allergy shots generally aren't as successful for mold as they are for other allergens like pollen, in part because there are so many types of mold.
- Be aware that many foods are fermented with fungi, including beer, bread, vinegar, soy sauce, and blue cheese. While some people with mold allergies can safely eat these foods, consult your doctor to find out whether these will be harmful to you, and take note if you have symptoms such as a rash, swollen throat, wheezing, or vomiting after eating them.
- Note that while some people are allergic to penicillin, which is derived from the *Penicillium* mold, that doesn't mean an allergy to mold will make you allergic to this antibiotic. Penicillin is highly purified and doesn't contain mold spores or protein. Tests for an allergy to penicillin are usually done by trial and error and involve skin and blood tests that aren't foolproof.

Nickel ALLERGY

PIERCED NOSES. Pierced eyebrows. Even pierced navels. These days, it seems many teenagers—and even some adults—are sporting more hardware than the local Sears. The recent piercing craze has sparked an upswing in nickel allergy—but not for the reasons you might think. You don't have to get pierced to become allergic to nickel. All you need to do is to wear a necklace or wristwatch with nickel in it.

"It isn't the actual piercing process itself. It isn't the actual blood exposure. It's the skin exposure," says Kevin Welch, M.D., assistant clinical professor at the University of South Alabama in Mobile and a dermatologist with the Medical Center Clinic in Pensacola, Florida. "You can develop the allergy just from prolonged contact of metal with skin."

No one is born with a nickel allergy, and you can minimize your risk of getting it by avoiding skin contact with nickel for ex-

tended periods of time. Once you do have the allergy, however, relatively brief contact with a metal containing nickel can trigger itching, burning, tiny red bumps, a rash, or even blistering eczema. That's why doctors call it contact dermatitis, and nickel allergy is second only to poison ivy as a cause of such skin afflictions.

In women, the most common cause of nickel allergy is earrings, followed by necklaces, largely due to the close and continuous contact these items have with the skin, says Ponciano Cruz Jr., M.D., professor and vice chairman of the department of dermatology at the University of Texas Southwestern Medical Center at Dallas.

In men, wristwatches are the most common cause. But with more men getting pierced and wearing more jewelry, Dr. Cruz says that the allergy is on the rise.

"Nickel allergy is very uncommon in

THE HIDDEN CONNECTION

Make Change If Your Food Contains Nickel

What's the first thing you think of when someone mentions the word *nickel*? For most people, it's probably coins or watches. But many common foods also contain nickel. Some research suggests that dietary nickel may be linked to hand dermatitis or eczema in those who are allergic. Some scientists theorize that a nickel-restricted diet might help people who are especially sensitive to the metal, but this is still being debated by experts. Until the issue is resolved, you might want to try following a low-nickel diet for a month or two and then gradually reintroduce the prohibited foods, doctors suggest. Of course, talk to your doctor first before trying this diet.

Foods to avoid include:

- Beans—green, brown, and white
- Buckwheat, millet, oatmeal, wheat bran breads and cereals, and multigrain breads
- Canned fruits and vegetables
- Chocolate and cocoa drinks, and tea from dispensers
- Figs, pineapple, prunes, and raspberries
- Kale, leeks, lettuce, peas, and spinach
- Nuts, baking powder, vitamins containing nickel, and fiber tablets containing wheat bran
- Salmon
- Shellfish such as shrimp, oysters, and mussels
- Sprouts

If you have a severe rash, you should also avoid the following foods, which contain smaller amounts of nickel than the foods listed above. These include beer, wine, herring, mackerel, tuna, tomatoes, onions, carrots, apples, and citrus fruits and their juices.

In addition, replace nickel-plated cooking utensils. You can use stainless steel pots and pans, except when you're cooking acidic foods that can leach nickel. Also, do not use the first quart of water from the tap because nickel may leach from pipes.

people who don't wear jewelry," adds Dr. Welch.

Fortunately, you don't have to avoid jewelry entirely. You just have to avoid items containing nickel. In general, jewelry labeled "hypoallergenic" is considered the least risky.

Dr. Cruz notes, however, that just because a jewelry manufacturer labels an item "hypoallergenic" does not guarantee that it is nickel-free. Indeed, hypoallergenic jewelry often is made of stainless steel that contains some nickel. Typically, this is safe because the nickel atoms are bound tightly to the steel, but some nickel might leach out with sweat or constant exposure.

All That Glitters . . .

Nickel allergy is common because the metal is common in objects used in everyday life, Dr. Cruz says. It can appear where you least suspect it, and the only way to know for sure that a metal is nickel-free is to use a nickel test kit, which can be obtained from a dermatologist or pharmacist.

Even gold is not an entirely safe choice. You can develop allergies to many metals, and in one study, gold was the second most common metal after nickel to produce allergies, at least in people who had their ears pierced. The total number of people with a gold allergy, however, was still relatively small.

"You can develop an allergy to 100 percent pure gold. It would look like a nickel allergy. But gold allergy is pretty rare," says Dr. Welch.

Further, gold jewelry is never 100 percent gold. It is always mixed with other metals to add hardness, and nickel is sometimes used.

Nickel even may be added to silver—especially "silver" coins, which are actually a nickel-copper sandwich. So simply handling coins can be a problem if you are allergic to nickel.

The Warning Signs

Most people who have a nickel allergy don't know it. "They know their problem is re-

Where's That Nickel?

If it's metal, it's suspect. Common objects that may contain nickel include earrings; watch backs, buckles, or bands; bra hooks or wire supports; necklaces; bracelets; rings; eyeglass frames; hair or eyelash curlers or hairpins; pants snaps, studs, or zippers; eye shadow; eating utensils; and coins.

lated to jewelry. Some may think it's the friction from the jewelry," says Dr. Cruz.

Your doctor can do patch tests to determine if you are allergic to nickel or gold, but most of the time this is unnecessary because the locations of the rash provide an obvious clue, Dr. Cruz notes.

The hands, wrists, ears, and stomach are the most common sites for nickel allergy, but any part of the body can be affected. Symptoms usually appear 24 to 36 hours after exposure. Even before a rash develops, you may notice itching or burning where there is contact with metal.

The earliest visible stage consists of small red spots or bumps, according to Dr. Welch, who says that he sees this in about two-thirds of his patients with nickel allergy. Avoid nickel, and the symptoms typically go away within a week.

Continued exposure to nickel can lead to tiny water blisters that aren't usually visible without magnification but make the skin moist and oozy. The skin may then peel off. If you remove the nickel at this stage, these symptoms can clear up in a day or two.

The most severe stage consists of a persistent rash that resembles a bad case of dishpan hands, with severe wrinkling and sometimes cracking or peeling skin. If the skin becomes raw, it may become painful. Ten to 20 percent of people with nickel allergy eventually develop this form of eczema. This condition takes about 10 days to heal, provided the skin does not become infected.

Symptoms may appear even where there is no direct contact with metal. Once a rash has developed in one location from contact with nickel, a rash can reappear in that spot later when another area comes in contact with the metal. And if you handle anything made of nickel, you can spread traces of the metal by touching other parts of your body, such as your eyelids, neck, or even your earlobes.

Born to Respond

While no one is born with a nickel allergy, some people are born with a predisposition to it. The reason is that they're born with T cells in their immune systems, waiting to attack nickel as if it were an invading enemy.

Once these T cells are exposed to nickel, your lymph glands gear up for war by cranking out carbon copies of the cells. The more you are exposed to nickel, the more T cells you make. And once you build this anti-nickel army, it never quite disbands. You are allergic for life.

So what can you do about it? If you reduce or eliminate your exposure to nickel soon after you first notice symptoms, you may be able to avoid developing more severe symptoms, according to Dr. Welch. On the other hand, the number of T cells you have may decline as your immune system weakens with age. As a result, your sensitivity to nickel may gradually diminish.

How Nickel Gets Under Your Skin

Workers in some jobs have a greater risk of nickel allergy, including hairdressers, retail clerks, caterers, domestic cleaners, and metalworkers. This is largely because their skin frequently gets roughed up on the job by chemicals, water, or just abrasion, Dr. Cruz says.

Yet even people who have healthy, intact skin can develop the condition, since nickel allergy is triggered by extended periods of metal-to-skin contact. The prob-lem begins when tiny bits of the metal get through the skin and make contact with the T cells in the lymph system, which is located just below the surface. When the surface of the skin is broken, even more nickel has a chance to get through. With piercing, for example, a thinner wall of skin covers the lymph system until the skin fully heals after a couple of weeks, Dr. Welch explains.

Even so, some people can cover themselves in cheap costume jewelry that is loaded with nickel and never develop the allergy. In fact, most people don't get it simply because they weren't born with nickel-sensitive T cells.

If you have been wearing jewelry for years and haven't developed the symptoms of nickel allergy, you probably don't need to worry about getting it. Since you don't know for sure if you are immune, however, it's still a good idea to remove jewelry when you don't need it and to wear hypoallergenic jewelry.

The Human Pincushions

Dennis Rodman, eat your heart out: Luis Antonio Aguero of Havana, Cuba, holds the dubious distinction of being the world's most pierced man.

According to *The Guinness Book of Records*, Aguero, as of last count, had acquired 230 piercings on his body and head, including a record 175 on his face.

But Elaine Davidson of Edinburgh, Scotland, holds the world record for most body piercings. Since 1997, she has acquired 462 piercings, 192 of which are on her head.

Nickel Allergy
ACTION PLAN

Once you have a nickel allergy, the only "cure" is to avoid touching anything with the metal in it—not an easy task.

If you don't already have a nickel allergy, you may want to take steps to avoid getting it. Try the following tips offered by Dr. Cruz and Dr. Welch.

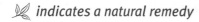 *indicates a natural remedy*

Prevention

- Buy nickel-free jewelry.
- If you must get pierced, have it done by a competent professional who uses stainless steel needles.
- For at least 2 weeks after piercing, use jewelry with posts made of surgical stainless steel, gold that is at least 14 karat, or plastic. You could even hold the hole open with a toothpick.
- Do not use sterling silver, gold plate, or gold-filled jewelry, at least initially after a piercing.

Treatment

- If you have symptoms of nickel allergy, eliminate contact between the metal and your skin.
- If the symptoms do not go away within a week, see a doctor. He can test you for nickel and other metal allergies. Be aware, however, that the nickel test is not 100 percent accurate and can sometimes produce false-positive results.
- Use jewelry labeled "hypoallergenic" or "nickel-free."
- To determine whether a metal contains nickel, get a nickel test kit from your dermatologist or pharmacist. The kit consists of two small bottles of clear liquids, one containing dimethylglyoxime and the other ammonium

hydroxide. If you put the two together on a metal containing nickel, they will turn pink.

🔏 Be careful with gold. Some jewelry is made of 9-karat gold, which can contain nickel and should be avoided. Use gold that is at least 14 karat; 18 karat is even safer.

🔏 Use solid gold, not plated or gold-filled jewelry, because the thin coating of gold can wear off, exposing nickel.

🔏 Get plastic sleeves to cover earring posts.

🔏 Coat metal that could come in contact with your skin, such as a bra fastener, with clear nail polish, paint, lacquer, or varnish.

🔏 Cover the back of your watch with adhesive tape or nail polish, or wear a sweatband under it. Another option is to get a watch with a plastic back.

🔏 Keep coins in a bag, purse, or wallet, rather than loose in your trouser pocket.

🔏 Wear cotton gloves when you handle things made of nickel at home or work. Use rubber or PVC gloves with cotton liners for wet work.

🔏 If you handle nickel, wash your hands before you touch other parts of your body, to avoid spreading the metal.

🔏 If you have a bad rash, protect your skin not only from nickel but also from other irritants to speed healing and to avoid infection. Wear gloves if necessary.

• Talk to your doctor or dermatologist about using special barrier creams, such as Ivy Block, that are available over the counter to help protect against poison ivy. They offer some limited protection against nickel.

• If you develop eczema, see a doctor. A steroid cream similar to hydrocortisone can help clear it up, but you must use prescription-strength formulations, such as clobetasol (Temovate) or fluocinonide (Fluocin), applied twice a day. If you have a widespread rash, a doctor may prescribe steroids in pills or shots, but this is rarely necessary.

• If the skin becomes crusted and yellow, weeps, or smells odd, see your doctor about getting antibiotics.

• Try an over-the-counter 1 percent hydrocortisone cream (such as Cortaid Maximum Strength Cream), which may help clear up a rash or itching, but don't use it for longer than the few days it takes for the rash to clear.

Fascinating fact!

Whether you get your earlobe or your eyebrow pierced, the risk of nickel allergy is about the same. But, oddly enough, the tongue appears to be immune. "I've never seen nickel allergy from piercing the mouth or tongue," says Ponciano Cruz Jr., M.D., professor and vice chairman of the department of dermatology at the University of Texas Southwestern Medical Center at Dallas. He theorizes that the gastrointestinal tract, which includes the mouth, tolerates nickel better than the rest of the body.

Pet ALLERGY

A TURTLE IS a man's best friend . . .

It just doesn't have the same ring to it as the old saying about dogs. But if you're a person with pet allergies, then befriending a reptile may not be such a bad idea. Every day, millions of us put up with runny noses, itchy eyes, and wheezy lungs just so we can enjoy the company of the furry members of our extended family—our pets.

Doctors have an easy solution to the pet allergies that plague our sinuses and attack our lungs: Just get rid of the pet, they say. But if you enjoy the company of one of more than 130 million domesticated animals that live in the United States, you'd probably be more willing to get rid of your doctor than your dog. "If you have an animal and you've become sensitized to it, the best thing to do is get rid of it," confirms B. Robert Feldman, M.D., associate director of the allergy division at the Children's Hospital of New York. "However, although

I've been making that suggestion for 37 years, almost nobody has taken that advice."

Allergies are caused by the production of certain antibodies. Because it takes a varying amount of time for people to develop antibodies and become sensitized to their pets, allergy symptoms can take a while to develop.

Finding a new home for your dog or cat might be the best solution to your allergy afflictions, but if you're one of the 44 percent of pet allergy sufferers who refuse to part with their pets, read on for some effective alternatives.

Causes of Pet Allergies

If the presence of your precious pet is causing you pain, you are not alone. Up to 15 percent of the general population and 30 percent of the allergic population have reactions to cats and dogs, with more people showing allergies to felines than canines. But these aren't the only creatures that can trigger your allergies. People also sneeze and sniffle around rodents, horses, cows, and birds.

The cause of your animal allergies may seem simple, but it's probably a bit more complicated than you think. Say you're at a friend's home, and his furry dog, Spot, is making your head swell up like a balloon. You look at the furniture, the carpet, and the air, and what do you see? Pet hair all over everything!

Using your best judgment, you can assume that the hair of this crafty canine is the cause of your misery. Close . . . but no doggie treat. "The hair is what people see, so that's what they expect to be allergic to," says Robert M. Zuckerman, M.D., an aller-

Saying Goodbye

You probably don't want to hear it, but there is one surefire way to alleviate the symptoms of your pet allergy: Remove the pet from your household. "Everything else is a distant second-best solution," says B. Robert Feldman, M.D., associate director of the allergy division at the Children's Hospital of New York. Once the pet is gone, so is the source of the allergy. It may take a few months for the allergens to subside to a non-irritating level, but after that, you should feel relief from your allergy symptoms.

Getting rid of such an important member of your household, of course, is easier said than done. "We tend to think that it's just a pet, but it's a lot more than that. It's a family member," says Bonnie Cushing, a family therapist in Montclair, New Jersey.

Cushing advises families to take the time needed to find a good home for their pet. "Network among your group of friends and try to find something that's close to home where you may even be able to go visit," she says. "It's worth taking the time to find your pet a good home because then you'll be assured of his future safety."

In addition, Cushing recommends that families honor the passage of their pet, just as they would a human being. To give your family's relationship with the pet closure, you could have a going-away party for him or just spend one last night enjoying his company.

People grieving over a lost pet also need to seek out the solace of friends who will understand and sympathize with their pain. "Connections with animals aren't honored the way that connections with people are," notes Cushing. "So people will grieve, and what will compound their grief is that they can't do it publicly." By discussing your feelings with sympathetic friends, you'll be able to work through your feelings of grief in a supportive environment.

gist and immunologist and associate professor of medicine at the Milton S. Hershey Medical Center of Pennsylvania State University in Hershey. In reality, a protein secreted by the sebaceous (oil-producing) glands and released with the dog's dander (dead skin cells) and saliva is the culprit. This protein, dubbed Can f 1 by scientists, is so tiny that it sneaks its way through fabrics and flows like air through an ordinary vacuum bag. So even when the hair is gone, tiny particles with the protein still hang around, waiting to land on your nose and eyes or be inhaled into your lungs.

If your allergy enemy is Garfield and not Snoopy, then a protein in cat dander and saliva, known as Fel d 1, is the source of your trouble. "The problem with cats is that the primary source of the allergen comes from the saliva," says Dr. Feldman. "They groom themselves, and when the saliva dries, it flakes off into microscopic particles that float throughout the house."

When Your Pet Is Just a Memory

Not only are the proteins of dogs and cats sneaky, they have a long shelf life as well. Even when the pet is removed from a home, it may take months before the number of allergens decreases to a harmless level. And in a modern well-insulated home or apartment, it may take years.

Just when you thought you couldn't hate these proteins more, recent studies have shown that they travel well, too. In 1996, researchers from the Johns Hopkins University School of Medicine in Baltimore

An Allergy for the Birds

A runny nose, itchy eyes, and asthma flare-ups are the most common signs of pet allergy, but bird lovers may be at risk for a much rarer and more dangerous allergic condition: hypersensitivity pneumonitis. This condition is sometimes called pigeon breeder's disease because it is most common among bird fanciers and breeders, people with a high exposure to the allergen proteins of birds.

Bird allergens can provoke pigeon breeder's disease in 5 to 20 percent of bird fanciers and breeders, and the results are not pretty. Symptoms such as fever, chills, chest tightness, fatigue, and coughing can result. Chronic cases can bring about the onset of even more serious conditions. This disease is rare, and it's usually not a concern for people who just own birds as pets. Be aware of the symptoms, though, and don't be afraid to talk to your doctor if they persist in the presence of your bird.

took dust and air samples from 40 homes without cats. Many of these homes harbored enough cat protein to cause allergic reactions. Why was the protein there? Doctors theorize that visitors probably transported it into the home, or a previous homeowner with a cat could have left the dander as a housewarming gift. "Cat dander is what is known as a ubiquitous antigen—it's everywhere," says Dr. Zuckerman. "Even people who don't own cats inhale cat dander in their everyday environment."

Beyond Morris and Fido

More than 39 percent of American households own a dog, while 32 percent have a cat. The American Humane Society currently estimates that 64.2 million cats and 62.4 million dogs are pawing around in our homes. Not surprisingly, our favorite pets are also our greatest causes of pet allergies, but they're not the only furballs causing problems. Keep in mind that any animal with fur or feathers can provoke allergy symptoms, and recently, certain rodents, such as guinea pigs and hamsters, have become increasingly popular as household pets.

Limited research has been done on the actual allergens released by hamsters, guinea pigs, and gerbils, but studies of mice and rats indicate that urine, not dander or saliva, holds most of the rodent allergens that make people miserable. And to make things worse, these urinary allergens can be easily carried around the house by airborne dust particles. If the urine of mice and rats causes people to react strongly, chances are that the urine of hamsters, gerbils, and guinea pigs will do the same. So take extra precautions such as wearing a mask and protective eyewear when changing the bedding in your pet's cage, or get a nonallergic friend or family member to do it, just to be on the safe side.

Symptoms of Pet Allergies

Imagine that it's springtime, and blossoms greet you everywhere you go. Of course, anybody who has experienced the symptoms of allergic rhinitis (hay fever) knows that with blossoms comes pollen—and with pollen come a runny, sneezing nose; itchy, red eyes; and even a wheezy chest.

Now imagine that these symptoms followed you inside and didn't haunt you just in the springtime, but all the time. You'd now know what it feels like to have full-blown pet allergies. In general, pet allergy symptoms mirror those of allergic rhinitis. People with severe pet allergies may even develop hives or an itchy rash after touching a pet.

By the numbers

44
Percentage of pet allergy sufferers who refuse to give up their pets

61
Percentage of American households with at least one pet

33
Percentage of American households with at least one child

Pet allergy reactions are similar to other allergic reactions because animal proteins affect the body in the same way that pollen, dust mites, or any other common allergen does. Once proteins from your dog or cat enter your body, they bind with white blood cells and cause your body to release the antibody histamine. When histamine is released—well, if you have pet allergies, you know the results all too well.

If you're a pet owner with asthma, the situation can be even grimmer. Doctors believe that people with asthma put themselves at even greater risk for asthma attacks if they share a home with a furry or feathery pet. Richard Lockey, M.D., director of the division of allergy and immunology at the University of South Florida in Tampa, once

treated a man with asthma who suffered a nearly fatal asthma attack while bathing his pet ferret.

When Your Pet Isn't the Culprit

The symptoms of pet allergy—especially for people with asthma—can be serious, so doctors always recommend getting rid of the offending pet. But before you kick out Fido or Fluffy, make sure that your pet is truly the source of the allergens—and not their flea powder or shampoo.

An 11-year-old girl died of a severe asthma attack just 2½ hours after washing her dog. The cause of the asthma attack,

Washing Away Your Sorrows

Some pet sprays and shampoos are advertised as being "miracle" products. Supposedly, these products remove dander and allergens from your dog and cat during the washing process.

What's the real scoop on these sprays and shampoos? They do, indeed, remove allergens—but not as effectively as you might think. "In one study, we wiped cats down with a damp cloth," says Judith Woodfolk, M.D., assistant professor of medicine at the Asthma and Allergic Diseases Center at the University of Virginia in Charlottesville. "We found that warm water alone was as effective as the pet shampoo." In addition, airborne allergen levels always returned to their previously high levels after about a week.

If you want to remove the greatest amount of allergens from your cat, says Dr. Woodfolk, you'll have to dunk him. Direct immersion of cats from the neck down in water for 3 minutes removed almost five times as much allergen as wiping. Of course, getting your cat to go along with this plan is another story.

Beware of Black Cats

Everyone's heard the old saying that letting a black cat cross your path is bad luck. Well, now it seems that there might actually be some truth to that superstition—at least if you're a person with allergies.

In a study conducted by the Long Island College Hospital in Brooklyn, people who are allergic to cats were found to be two to four times more likely to have severe reactions to dark-haired cats than light-haired ones. The results of the questionnaire were surprising to the researchers, but the size of the survey (321 patients) gives the results some statistical validity.

"We just put this study together as a lark," admits Clifford Bassett, M.D., assistant clinical professor of medicine at the State University of New York in Brooklyn and one of the study's authors. "We didn't expect to find any significant results when we decided to look at whether the color of the cat influenced allergic symptoms, but lo and behold, we found a strong statistical significance that this was the case—the darker the color, the more allergy-related symptoms were involved."

The survey was composed of entirely cat-allergic individuals, with an equal number of dark-haired-cat owners and light-haired-cat owners. Thirty-five of the survey participants were cat-allergic individuals who did not own a cat. Along with the color of the cat, the survey examined the kind of symptoms patients developed, the severity of the symptoms, and the frequency of the symptoms. The study also found that pet owners who allowed their cats in the bedroom were 20 times more likely to develop severe allergic symptoms than those who did not.

When the survey results started pouring in, researchers were astounded by what they discovered. "The findings are really surprising," says Shahzad Hussain, M.D., a chief fellow of the department of allergy and immunology at Long Island College Hospital and one of the study's authors. "As to why these people with dark-haired cats are reporting more allergic symptoms, we've speculated, but we don't know the answer. Maybe there's something in the cat's hair."

While interesting, the study results are based on a questionnaire, not solid clinical research. The researchers' next step is to measure the amount of Fel d 1, the allergy-causing protein in cats, produced by dark-haired cats and light-haired cats. In the meantime, however, you may be wise to heed the wisdom of the ages—and prevent a black cat from crossing your path.

however, was not dog allergen but pyrethrin, a common insecticide and an ingredient in the dog's shampoo. It was the first documented case of an allergic reaction to pyrethrin. While tragic situations such as this are rare, they serve as evidence that the cause of allergies may not always be what it seems.

Before removing a suspect pet from your home, be sure to see your doctor about an allergy test. You just might save yourself some heartache.

Hypoallergenic Pets?

Suppose you had to part ways with your precious long-haired cat or your beloved Old English sheepdog because your allergy symptoms made you miserable. Are you destined to live without an animal friend for the rest of your days?

Although most doctors will tell you that the notion of a hypoallergenic dog or cat is a myth, some people have found relief from their allergy symptoms while still enjoying the company of certain breeds. The hairless sphynx has kept some cat owners relatively sneeze- and sniffle-free, and poodles and bichon frise breeds have done the same for some dog lovers. "Dogs with more hairlike coverings as opposed to furlike coverings seem to be less allergenic," says Dr. Zuckerman.

Simple mathematics does give you one advantage when it comes to choosing a pet. "The larger the animal, the greater the area

of skin which exists, and the more dander that will be produced," notes Dr. Feldman. "If you have a Chihuahua, you're going to have a lot less dander than if you have a Great Dane." Of course, most allergists will tell you that buying a different breed of dog or cat is no guarantee that you will not have any symptoms.

Fish and reptiles may lack the charisma of fur-bearing pets, but their absence of allergy-causing protein and dander can be a pet lover's dream. Remember our friend the turtle? He can provide hours of entertainment without provoking a single sneeze. Fish, hermit crabs, lizards, and snakes are other popular hypoallergenic alternatives. Before you rush to the store to buy an iguana, however, keep in mind that all reptiles are a source of salmonellosis. In fact, reptiles actually can take credit for around 93,000 cases of salmonella infections a year. To prevent catching salmonella from your wrinkly pet, wash your hands after handling it and keep it away from areas where you prepare food. Since young children are at an increased risk of complications from salmonella, you probably shouldn't have a reptile in your home at all if you have a child who is younger than 5 years old.

Finally, if cats and dogs make you wheeze and fish and reptiles hold no charm for you, there is one pet out there that is 100 percent hypoallergenic. And on top of that, it will never shed, will never make a mess, and doesn't even need to be fed. What is this miracle pet, you ask? It's the Pet Rock.

Pet Allergy
ACTION PLAN

Despite the most sincere warnings from the doctor, some people would rather put up with allergies than let their pets go. If your love for your pet fits this description, then you need to do the next best thing: Make your home as allergen-free as humanly possible.

Prevention

- Keep your pet outside. This won't completely reduce your exposure to allergens, but it will help.
- If keeping your pet outdoors is not an option, then secure an area of your house for your pet, and try to restrict it to this area most of the time. You may have better luck arranging this if you have a dog; cats are free-roaming and won't put up with being confined to one room.
- Make sure that the area of the house where you keep your pet will be easy to clean and has little furniture and carpeting.
- No matter how territorial your cat may be, never allow him to stake his claim in the bedroom. Ideally, the bedrooms should be absolutely off-limits to the dog or cat. The particles that carry animal allergens are so small that they can seep right into your comforters, sheets, and pillow covers.
- Animal proteins tend to be particularly "sticky" allergens, so it's inevitable that some allergens on your clothes or floating through the air will make their way to your bed. To prevent pet dander from making its home there, encase your pillows, mattress, and box spring in plastic or allergen-proof covers and then place your regular pillow and mattress covers over them.
- For extra protection, get a large allergen-proof mattress encasing to place over the entire bed during the day. They are available for as little as $7 for a pillow encasing and as much as $99 for a king-size mattress encasing.
- Wash your covers, comforters, and sheets twice a week in hot water for the best results, recommends Dr. Zuckerman. Washing your bedding frequently is an important step in allergen-proofing your bedroom. You can purchase an allergen-free laundry additive, but hot water alone is equally effective.
- Regularly clean drapes and furniture and keep stuffed animal collections in

a glass case. Just as your bedding can be a reservoir for all sorts of nasty pet allergens, so can many other household items, such as carpeting, upholstered furniture, drapes, and even stuffed animals.

• Use a specialized filter to clear pet allergens from the air. Because the parti-

When You're Allergic to an Uninvited Guest

Quick quiz: What's the most common animal living indoors with man?

Surprisingly, it's not a dog or a cat, but the mouse, if you include commercial buildings, says Bobby Corrigan, an urban rodentologist with a doctorate from Purdue University in West Lafayette, Indiana, who now advises large corporations, cities, and schools on controlling rodents.

Whether they share your home or workplace, rats and mice can trigger allergies and asthma attacks much as dogs, cats, cockroaches, or dust mites can. And since the allergen is in the rodent's urine, it can spread widely through your home as it evaporates. Even 3 years after it has dried, it can continue to trigger allergies, says Peyton Eggleston, M.D., professor of pediatrics at the Johns Hopkins University in Baltimore.

Rodents seem to be a growing problem in all regions of the United States, according to Corrigan. Deterioration of inner cities and cutbacks in municipal programs may be one reason. Urban sprawl may be another. When you cut down the woods and meadows to put up houses and condos, where are the mice going to move? In with you.

Further, since a mouse can fit through a hole as wide as a pencil, rodent-proofing your home isn't an easy task. If you determine that you already have rodents in your house, the first step is to seal any holes so that new ones won't get in. Plug any quarter-inch or larger holes into your home with a silicone sealant, plaster, or cement that is appropriate to the surrounding material—not latex caulk. If the seal doesn't allow air, odors, and heat through, rodents won't try to gnaw through it. Also, look for holes around pipes.

In addition, look for light leaking through exterior doors, especially garage doors, and seal with metal-edged weather stripping. Obviously, keep your garage door closed.

Your next step is to make your home as inhospitable as possible to rodents. Do this by clearing out clutter in your garage and basement to eliminate hiding places, keeping all garbage in tightly covered metal cans, and not leaving pet food out at night.

Finally, as unpleasant as it is, you'll need to exterminate any rodents who refuse to find a new home. When you've determined that you're finally rid of the pests, thoroughly vacuum and wash all surfaces and steam-clean carpets to remove allergens.

cles that carry animal allergens are so tiny, they hang in the air for a long time, which makes HEPA (high-efficiency particulate air) filters very effective. In a study of nine homes with dogs, a HEPA filter reduced dog allergens in the air by 90 percent when the dog was not in the room and 75 percent when it was present. The filters are available from $45 and up in major retail stores.

"It's helpful to have an electronic air cleaner with a HEPA filter in the bedroom," says Dr. Feldman. "For most people, the bedroom is the one area of the house where they spend the most time."

- Hardwood and tile floors are preferable to carpeted ones. But if you can't tear up your carpet and install hardwood flooring, you can make a difference by doing a thorough job vacuuming.
- To trap the tiny particles that carry pet allergens, add a few simple attachments to your vacuum. "We found that vacuum cleaners that incorporated a HEPA filter, or a high-quality secondary filter, along with a double-thickness dust bag worked the best," says Judith Woodfolk, M.D., assistant professor of medicine at the Asthma and Allergic Diseases Center at the University of Virginia in Charlottesville. These filters, which attach easily to your ordinary vacuum, are available for about $7.
- To temporarily remove some of the allergens, wipe your pet down with a warm, damp washcloth at least twice a week.
- If you can get your cat to cooperate, immersing him from the neck down

The Miracle Cat-Allergy Cure?

A "cat challenge room" may sound like a frightening adversary to people with cat allergies. But thanks to a drug already helping people with asthma, the room proved to be not much of a challenge at all to participants in one study.

In the study conducted by scientists at the Johns Hopkins University in Baltimore, 18 people were given either zafirlukast (Accolate), a prescription asthma drug taken in pill form, or a placebo (a fake pill). The participants then spent an hour in the "cat challenge room," a room with 10 to 100 times the level of cat allergen that you would normally find in the home.

The results were pretty promising. Zafirlukast not only reduced shortness of breath and wheezing in participants but also cleared up their runny noses. And because the drug is a pill, puffing on an inhaler to prevent cat allergy could soon be a practice of the past.

THE HIDDEN CONNECTION

Goose Down and Allergies

Even if there isn't a pet in sight, you could still be bombarded by animal allergens from some common household items.

One of the common criminals lurking around the house is goose down, a popular filling for comforters and pillows. When feathers seep through their fabric coverings, they have the potential to pester your sinuses just like plumage from Polly's cage. "It all depends on the quality of material used in the coverings," says Robert M. Zuckerman, M.D., an allergist and immunologist and associate professor of medicine at the Milton S. Hershey Medical Center of Pennsylvania State University in Hershey. "Still, I recommend plastic encasements for your quilts, mattresses, and pillows to prevent feathers from flying out."

What about animal products like pelts, fur coats, and sheepskin blankets? In this case, your allergies probably aren't being affected. "With pets, it's usually living skin that flakes off and becomes a problem," says Dr. Zuckerman. "The tanning process really takes care of this with furs."

Still, one study suggests that animal skins, when used as bedding, may trap more allergens ordinarily found in the home than other types of bedding.

in warm water for 3 minutes is the most effective way to remove allergens.
• Consider purchasing a more hypoallergenic pet, such as a hairless sphynx cat or a fish.

Treatment

• Discuss with your doctor what type of antihistamine, internasal steroid spray, or immunotherapy would be appropriate for you.
• Zafirlukast (Accolate), a prescription asthma medication given in pill form, has shown great promise in combating the symptoms of cat allergy.
• If you're still experiencing symptoms despite your best efforts at reducing the amount of allergen in your home and taking the medication your doctor recommends, you may want to seriously consider removing your pet from your home. Sometimes this is the only way to relieve symptoms.

Physical
ALLERGY

CHANCES ARE, you're not happy when your body responds to pollen, pet dander, and other allergens with a runny nose, a wheezy chest, and a breakout of hives. But, hey, it could always be worse. What if the glorious sun and tranquil water made you erupt in itchy, red welts, or a bright winter's day brought you to your knees, wheezy and short of breath?

Reacting this way to the glory of nature doesn't seem fair. But for people with physical allergies, it's something they have to fight against every day of their lives. Loosely defined, physical allergy is a condition in which the body reacts to physical stimuli such as cold, heat, light, or minor injury. Like a veteran actor, physical allergies can take many forms, but they most commonly manifest themselves as hives, skin blotches, or itching. And like that same veteran actor, they might get testy if you don't treat them properly.

Welts, Blotches, and Hives . . . Oh, My!

Essentially, *urticaria* is your doctor's fancy word for hives, the itchy, red welts that appear on your skin. If you haven't gotten them before, one of your friends probably has. One in five of us gets them at some point. And three out of every 20 of these blotchy breakouts are caused by a physical irritant. "People will get urticaria from various stimuli, which include cold, heat, water, vibration, sun, and pressure," says Daryl Altman, M.D., an allergist/immunologist at Allergy Associates in Baldwin, New York. "Those are the big ones."

Take your thumbnail and stroke it firmly across the surface of your skin. The stroke will produce a white line, then a red line, and then a slight swelling. This reaction is considered normal. If, however, you're like 2 to 5 percent of the population, the response is exaggerated to the

THE HIDDEN CONNECTION

Sunscreens and Dermatitis

Similar to solar urticaria, photoallergic contact dermatitis causes red rashes, swelling, and blistering on areas of the skin that are exposed to sunlight. But unlike solar urticaria, the sun doesn't cause this rare form of dermatitis. Instead, your body has a skin reaction to a chemical when exposed to a specific wavelength of sunlight.

"If you're exposed to the allergen and the sun at the same time, then you'll get a reaction," says Daryl Altman, M.D., an allergist/immunologist at Allergy Associates in Baldwin, New York.

Common causes are aftershave lotions, sunscreens, perfumes, and oils. "Some people will put on a sunscreen with para-aminobenzoic acid (PABA), go to Cancun, and develop a terrible red rash when they have sunlight exposure. Once the rash has developed, it will likely persist for days, whether or not you are exposed to sunlight," reports Mark Dykewicz, M.D., associate professor of internal medicine and director of the training program in allergy and immunology at St. Louis University School of Medicine.

If you develop photoallergic contact dermatitis, your best bet is to identify the source of your irritation and quit using it. And be sure to contact your allergist or dermatologist. "This condition is not responsive to antihistamines. You should use a topical steroid or may even need a systemic steroid if your symptoms become severe," says Dr. Dykewicz.

point where welts show up on the stroke line.

This is *dermographism*, states Mark Dykewicz, M.D., associate professor of internal medicine and director of the training program in allergy and immunology at St. Louis University School of Medicine. The most common of the physical allergy forms, dermographism develops when pressure is applied to the skin from clothing, chairs, toweling off after a shower, or—the most unfair of all—passionate embraces from your sweetie. Common among younger people, the hives of dermographism usually clear up in about a half-hour, and the disease itself usually goes away completely after a year or two.

If touching doesn't get you, then

sweating just might. *Cholinergic urticaria* is triggered by perspiration as well as emotional stress or by hot or alcoholic beverages. It's a common condition of young adults and affects up to 15 percent of adults. "Most kinds of physical urticaria produce the same type of hives," says Dr. Altman. "Cholinergic urticaria produces hives that tend to be smaller: little red dots instead of big red blotches." The midsection and arms are the likely targets, and again, young people are its favorite victims.

Here's another quick skin test for you. Put a few ice cubes inside a wet towel and place the towel on the back of your forearm. Let it melt there for about 4 minutes. If the area, including where the water ran off your arm, swells and gets itchy, then you may have *cold urticaria*. This condition can be dangerous. In rare instances, patients with cold urticaria have gone into anaphylactic shock and died while swimming, states Dr. Altman. It's important to add that although there is a possibility of anaphylactic shock, it is extremely rare in someone who has never had this type of reaction before.

In addition to cold urticaria, there are several other rare forms of physical allergy, including *solar urticaria* (reaction to sunlight), *heat urticaria* (reaction to heat or hot water), *delayed pressure urticaria* (reaction to sustained pressure), *vibratory urticaria* (reaction to vibration), and *aquagenic urticaria* (reaction to water).

With most of these conditions, hives usually go away 30 minutes after they develop. Delayed pressure urticaria, however, causes hives 4 to 6 hours after pressure is applied to the skin and may persist for many hours. See your doctor if you're concerned about any of these conditions—and see the Action Plan on page 371 for quick relief.

Exercise, Cold Air, and Asthma

Blotches, bumps, and welts aren't the only ways that physical allergies can affect the body. Consider this scenario: You're taking a jog on a cold January morning. This may seem like a good idea at first. The scenery, with the leafless skeletons of trees and the smattering of snow on the ground, is breathtaking. But for someone with asthma, the air can quite literally be breathtaking, too.

"When most people with asthma are studied, the majority of them will have a worsening of their symptoms when they're exposed to cold air," says David Khan, M.D., assistant professor of allergy and immunology at the University of Texas

By the
numbers

10–20
Percentage of
the population
that will develop
hives at some
point in their lives

5
Percentage of
the population
that will develop
dermographism
at some point

15
Percentage of
cases of hives
caused by a
physical irritant

Southwestern Medical Center at Dallas. "Winter weather obviously brings out that problem."

The cold air does not directly cause asthma symptoms, explains Dr. Khan. Instead, researchers have theorized that the cold air triggers the body to increase bloodflow to the airway. In some cases, this increased bloodflow can result in swelling—not a very pleasant scenario for someone with asthma who may already have difficulty breathing.

When you combine the effects of cold air and intense exercise, the problem is magnified. "Those are actually elements we use in the laboratory for our research models," says Dr. Khan. "We have patients run while breathing in extra-cold air. and it's the combination of the two that triggers their symptoms."

Ozone and Asthma: A Modern Problem

As if cold air weren't enough, modern society has found a way to make sure our lungs suffer in warm weather as well.

Many people cough, have shortness of breath, and wheeze in the summer months because of the harmful effects of ozone, a form of oxygen that is the main component of smog. The hydrocarbons choked out by cars, factories, and construction equipment react with sunlight to produce ozone, so not surprisingly, urban areas have the most dangerous levels.

High levels of ozone affect everyone, even conditioned athletes. But they take their biggest toll, perhaps, on those who already have lung problems. "In people who have allergic asthma or allergic rhinitis (hay fever), having ozone and allergy is a double whammy," says David Khan, M.D., assistant professor of allergy and immunology at the University of Texas Southwestern Medical Center at Dallas. "The ozone augments the influence that the allergy is having on the asthma."

The current federal health-based air-quality standard is 0.12 parts per million of ozone, but studies have shown that even levels lower than that are dangerous. Your best bet on high-ozone days is to stay indoors and filter air coming into your house through an air conditioner. Also, stay on top of pollution alerts put out by public health authorities in the newspaper or online.

Physical Allergy
ACTION PLAN

Obviously, the best way to avoid developing physical urticaria is to avoid the irritant—whether it be pressure, sweat, heat, cold, water, or sunlight. Here are some tips to help you do just that, as well as strategies for relief when you do experience symptoms.

🌿 *indicates a natural remedy*

🌿 For dermographism or other kinds of pressure-induced urticaria, avoid tight belts, bra straps, or other articles of clothing that apply pressure to the skin.

🌿 If you have cold urticaria, dress warmly or stay indoors. Don't go swimming in a cold swimming pool.

🌿 Sometimes urticaria can make sunlight your enemy. Cover up adequately or use sunscreen.

🌿 Some types of physical urticaria are stress-related, so try tai chi or meditation. Though there's no medical data to support it, these methods of stress reduction have proven helpful for some.

🌿 Take a 400-milligram tablet of quercetin twice a day between meals. Available at health food stores, this bioflavonoid is effective in reducing allergic responsiveness, states Andrew Weil, M.D., director of the program in integrative medicine and clinical professor of medicine at the University of Arizona College of Medicine in Tucson.

🌿 Add garlic, onions, chamomile, and licorice to your diet. All four can make histamine production drop. Histamine is one of the inflammatory chemicals that is responsible for allergy symptoms.

🌿 For soothing relief, try Aveeno Daily Moisturizing Bath. This product can do the trick because it is made with natural colloidal oatmeal, says Dr. Altman.

• Consider oral antihistamines, which are often the best way to keep hive production under control. Some good ones are cyproheptadine (Periactin), chlorpheniramine (Tussi-12), and diphenhydramine (Benadryl). Less-sedating antihistamines, however, such as cetirizine (Zyrtec), fexofenadine (Allegra), and loratadine (Claritin), also work well and are being used more often, says Dr. Altman.

- Some types of urticaria may be a sign of a serious underlying illness such as cancer. Consult your physician if you're at all concerned about your symptoms.

Beat the Cold Air

- Make friends with your scarf. Not only will a scarf increase the temperature of the air that first enters your lungs, but it also increases the local humidity as you exhale, creating an environment of warm air entering your airway.
- If you want something a little more stable than a scarf, buy a cold-air mask that completely covers the mouth and nose. These masks are available online for around $13.
- Before participating in exercise or physically strenuous activities, spend time warming up to avoid exercise-induced asthma.
- When you first step into the frozen tundra, adjust to the climate for a few minutes before starting into a full-fledged workout. Do the same after your workout before you head back into your warm, cozy home.
- Take two puffs on an inhaler of albuterol (Proventil) or cromolyn (Intal) 15 to 30 minutes before heading outdoors. This usually holds off asthma symptoms, states Dr. Khan. Salmeterol (Serevent) and nedocromil (Tilade) are other effective inhalers for preventing asthma.
- Consider oral prescription drugs. Zafirlukast (Accolate) and montelukast (Singulair) are effective oral pill medications used to prevent exercise-induced asthma, states Dr. Khan.

Poison Plant
ALLERGY

JACK WRIGHT WILL never forget his sixth-grade summer. While "roughing it" in the woods of northern California, Jack picked the wrong leaf for the wrong job. A few hours after using a shiny green leaf for toilet paper, he had a very itchy rash in a very private place. "I took only one leaf, but that plant sure got its revenge," says Jack, a high school history teacher in Chesapeake, Virginia.

Just as a cactus has spikes and mistletoe has toxic berries, poisonous plants have adapted an effective survival strategy. Contact with any part of a poisonous plant causes an itchy, red, blistery rash. In fact, contact with the poisonous trio—ivy, oak, and sumac—is the single most common cause of allergic reactions in the United States. Each year 10 million to 50 million Americans develop an allergic rash after contact with these poisonous plants.

According to the American Academy of Dermatology, about 85 percent of people are susceptible to becoming allergic to poison ivy, oak, or sumac, but rarely on their first exposure to the poisonous plant.

These itchy rashes are caused by contact with urushiol, a colorless to slightly yellow oily ingredient found in the sap of all three poisonous plants. Although an intact plant is incapable of triggering an allergic reaction, when the fragile leaves, roots, or stems are damaged, the sap containing this oil leaks out. And it's persistent stuff: It can stick on objects such as clothing, boots, and dog fur, staying active for months. It can even trigger a reaction a year later. Even airborne urushiol particles, such as those from burning plants, can cause a rash.

Luckily, nature has given us an edge. Like invisible ink in reverse, urushiol turns brownish black after exposure to air, making it easier to spot. Since oily black spots on a plant are a good indication that it is a poison plant, sensitive people should avoid touching any plant with these spots.

Just as cactus spikes don't hurt if you don't touch them, an intact poison plant won't trigger an allergic reaction. But damage a part of it, and you'll pay! Pulling weeds or cutting a plant while mowing releases the urushiol. A hiker's leg, a child's lost ball, or a gardener's tool can break a stem and allow urushiol to seep out. Even a gust of wind or a spider's kiss may be enough to crack a leaf and allow the sap to leak.

One of the major problems with poison plants is that they're so ubiquitous. Poison plants spread like the weeds they are and grow almost everywhere in the United States. Your only possible escape is to move to Hawaii, Alaska, or some desert areas of Nevada, says Alan Kling, M.D., clinical assistant professor at Mount Sinai School of Medicine in New York City. Poison ivy usually grows east of the Rocky Mountains and in Canada. Poison oak grows in the western United States, Canada, Mexico, and in the southeastern states. Poison sumac grows in the Northeast, Midwest, and in swampy areas of the southeastern states.

Regardless of how difficult they are to evade, the best defense against uncom-

fortable and temporarily disfiguring poison plant rashes is to learn to recognize

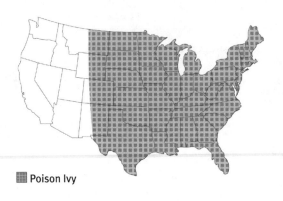
Poison Ivy

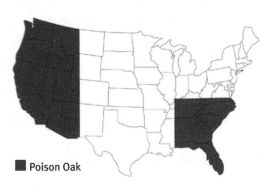
Poison Oak

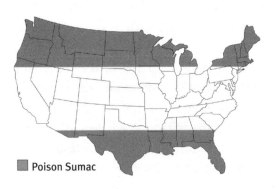
Poison Sumac

the plants and avoid contact with them. Sadly, this isn't a simple task. These tricky plants *look* different in different parts of the country. Take poison ivy, for example. In the East, Midwest, and South, it grows as a vine. But in the far northern and western United States, Canada, and around the Great Lakes, it grows as a shrub. The good news is that everywhere it grows, each leaf has three leaflets. It can also be identified by the distinctive hair that grows on its fruit, trunk, and leaves. Poison ivy is easily recognized in the spring because it has yellow or green flowers or white berries. The leaves are just as easy to spot in the fall because they turn red.

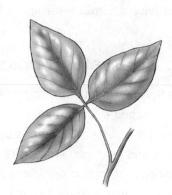

Poison ivy

Poison oak, too, looks different in different places. In the West, this plant may grow as a high-climbing vine or tall shrub, but in the East, it grows as a low shrub. Its notched leaves look like those of the common white oak tree. The yellow berries grow in clusters and are all green in summer and off-white in winter.

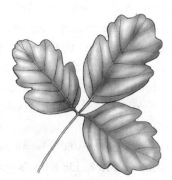

Poison oak

Poison sumac is the one consistent poison plant. Each leaf has 7 to 13 leaflets. This tall shrub grows in peat bogs in the Northeast and Midwest and in swampy areas in parts of the southeastern states. It's sometimes called poison elder or poison ash because it resembles these plants. It sports green berries in summer that turn yellow-white.

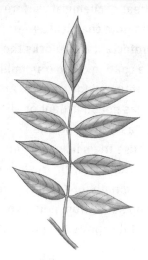

Poison sumac

If you are sensitive to one of these three plants, you are sensitive to all of them, Dr. Kling cautions. That's because although the plants may look different, they're from the same plant family. Also, because they all have the same urushiol, the allergenic component of the plant's resin, the itchy rash they cause is similar.

Poison plant rashes usually begin as blisters that sting and itch, Dr. Kling says. The blisters often appear in thin lines where your skin has brushed against the plant. Later, the blisters break and weep a clear yellow fluid. As the fluid dries, it crusts on your skin, looking sort of like crumbly amber. The rash should heal and disappear in about 10 days.

Who's at Risk?

About half the people who are exposed to poisonous plants will break out in a rash. Interestingly, people who are immunodeficient, such as those with leukemia or AIDS, may actually be less susceptible.

Seniors also have an edge. They seem to get poison plant rashes less often, as do those who have asthma, allergic rhinitis (hay fever), and other types of allergies. This may be because these people have diminished immune function or because they're simply less likely to be working or playing outside, making them less likely to come in contact with the nasty plants.

Sensitivity declines with age. Children

Army Develops New Defense against Urushiol

The threat of chemical warfare is very real to the U.S. Army. In an effort to protect soldiers from chemical agents, Army researchers developed a Teflon-like topical skin protectant that blocks the absorption of a variety of substances. When applied, a coating 0.1 to 0.15 millimeter thick is formed, and in animal studies its effects continued for 4 hours. After study results showed that topical skin protectant (TSP) was not an irritant or allergen for people, the Army was anxious to see if TSP worked as well on people.

Because trials using chemical warfare agents would be unethical, the Army tested TSP with urushiol on 81 enlisted volunteers. The results were encouraging both for soldiers threatened by possible chemical warfare and for civilians who suffer from poison plant rashes. The analysis revealed that TSP was successful in protecting the volunteers from high and low concentrations of urushiol.

who are sensitive to the poisonous plants will probably find that their sensitivity decreases by half by the time they reach young adulthood, as long as they aren't exposed repeatedly.

Never assume that you're one of the lucky ones who are immune to these plants. You may have an allergic reaction this year but walk away unscathed the next. Your body's reaction to these plants can change suddenly; therefore, it's unwise to assume that you're permanently insensitive if you don't develop the symptoms after your first contact.

What's Going On in Your Body?

The itching, blistering reaction you get from poison plants is caused by a T-cell response to the urushiol.

Within minutes of coming into contact with your skin, the oil begins to penetrate it. If you're sensitive to it, a reaction will appear as a line or streak of rash, usually within 12 to 48 hours. The rash can break out as early as 6 hours after exposure or as late as 3 days after. Since the yard work you did on Sunday could be a distant memory by Wednesday, identifying a poison plant rash can take some pretty good detective work.

More often than not, the rash appears on areas of your body where the skin is thin, such as your face. Developing a rash on the palms of your hands or the soles of your feet, where the skin is thicker, is very unlikely. Regardless of what your friends or family may tell you, rashes do not spread. Although it is common for new rashes to appear, they are more accurately attributed to how quickly your body absorbs the urushiol. Since urushiol is absorbed more slowly into skin that is thick, you may develop new rashes at a later time on those areas.

While your hands aren't likely to break out in a rash themselves, they are often the transfer agents for the allergenic oil. Many times a rash that develops on the face or arm may resemble a handprint, and linear lesions may trace the marks of scratching fingers.

Perhaps the best thing about poison plant rashes is that once you've had one, it's likely to motivate you to learn how to identify the plants and avoid them like the plague in the future.

Poison Plant Allergy
ACTION PLAN

In the case of poisonous plants, the best defense is avoidance. If that's not possible, some over-the-counter products can help to protect you from urushiol, the allergenic component of the plant's sap.

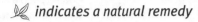 *indicates a natural remedy*

Prevention

- If you're going to be where poisonous plants grow, wear long pants, long sleeves, boots, and gloves. If you need to touch the plants, wear vinyl gloves. Urushiol can soak through cloth and rubber, but vinyl stops it in its tracks.
- Apply IvyBlock, a protective cream containing bentoquatam. It is designed to be put on your skin *before* you go out in the woods. It prevents urushiol from penetrating your skin by creating a claylike barrier, according to Andrew Weil, M.D., director of the program in integrative medicine and clinical professor of medicine at the University of Arizona College of Medicine in Tucson. IvyBlock isn't going to help you get dates, though. Once it dries, the cream leaves a faint white coating.
- Consider another over-the-counter product, Tecnu Oak-N-Ivy Brand Outdoor Skin Cleanser, which will remove the urushiol from your skin up to 8 hours after contact. If you're highly allergic to poison plants, keep this product handy and take it with you on outdoor trips, says Dr. Weil.

Treatment

If you mistakenly come in contact with a poison plant, you still might be able to avoid a rash if you act quickly. And if you do get a rash, there are a number of natural and conventional remedies that can help to ease the itch.

Making Contact

Wash all exposed areas with cold running water. This can keep the urushiol from contacting your skin. Head for the nearest stream, lake, or garden hose. If you can get there within 5 minutes, water may be all you need. If it's longer than a few minutes away, use soap, too, since you can wash the oil off with soap and water as long as you do it within the first 30 minutes, states Dr. Weil.

🌿 If you're a bit slower on the uptake, grab a bottle of rubbing alcohol. Gently cleaning your skin with rubbing alcohol will dissolve the resin. More great news: Beer and other alcoholic beverages work, too. After applying the alcohol, rinse your skin thoroughly with water. Even if you can't tend to exposed areas right away, you may still be able to minimize the rash by treating it within 2 hours, recommends Dr. Weil.

When the Best Laid Plans Fail

Although people who *know* they are about to enter an area thick with poison plants might arm themselves with a barrier lotion, most contacts with the plants are not anticipated. It's usually that spontaneous hike in the woods that leads to the itch.

The truth is, even if you do nothing to ease your symptoms, a mild plant rash will resolve itself in about 2 weeks. If the discomfort is just too much to ignore, here are some treatments to ease your itching and scratching.

🌿 The best treatment is to run hot water—make it as hot as you can stand—on the affected areas for at least 3 minutes or as long as you can tolerate it without burning your skin, says Dr. Weil. The itching will briefly become more intense, and then it will stop for several hours, as if the nerves responsible for conveying the sensation to the brain become overloaded and quit. As soon as the itching starts again, go back to the hot water. The itching reaction will respond quickly, and your skin will return to normal much faster than it would otherwise. This technique should not be done if your skin is open or peeling.

🌿 Have witch hazel astringent handy. Distilled from the witch hazel shrub, which grows wild in the Northeast (probably right next to a hairy poison ivy vine), witch hazel astringent soothes poison ivy blisters. Pour the solution onto a clean cloth or gauze pad to make a wet dressing. Carefully pat the area, then remove the cloth and allow to air dry. Don't leave the dressing on until it dries, or it may stick to the skin. According to Dr. Weil, it soothes, cools, cleans, relieves itches, and is a truly useful all-around astringent.

By the
numbers

1
Percentage of people who are totally immune to poison ivy

15
Ranking of poison ivy, poison sumac, and poison oak among the most common causes of allergic reaction in the United States

10–50
Millions of Americans each year who develop an allergic rash after contact with these poisonous plants

✻ You can dry up the blisters with baking soda mixed with a little water, Dr. Weil says. Just pat it on and wait for it to dry. A mixture of half vinegar and half rubbing alcohol also is an excellent remedy. Be aware, though, that it will sting, and be careful not to get it into your eyes. Another alternative is to rub on a mixture of equal parts buttermilk, vinegar, and salt.

✻ Try another home remedy that Dr. Weil recommends: Mix just enough clay and water to form a spreadable paste. Once the paste is applied to the affected areas, allow it to dry.

✻ Crush whole fresh plantain or jewelweed and rub the juice on affected areas. Since the juice is clear, just leave it on until the next time you wash. These herbs may have a soothing effect similar to that of the compresses that have long been recommended by physicians for patients suffering from an itchy rash, says Dr. Weil. Conventional doctors contend that there is no scientific evidence to support the use of any herbal remedies, despite anecdotal reports that plants like plantain and jewelweed ease discomfort.

• Know that over-the-counter products such as hydrocortisone creams have little effect on rashes. Instead, relieve the itching by taking cool showers and applying calamine lotion or soak a mini-compress in Burrow's solution, which is available in drugstores as Domeboro Astringent Solution. You may ease unpleasant itching and blisters simply by taking a lukewarm bath treated with a solution of baking soda or oatmeal.

• Resist the urge to use itch-control products like antihistamines, which don't help much, states Dr. Weil.

✻ Also resist the urge to scratch. You won't spread the rash by scratching the blisters, but bacteria under your fingernails could cause an infection.

At the Doctor's Office

When exposure to a poisonous plant causes extreme symptoms, medical treatment is necessary.

• In severe cases of hypersensitivity, a severe rash, blisters, and extreme swelling can develop on the arms, legs, face, and even the genitals. If you develop any of these symptoms, see your doctor immediately.

• If you are known to have severe reactions to poisonous plants and have come in contact with them, consult your doctor immediately. A prescription cortisone cream may stop your body's severe reaction. Use it for as long as prescribed, or the rash may return.

SINUSITIS

WITH MORE THAN 350 MILES of connected chambers and passageways, the Mammoth Cave system in Kentucky is the longest in the world. Water flows steadily through the limestone caverns, and air wafts through the dark tunnels linking the chambers.

To better understand your sinuses and nasal passages, you can think of them as a type of cave system, admittedly on a much smaller scale. In this analogy, it is common-cold viruses, bacteria, and allergy triggers such as pollen that venture through the dark passageways rather than determined cave explorers. And when these microscopic nuisances make their way up your nose, you could wind up with a case of sinusitis.

Your symptoms could range from the fever, coughing, and yellow mucus that are the hallmarks of a hot, acute case, to the lingering postnasal drip and fatigue found in a smoldering, chronic case.

Let's venture into the caverns of your sinus system together to see how and why sinusitis strikes.

The Science of Sinusitis

A sinus is simply a hollow air pocket, of which we have dozens scattered throughout our bodies. But generally when we talk about sinuses, we're referring to the paranasal sinuses buried behind the face and forehead.

The paranasal sinuses are four pairs of open spaces, lined with mucous membranes, that are situated in the bones of the head surrounding the nose. The frontal sinuses are above the eyes in the brow area, the maxillary sinuses are in each cheek, the ethmoids are behind the bridge of the nose and between the eyes, and the sphenoids are behind the eyes.

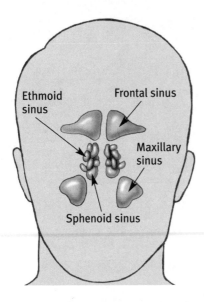

Ethmoid sinus

Frontal sinus

Maxillary sinus

Sphenoid sinus

Experts believe that one of the reasons we have sinuses is to lighten the weight of our skulls (it's apparently better to be an airhead than a bonehead!). These pockets also help warm, filter, and humidify the air we breathe; improve our ability to smell; and help us pronounce certain sounds while speaking. They also churn out a steady flow of mucus, which normally is very useful in keeping nasal passages clean, but is a dangerous ingredient when the sinuses stop working properly.

If you venture into enough real-life caves, you'll eventually have to squeeze through a tiny opening linking one room to another. That's how your sinuses are designed, too. Your nostrils head back into an open passage that leads to your throat. The sinuses are linked to this nasal passage by tiny openings called ostia, which are the size of pinholes.

The mucus your sinuses create must escape through these small openings and head back toward your throat or out your nose. To get it there, a vast number of cilia, microscopic hairlike projections in the mucous lining of each sinus and the nose, beat in unison to push the mucus along.

As it goes, the sticky fluid captures dust and bits of airborne clutter that you inhale through your nose and carries them to your throat, where you swallow them, and then the acids in your stomach destroy them. When the system works properly, air and fluids pass freely through the nose and sinuses, and everyone is happy.

But sometimes rhinitis—which is an inflammation in the nose—will cause the lining inside the nasal passages to swell,

Feel Your Pain

Depending on which sinus is affected, your body may send different signals indicating that you have sinusitis. Note here the specific sinuses and their related symptoms.
- Maxillary: Toothache or pain over the cheekbone
- Ethmoid: Pain or pressure near the inner corner of the eye
- Frontal: Major headache and tenderness near your forehead
- Sphenoid: Major headache in several spots or at the back of your head

Learn the Signs of Rhinitis and Sinusitis

If you're prone to fits of allergic rhinitis, or hay fever, you may have trouble distinguishing its common symptoms from those of sinusitis. Here's a handy way to sort them out. The number of shaded squares indicates the degree to which the symptom is associated with the particular condition. The more shaded squares, the more severe the symptoms are likely to be.

	Rhinitis	Sinusitis
Congestion	■ ■ ■ ■	■ ■ ■ ■
Sneezing	■ ■ ■ □	■ □ □ □
Itching	■ ■ ■ □	□ □ □ □
Clear discharge	■ ■ ■ ■	■ □ □ □
Discharge containing pus	■ □ □ □	■ ■ ■ ■
Postnasal drip	■ ■ □ □	■ ■ ■ ■
Headache	■ □ □ □	■ ■ ■ □
Facial pressure	■ □ □ □	■ ■ ■ ■
Loss or impairment of the sense of smell	■ ■ □ □	■ ■ ■ ■
Cough	■ □ □ □	■ ■ ■ □
Throat clearing	■ □ □ □	■ ■ ■ □
Fever	■ □ □ □	■ ■ □ □

pinching shut those ostia leading to the sinuses. Rhinitis can be triggered by allergies (when it's known as hay fever), viruses like the one that causes the common cold, cigarette smoke and strong fumes, and cold air.

If you're allergic to pollen, mold spores, and pet dander, breathing in these allergens could trigger your rhinitis. (You might want to look at Hay Fever on page 307 for more detail on this process and other issues discussed in this chapter.)

With the normal flow of air and mucus interrupted, things can turn ugly. When the ostia swell shut, air and mucus get trapped in one or more sinuses. The bacteria that normally live quietly in the area find this fluid to be a great place to start multiplying rapidly. As the fluid thickens, your cilia struggle to push it away, damaging them.

At this point, you officially have sinusitis, which is defined simply as an inflammation of the sinuses. Pressure can build in the closed-off sinus to cause pain, or a vacuum can form that tugs on the lining with even more pain.

If you have acute sinusitis—which can last from 2 to 3 weeks or linger as long as 8 weeks—you'll probably cough a lot and notice thick yellow mucus coming from your nostrils or going down the back of your throat. You may also have a fever; headache; tenderness in your face, which might get worse when you lean forward; and pain in your upper teeth.

If it's sinusitis from a cold virus, the congestion and pain hit just as you're feeling better from the cold.

If you have chronic sinusitis—which drags on for 3 to 8 weeks and can even linger for months or years—you'll probably have congestion and postnasal drip, with possible bad breath, poor ability to smell, sore throat, headache, and fatigue.

A chronic case that doesn't want to go away can be due to several factors, including:
• An acute infection that wasn't treated properly
• Airborne allergens that keep the sinuses from being able to properly drain
• Structural defects that prevent drainage, such as polyps, a deviated septum, or too-small ostia
• Fungal growth in the sinuses

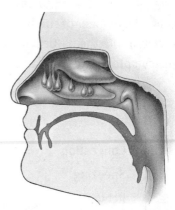

Nasal polyps look like teardrop-shaped lumps in the lining of the nasal passages.

While avoiding long-term discomfort is a good enough reason to act quickly to eradicate sinusitis, infrequent but serious complications make sinusitis a disease you don't want to ignore. In rare cases, a sinus infection can erode surrounding bone, damage the eyes, or get to the brain, where it can cause meningitis or an abscess.

Fortunately, just as spelunkers have all types of flashlights, ropes, and other equipment to conquer even the most intimidating of caves, we have a wide variety of tools to open up our sinuses and bring them back to normal. These range from conventional approaches, like antibiotics, decongestants, and surgery, to simple self-care options, like saltwater rinses, papaya tablets, and even a hot bowl of homemade chicken soup. Let's see how they work.

Conventional Treatment Options

Conventional medicine has the benefit of a wide range of both prescription and over-the-counter medications to help relieve the symptoms of sinusitis. In cases where these drugs fail to successfully treat sinusitis, surgery may offer another alternative.

Antibiotics. These bacteria-killing drugs are an important tool for fighting sinusitis, since they can stop an infection before it progresses to a serious complication. They typically shouldn't be used, however, as the sole weapon against sinusitis. To explain why, Terence Davidson, M.D., an otolaryngologist and professor of surgery at the University of California, San Diego, uses a kitchen-sink metaphor: The sink drains through a fairly thin pipe. When gunk blocks the pipe, the sink backs up with foul-smelling water. Pouring bleach into it—the equivalent of taking an antibiotic—will clean up the water, but it won't fix the underlying problem of the plugged drain. In the sinuses, you have to both get rid of the infection and open up the drain.

Antibiotics are more likely to help a case of acute sinusitis than a chronic one. If your doctor prescribes antibiotics, you'll most likely need to take them for at least 2 weeks for acute sinusitis and at least 3 weeks for chronic sinusitis. In either case, you should keep taking the antibiotics for 7 days after you stop having symptoms. This is to help ensure that all the bacteria have been rooted out, so no remaining ones will be left to develop resistance and rise up again.

Because antibiotics have been used excessively and inappropriately, some of the bacteria that commonly cause sinusitis have become resistant to some antibiotics like penicillin and amoxicillin. Because older, less expensive antibiotics have started to wear out their usefulness, you may need to step up to newer, pricier, more high-powered types to knock the bacteria out.

Work carefully with your doctor if you require antibiotics. These drugs come with a price: Because they can cause bacteria in your sinuses to become resistant, they can contribute to a chronic case of sinusitis, according to Robert Ivker, D.O., assistant clinical professor in the department of family medicine and clinical instructor in the department of otolaryngology at the University of Colorado School of Medicine in Denver and author of *Sinus Survival*. They also destroy the friendly bacteria in your digestive and respiratory tracts that keep the areas healthy and in balance with yeast and other fungal organisms. Overuse of antibiotics can result in a yeast overgrowth that is often present in most severe cases of sinusitis.

Finally, antibiotics can also weaken the immune system by keeping it from fighting its own battles—and by possibly leaving you with bacteria resistant to antibiotics, says Andrew Weil, M.D., director of the program in integrative medicine and clinical professor of medicine at the University of Arizona College of Medicine in Tucson.

Decongestants. These drugs, some of which are over-the-counter and some of which are prescription, may be helpful in reducing the swelling and pressure in your nasal area. They come in styles that you take by mouth or spray up your nose. Both of these, however, can potentially cause side effects.

Oral forms can cause increased blood pressure, agitation, insomnia, irregular heartbeat, and urinary retention. While the nasal sprays go to work in minutes, they can have a rebound effect that leaves you even more congested if you use them for too long—more than 3 or 4 days at a time.

Mucolytics. These are drugs that you take by mouth to thin mucus, typically so you can cough it up out of your lungs more easily. A common one is guaifenesin, found in drugs like Robitussin. Guaifenesin may be useful in thinning the mucus in your sinuses, too, though this is still unproven and requires a high dose of the drug.

Guaifenesin tends to make you very thirsty, which is a side benefit in this case; drinking plenty of water is a good idea when you have sinusitis because it keeps your body well-hydrated.

Nasal corticosteroids. Since sinusitis is an inflammatory disease and nasal steroid sprays reduce inflammation, it makes sense that these would help treat sinusitis. But researchers have had a tough time proving this to be true.

The drugs are very useful for treating allergic rhinitis because they make the mucous lining in the nose react less violently to allergens and cut down on the cells that rush to the area and create inflammation. But since the drugs have a hard time making it through the tiny holes into the sinuses, it's hard to tell just how much help they are to them.

Since they're regarded as safe, however, doctors readily recommend using these drugs as a useful ingredient in treating sinusitis.

Antihistamines. Experts warn that antihistamines aren't a good choice for treating acute sinusitis unless you have extreme allergies, since these drugs dry out and thicken the mucus in your nasal passages, giving the troublesome bacteria an even better environment to breed.

If you take them to help manage allergic rhinitis, however, antihistamines can keep your nose in working order so you don't get sinusitis in the first place.

Surgery. If you can't shake your sinusitis, you may need surgery to get your sinuses back to normal.

Working through your nostrils with the help of a tiny telescope called an endoscope, a surgeon can correct your septum, the wall between your nostrils, if it's crooked enough to impair the mucus flow through the area. Surgery can also widen the opening to a sinus and remove polyps, which are fluid-filled growths that can droop from the walls of your nasal passages and cover an opening to a sinus.

These surgeries won't make you sinusitis-proof, but afterward your sinuses will drain better and be better accessible so you can treat your symptoms more easily when they strike again.

Alternative Treatment Options

Doctors familiar with alternative or holistic options often bemoan the fact that practitioners with a conventional philosophy tend to focus just on drugs and surgery to cope with sinusitis. The truth is that 40 percent of people with sinusitis will heal on their own without antibiotics. Plenty of nondrug options can help clear out infection, open your nasal passages, and increase your chances of being one of the people who can get better without the bacteria-killing drugs.

Here are some of the self-care methods that you can use to prevent or get rid of sinusitis symptoms.

Nasal washing. This approach, which is a key way to naturally manage allergic rhinitis, is also important in battling sinusitis.

"I've been using it for about 15 years. It really is an alternative-medicine treatment that is useful," Dr. Davidson says. "About half the patients I give it to stay on it for life and say that it has made a major difference in their lives."

Using any of the systems of getting salt water into your nose, where it washes away pus and debris, is better than not doing it, Dr. Davidson says. By washing the stuff out of your nose, you can reduce your need for antibiotics. Options include a neti pot, which looks like an Aladdin's lamp with a spigot to pour the water into your nose, and a rubber bulb syringe to suck up water and squirt it in. (To learn more about nasal washing in general, see Hay Fever on page 307.)

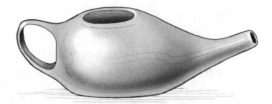

A neti pot can help clean your nasal passages.

Dr. Davidson prefers, however, "pulsatile irrigation," which you can achieve by using a Waterpik (normally used to clean teeth with jets of water) with an attachment that fits into your nostril. When you properly adjust the pressure, the rapid pulses of water dislodge the sticky mucus deep in your nose better than a steady stream, he says.

These devices may carry an extra benefit, according to Murray Grossan, M.D., an otolaryngologist with Cedars-Sinai Medical Center in Los Angeles, who developed a type of nasal irrigator attachment. The cilia in the sinuses and nose wave at 16 beats per second to move mucus along. His irrigator pulses at 20 beats per second, stimulating damaged or sluggish cilia to keep their normal rhythm, he says. (For information on ordering this product, see the Resource Guide on page 497.)

Aside from these benefits, washing allergens out of your schnozzle before they spark congestion and inflammation can help you avoid a case of sinusitis before it even gets started.

Avoidance of allergens. Since many sinusitis episodes begin after a bout of allergic rhinitis, it makes sense to do all you reasonably can to avoid exposure to the triggers—like pet dander, mold spores, pollen, and dust mites—that make your nose congested.

Olive leaf extract. Robert Rountree, M.D.,

a holistic physician in Boulder, Colorado, and coauthor of *Immunotics*, often recommends olive leaf extract as a natural antibiotic for people with sinusitis. This herbal supplement comes in capsule form.

Dr. Rountree often suggests taking one or two 500-milligram capsules of this extract every 4 to 6 hours, up to eight capsules a day, in addition to performing nasal washes,

Choose Your Weapon

If you want to rinse debris from your nasal passages with salt water, doctors often recommend low-tech but effective ways to do it.

Diane G. Heatley, M.D., associate professor of pediatric otolaryngology at the University of Wisconsin in Madison, conducted a study comparing two common methods, neti pots and bulb syringes, for chronic sinusitis.

The neti pot looks like a little Aladdin's lamp, which you fill with salt water and pour into your nose through the spout. A bulb syringe is a hollow molded-rubber ball with a spout, which you use to suck up water and squirt it into your nose.

Her study found that the devices are equally effective, and participants were almost evenly divided on which one they preferred. "In my own mind, just getting saline into the nose is helpful, so I would tell people there are several different ways to do it. People are going to have preferences," Dr. Heatley says. If one way doesn't suit you, give the other a try.

Follow a few caveats, however, to use either device more safely. First, some neti pots are made of ceramic or porcelain, which works fine, but since they're often clutched with wet hands over a sink, the danger of a dropped pot shattering is a possibility. So handle them with care. Because she works with kids, Dr. Heatley developed a plastic neti pot, called Sinucleanse, to address this issue. (For information on ordering this product, see the Resource Guide on page 497.)

Also, be sure to put your pot in the top rack of your dishwasher each week, and don't share it with family members. And if you use a bulb syringe, stick it in the dishwasher or in a pot of boiling water every week to sterilize it, or just buy a new one every few weeks. Using it for too long without cleaning it can lead to fungus growth inside.

to chase out sinusitis without having to use prescription antibiotics. If you do not see any improvement in 10 days, he recommends that you try something else.

Sinus Survival Botanical Nasal Spray. Another product Dr. Rountree recommends is Sinus Survival Botanical Nasal Spray, which Dr. Ivker helped to develop. It helps moisten your nasal membranes and loosen mucus. In addition, it contains aloe vera, goldenseal, grapefruit seed extract, and selenium, which heal the membranes and fight microbes and allergens. Use several sprays in each nostril every 2 hours until your infection clears. (For purchasing information, see the Resource Guide on page 497.)

Proper nose-blowing. Honking your nose like Louis Armstrong blowing his trumpet is very bad for your sinuses. Hard blowing builds up so much pressure in the nose that you can drive pus up into your sinuses and even your middle ear, Dr. Grossan says. The key is to blow gently when you need to clear your nose. This is the most important thing you can teach your children in order to help them avoid sinus and ear problems.

Steam. When steam wafts up into your nasal passages, it moistens them and helps liquefy mucus, which may leave you less congested. One way to use steam to your advantage is to boil water in a pot and, after carefully removing it from the heat and covering your head with a towel, lean over the pot for about 10 minutes, forming a tent with the towel to hold in the steam. Just be sure to keep far enough away from the steam to avoid burning yourself, and never inhale steam directly from a boiling pot. A long, warm shower can also work.

Certain aromatic ingredients can aid even further in the opening of your nasal passages if you allow them to simmer in the pot and release their aromas with the steam, says Dr. Rountree. Try adding one of the following: oil of thyme, oil of lemon balm, or oil of rosemary, or fresh rosemary, fresh oregano, or sage. If you tend to have strong allergic reactions, Dr. Rountree recommends that you only use a drop or two of the oil the first time and only increase the amount as you can tolerate it.

Warm compresses. Drape a warm washcloth over your forehead or cheeks to relieve sinusitis pain. You can also dip the cloth in water that contains the previously mentioned aromatic ingredients but has cooled slightly for an even more soothing treatment, Dr. Rountree says.

Herbs. Dr. Rountree recommends several herbs that kill bacteria or boost your immune system to better fight sinusitis. For example, you can take capsules containing garlic extract, or just add garlic to food for its antimicrobial properties. Berberine, goldenseal, astragalus, and echinacea are all useful herbs for bolstering your immune system, he says. Dr. Rountree usually recommends using 15 to 20 drops of an alcohol- or glycerine-based tincture that contains one or more of the herbs four times a day for 7 to 10 days.

Avoidance of dairy products. Since milk

and dairy products can thicken your mucus, try to avoid them when you're battling sinusitis or trying to avoid it. Dairy is also the most common food allergen responsible for causing allergies, sinusitis, and asthma.

Avoidance of irritants. Try to avoid fumes that can irritate your nose and cause congestion. Cigarette smoke is the main offender, but you should also try to avoid perfumes and household cleaners if they bother you.

Relaxation. Rest and relaxation are particularly important for your body when it's under the stress of a condition like sinusitis.

When Diane G. Heatley, M.D., associate professor of pediatric otolaryngology at the University of Wisconsin in Madison, was comparing methods of nasal irrigation for chronic sinusitis, she added hand and foot reflexology as a control, or a method with no effect, to compare to the others. To her surprise, patients reported that it made them feel just as good as nasal washing. She isn't recommending reflexology until she researches it more, but she thinks the simple act of rubbing patients' hands and feet for 10 minutes may have reduced stress levels enough to help them feel better.

Getting at least 8 hours of sleep a night—or enough that you don't need an alarm clock to wake up—is important for maintaining a strong immune system. So is keeping your stress levels in check. (For more ways to relieve stress, see Allergy-Free Stress Busters on page 173.)

Water. By drinking as much water as you can tolerate—even up to 20 glasses a day—

you can help liquefy your mucus and help it drain better, suggests Wellington Tichenor, M.D., an allergist in New York City.

Chicken soup. The stuff mom used to ladle out for you when you were sick packed more power than she knew: Chicken soup has even made it into a textbook on treating respiratory diseases.

Here's why: Hot chicken soup replaces fluids. The steam wafting off it and the spicy peppers you can stir into it help loosen congestion. For an even bigger nose-opening kick, you can add some horseradish root, which some people report loosens their congestion. Finally, garlic has decongestant, antibiotic, and antiviral properties, and onion also works against viruses.

Papaya and pineapple enzymes. Enzymes from papaya and pineapple—papain and bromelain, respectively—can dissolve the proteins in the thick mucus in your nasal passages and sinuses, making the goo break up, Dr. Grossan says. (He developed his own line, called Clear-Ease, that combines both these enzymes.) This gives your cilia an environment in which they can function normally. Clear-Ease is a calibrated mixture of papain and bromelain. Eating papaya and pineapple won't accomplish the same thing as taking one Clear-Ease three times a day for 2 to 3 weeks to help ease sinus pain and swelling. The trick to using these tablets is to let them dissolve in your "buccal pouch," or the space between your cheek and gum. (For information on where you can purchase this product, see the Resource Guide on page 497.)

Sinusitis Allergy
ACTION PLAN

If left untreated, sinusitis can have serious complications. Of course, it's best to avoid getting the condition altogether; when that's not possible, check out the treatment tips below.

 indicates a natural remedy

Prevention

- Avoid the allergens that trigger your allergic rhinitis whenever possible, and try to keep the rhinitis under control when symptoms do arise so that it doesn't lead to sinusitis.
- Blow your nose gently to avoid pushing pus into your sinuses.
- Avoid cigarette smoke and other fumes that irritate your nose.

Treatment

- Consult your doctor when you have sinusitis symptoms. Left untreated, it can turn into a nasty, and even dangerous, illness.
- Your doctor will likely want to put you on antibiotics. Work with your doctor to make sure there isn't a better alternative in your case. If there isn't, be sure to take all the pills that are prescribed to lessen your chances of leaving drug-resistant bacteria in your sinuses.
- During sinusitis, flush out your nose with salt water using a neti pot, a bulb syringe, or a Waterpik with a nasal attachment one to three times a day.
- If you use spray decongestants, be sure not to use them for more than 4 days. Using them excessively may give you congestion.
- You may benefit from drugs that thin your mucus and from nasal corticosteroid sprays that lessen inflammation in your nasal passages and sinuses. Talk to your doctor.
- Antihistamines are useful to combat the effects of allergies, but don't take

them just to try to treat sinusitis. They can make it even worse.

🌿 Try taking capsules containing olive leaf extract, for its antibacterial use. Dr. Rountree suggests taking one or two 500-milligram capsules of this extract every 4 to 6 hours, up to eight capsules a day, in addition to performing nasal washes.

🌿 Spray your nose with saline spray every 2 hours. One such spray is Sinus Survival Botanical Nasal Spray, which contains herbs that may help fight sinusitis. (For important information on saline sprays, see "Be Careful with Store-Bought Sprays" on page 323.)

🌿 Twice a day, breathe steam through your nose. You might try adding aromatic ingredients to the water for additional aid in opening your nasal passages. These ingredients include oil of thyme, oil of lemon balm, or oil of rosemary, or fresh rosemary, fresh oregano, or sage.

🌿 To relieve pain, soak a washcloth in warm water and lay it over your cheek or forehead.

🌿 Take the following herbs, as recommended by Dr. Rountree and also Dr. Ivker, coauthor of *The Complete Self-Care Guide to Holistic Medicine*.

- Garlic: 1,200 to 2,000 milligrams three times a day
- Goldenseal or berberine: 200 milligrams three times a day or 20 drops of tincture four or five times a day
- Echinacea: 200 milligrams three times a day or 25 drops of tincture four or five times a day
- Astragalus: 500 to 1,000 milligrams every 4 to 6 hours or 15 to 30 drops of tincture four times a day

These herbs can be taken together for 7 to 10 days until your infection resolves and your mucus is clear again. If your mucus remains a yellow-green color after that time, Dr. Rountree suggests trying something else.

🌿 Avoid dairy products when you have sinusitis.

🌿 Be sure to get plenty of rest and avoid stress as much as possible.

🌿 Drink as much water each day as you comfortably can.

🌿 Fix yourself a bowl of spicy, garlicky chicken soup.

🌿 Three times a day, melt a tablet of papaya or papaya/bromelain enzyme in your mouth.

- If you require surgery, be sure it's used as a last resort after you've taken all the other steps that may be effective.

Stinging and Biting Insect ALLERGIES

A STING FROM A SINGLE insect can kill you. But predicting who will have an anaphylactic reaction—and which critter will cause it—is like playing insect roulette. "You don't know you have the allergy until you have the reaction," says David B. K. Golden, M.D., associate professor of medicine at the Johns Hopkins University in Baltimore who specializes in research into anaphylaxis and insect sting allergies.

Considering that approximately four million insects commonly live on a single acre, a little paranoia is probably not such a bad thing.

A survey found that 3 percent of people have had a severe reaction to an insect sting, according to Dr. Golden. The survey also found, however, that 9 out of 10 of them did not go to their doctors afterward for help. "Most people are not scared, but they should be," he notes.

Free from Fear: EpiPens and Venom Immunotherapy

If you or your children do not have this allergy, you can reduce your odds of getting it by taking some simple precautions to avoid getting stung. And if you are one of the 3 percent who do have a severe allergy, there are medical treatments that minimize the danger.

Your doctor may recommend that you carry an EpiPen Auto-Injector, a hypodermic needle of epinephrine that you can administer yourself. If you do have an anaphylactic reaction, this will buy you time to get to an emergency room, where doctors may also administer oxygen and intravenous fluids. Other medications are sometimes used, including steroids and antihistamines, says Dr. Golden. The EpiPen Jr. is available for children who weigh 25 to 50 pounds.

EpiPens are available only with a doctor's prescription and are expensive, but most insurance plans may cover EpiPens, he notes.

A preventive treatment is venom immunotherapy, or VIT, which desensitizes you through gradually increasing doses of insect venom given over 2 to 6 months, followed by maintenance injections every 4 to 8 weeks for 3 to 5 years. These shots can virtually cure you of your insect allergy, freeing you to venture outside without fear, says Dr. Golden. "As long as you're on the shots, you are so well-protected that you really don't have anything to worry about. The amazing thing is that even if they get stung long after they stop the shots, most people have little or no reaction."

VIT is available for the most common insect allergies: yellow jackets and other wasps, hornets, bees, and fire ants. While on this treatment, 98 percent of people have no severe allergic reactions to insect stings, and about 90 percent have no problems from fire ant stings, states Dr. Golden. The risk of an allergic reaction after stopping VIT increases very slightly, so some people may want to either stay on shots every couple of months or carry an EpiPen.

Older adults, especially those with other medical problems, are at the greatest risk for a life-threatening reaction and should be immunized with VIT. Insect allergies in children under age 17 are not usually life-threatening—no blood pressure drop, no throat tightness, and no breathing problems, says Dr. Golden. "A research study shows that when those children are stung again, only 10 percent will have hives, and only one child in the study developed more severe symptoms. These children with non-life-threatening reactions do not need to be immunized," states Dr. Golden. Children may still need to carry an EpiPen, however, so talk to an allergist.

Know Your Enemy

Insects that sting are far more likely to cause allergies and anaphylaxis than insects that bite. Only some biting insects, such as mosquitoes, blackflies, deerflies, and bedbugs, can trigger allergies, mainly to their saliva. These bites usually cause only local swelling; anaphylaxis is rare, though possible.

In the case of allergies to fleabites, however, you may experience hives, typically around your ankles or lower legs. The rash may start to spread, or you could break out all over. This allergic reaction can last for months but will begin clearing up within days after you start taking oral antihistamines.

Of the stingers, the main problem in

North America are the ones belonging to the order Hymenoptera, which includes yellow jackets and other wasps, hornets, bees, and fire ants. Of the flying insects, yellow jackets are a far bigger problem than honeybees.

But if you live in fire ant country, including much of the South, watch your

Skeeter Syndrome

If you're allergic to mosquitoes, a bite can produce large swelling that may resemble an infection such as bacterial abscess cellulitis, complete with low-grade fever. But the swelling starts quickly after the bite, usually too soon for an infection, and antibiotics are ineffective.

Skeeter syndrome can cause half of the face to swell up bright red or even an entire arm or leg to become inflamed. Children or adults who have not been exposed to the local mosquitoes before seem to be at greatest risk, as well as people who have HIV.

If you have skeeter syndrome, treatment with an oral antihistamine as soon as possible after the bite to reduce itching and redness is generally considered safe and effective. You can also take antihistamines before outdoor activity and apply over-the-counter or prescription steroid creams after a bite to prevent severe swelling.

Most people grow out of the hypersensitivity as they grow older and have experienced more mosquito bites. But anaphylaxis is possible, though rare, and should be treated immediately.

Get prompt medical help if the swelling worsens despite your taking antihistamines and applying topical steroids or if you have flulike symptoms. Talk to an allergist about your options if you have persistent problems or if you are unsure of the cause of your allergy.

Pesticide sprays used to control mosquitoes, such as synthetic forms of pyrethrin or malathion, can sometimes produce allergic reactions, including difficulty breathing, cautions Jim David, mosquito control director for the St. Lucie County Mosquito Control District in Fort Pierce, Florida. Notify your local mosquito control or health department if you are severely allergic. Be aware that synthetic forms of pyrethrin, such as allethrin, permethrin, and resmethrin, are used in mosquito coils and plant sprays.

toes; stings from fire ants are far more common than stings from yellow jackets.

The First Sting Is a Freebie

You are not born with insect allergies, and only about one in five people has the potential to develop an insect sting allergy, says Jerome Goddard, Ph.D., clinical assistant professor of preventive medicine at the University of Mississippi Medical Center in Jackson and a medical entomologist with the Mississippi State Department of Health.

Your first sting will probably not cause an allergic reaction, so don't assume that you're safe if it doesn't. "Often, you get stung by a lot of insects the first time, and then the next time you are stung you may be allergic," explains Dr. Goddard.

You may, however, need medical attention for reasons other than allergies. People can die from multiple stings just because of the massive amount of venom injected into their bodies. And insects can spread diseases that may require antibiotics.

In addition, you may be cross-reactive. This means you could have an allergic reaction the first time you are stung by a particular type of insect if you have already encountered one with a similar venom, say, a hornet and a yellow jacket.

If you do develop an allergy, don't panic. Unlike food allergies, once you first demonstrate an allergic reaction to an insect sting, later reactions to other stings do not generally become progressively worse. "Whatever you had the first time is probably the severity you will have in the future," says Dr. Golden. Further, just because you react once doesn't mean you will react the second or third time, he adds.

Discuss any allergic reaction with your doctor, and bring the insect with you, if possible. An allergy test can help determine what caused your reaction, but many

Jeepers Creepers!

Most caterpillars are harmless to humans. But some have venom in their spiny hairs that can trigger an allergy, says Jerome Goddard, Ph.D., clinical assistant professor of preventive medicine at the University of Mississippi Medical Center in Jackson and a medical entomologist with the Mississippi State Department of Health.

Four common species to watch out for are the saddleback caterpillar, the IO moth caterpillar, the brown-tail moth caterpillar, and the puss caterpillar.

Unfortunately, you don't necessarily need to touch the caterpillar to get a reaction. Sometimes millions of stinging larvae are emerging, and their hairs can be carried by the wind, causing skin rash, asthma, or respiratory irritation.

people test positive after a sting even if they had no reaction, says Dr. Golden.

Insect Behavior 101

The best way to avoid potentially troublesome insects is to learn their habits and favorite hangouts. That way, you can make sure you are where they are not. Keep in mind that most flying insects are not out to get you; they are much too busy chasing pollen or prey, says Dr. Goddard. "Away from the nest, they're really not very dangerous."

But if you are careless, you can make any insect mad, especially yellow jackets and hornets. Read on to learn the personalities of the most common stinging insects.

• **Bees**

"Bees are really pretty docile," says Dr. Golden. "Kids get stung by honeybees because they run around barefoot and step on them. Adults usually don't get stung." The result: "Only about 15 percent of our patients are allergic to honeybees," he says.

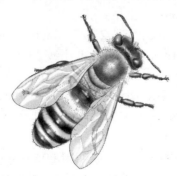

Honeybees are covered with short, dense golden brown and black hair. Their abdomens are striped.

Bumblebees are even less aggressive and less abundant than honeybees and so are less likely to produce allergies. But because they nest in the ground in places like piles of grass clippings, mouse nests, or building insulation, you could accidentally rouse them to anger while mowing the lawn.

Our docile honeybees have an evil twin called the Africanized honeybee. These "killer bees" are found primarily in southern Texas, but they can also be found near the Mexican border in New Mexico, Arizona, and California. They're expected to gradually move northward.

The venom of killer bees is not more toxic than that of domestic bees, but they are more likely to attack with little provocation. When they defend their colony, they attack in swarms that can inflict 400 to 1,000 stings—enough to kill you from the toxin alone or from an overdose of histamine produced by your own body.

• **Wasps**

Most wasps are loners and don't sting. But social wasps, ones that form nests, will sting, especially in defense of their colony. The main ones to worry about are paper wasps, yellow jackets, and hornets.

Dr. Golden says that about 85 percent of his patients with insect allergies are sensitized to yellow jackets. And once you become allergic to yellow jackets, you may have cross-reaction allergies from other stings.
• Hornets and yellow jackets are almost 100 percent cross-reactive.

• Paper wasps are about 50 percent cross-reactive with hornets and yellow jackets.
• Bees and yellow jackets are not cross-reactive.

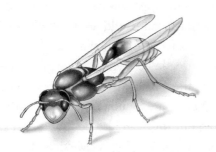

Paper wasps are reddish brown with yellow circles on their backs. They have longer legs and more slender bodies than yellow jackets and hornets.

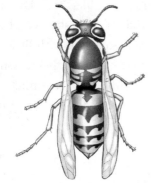

Yellow jackets are wasps with definite waists. They are black and yellow or black and white.

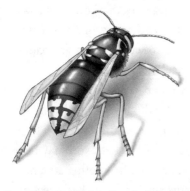

Hornets are large, with black and white markings on their heads and bodies.

• Fire Ants

If you live in fire ant country, odds are more than 50-50 that you will get stung at least once each year. Imported fire ants are a huge problem in states along the Gulf Coast, as well as Puerto Rico, and can be found as far north as Maryland and as far west as Texas and parts of California. They are native to South America.

Once imported fire ants inhabit an area, their numbers can quickly grow. A single nest can have 10,000 ants after a year, 60,000 ants after 2 years, and 200,000 ants after 3 years. And heavily infested areas can have 50 to 400 or more mature colonies per acre.

"Fire ants are the leading cause of anaphylactic reactions in children in our region. Even if you put all the flying insects together, the incidence of anaphylactic reactions from fire ants is probably three to four times higher, and they produce a more severe reaction," says Shih-Wen Huang, M.D., professor of pediatrics in the division of immunology and allergy at the University of Florida College of Medicine in Gainesville.

A survey of 2,022 doctors in 13 southern states found they had treated 20,755 patients for fire ant stings of varying severity, says Dr. Goddard. Of these patients, 413 suffered anaphylactic shock, or about 2 percent.

Imported fire ants need no provocation to sting, and once on you they will sting repeatedly. About 60 percent of bites are on the feet, but they can occur anywhere. "I've seen kids bitten on the face because an ant dropped from a tree," reports Dr. Huang.

The large amount of venom in massive attacks can be life-threatening. If you are allergic to fire ants, though, it doesn't take that much venom to send you to the hospital. The exact amount is unclear because the amount of venom injected varies with fire ant stings, says Dr. Golden.

Fire ant colonies can be destroyed safely with slow-acting pesticides that use growth hormone regulators to target only ants, says Anita Neal, an environmental horticulture agent at the St. Lucie County Cooperative Extension at the University of Florida Institute of Food and Agricultural Sciences in Fort Pierce. "You're not harming the environment," she assures.

Some of the safer products found in the marketplace are bait forms, which are chemicals incorporated into attractants, targeting specific pests. An example is a product on the market called Amdro (hydramethylnon), which attracts the ant and, once consumed, is shared throughout the mound (ants being social insects), acting as a stomach poison. This product acts on ants only. Your local extension agent can advise you of the current products available and their mode of operation, says Neal.

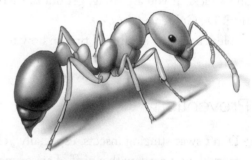

Fire ants are reddish brown ants that are smaller than carpenter and pharaoh ants.

Steer Clear of Stinging Ants

In addition to imported fire ants, other stinging ants, including harvester ants and two species of native fire ants, are found throughout the United States. If they sting, they can potentially trigger an allergy, says Sanford Porter, Ph.D., a research entomologist with the USDA Research Center in Gainesville, Florida.

Harvester ants can grow from ¼ to 1 inch long, and a sting from one can raise a painful but nonallergic welt 2 to 3 inches across that lasts for several days. Harvester ants can be found in colder climes, including mountainous areas like Utah and Colorado.

Fortunately, most of your garden-variety ants produce only a harmless bite that feels like a tiny pinch. So don't go exterminating ants at random, advises Dr. Porter: Killing off harmless ants just makes it easier for stinging ants to move in.

Stinging and Biting Insect **ACTION PLAN**

A little common sense goes a long way toward avoiding insect stings, says Dr. Golden.

For example, most people apparently develop their allergies after a multiple-sting encounter. When some bees and yellow jackets sting you, they also put down an "X marks the spot" pheromone that tells their buddies to come and attack. "If you are stung, get out of there fast, before reinforcements arrive," Dr. Golden advises.

Here are some additional tips on how to avoid getting stung.

Prevention

- Don't swat stinging insects, especially yellow jackets. If one gets in your face, blow it away with a puff of air, or move away slowly.
- Stinging insects will attack when they perceive that their nest is endangered. Avoid crossing flight lines to and from the nest.
- Hitting a nest with a ball or rattling one with a lawn mower will rile insects, so periodically survey your property for nests. Yellow jacket nests are sometimes underground. You can locate underground nests by observing flight lines of workers entering and leaving the nest opening.
- Do not destroy a nest or hive unless necessary. Talk to your cooperative extension agent to determine if it is a stinging insect and in a threatening location. If it must be removed, have a professional do the job.
- Yellow jackets are attracted to food and sweets. At picnics, drink out of clear plastic cups and look before you drink.
- Keep garbage cans tightly covered.
- Do not go barefoot in warm weather. Bees often feed on flowers at ground level.
- Stay on well-established trails when hiking in the woods.
- Close your windows and use air-conditioning while driving. Insects can

bounce from the mirrors into open windows. In addition, close the windows when you park your car, particularly during the warm months, since bees and other insects can fly in and surprise you.

- If you are stung and a hive is nearby, run.
- After a nest has been disturbed, stay clear of it for at least 2 weeks.
- If you'll be venturing where you know there are a lot of mosquitoes, apply a light spray of mosquito repellent directly to your clothes and hat, and as necessary to exposed skin, but not under clothing. Mosquito repellents containing DEET are generally safe for adults when used as directed and are the only repellents recommended for use because of their proven effectiveness.
- Ask your garden center for a natural alternative to DEET. Some people report success with products containing geraniol, an extract of lemongrass.

Treatment

- A normal insect sting will typically cause some pain, swelling, itching, and redness in the immediate area that last from a few hours to a few days. If

Get Out Those Hawaiian Shirts

It's a myth that if you look like a flower, you'll get stung by a bee.

In fact, dresses with floral patterns or bright colors do not increase your risk of being stung, says Nancy Breisch, Ph.D., an entomologist with the University of Maryland in College Park. "Their eyesight is much different than ours, and they use visual cues in the ultraviolet rays we can't perceive."

In addition, contrary to popular belief, wearing your favorite perfume or cologne will probably not increase your chances of getting stung. "Almost everyone wears multiple scents that would be very apparent to insects," says Dr. Breisch. "Our shampoos, conditioners, deodorants, makeup, laundry detergents, fabric softeners, and various skin products make us reek as far as insects are concerned. Our fashion choices are more or less irrelevant."

Another common myth is that bees cause most stings. In truth, yellow jackets (which are a type of wasp) sting the most. Unfortunately, people call anything that stings a bee, which gives docile bees a bad reputation.

your symptoms seem unusual, talk to your doctor or call 911, or the emergency number for your community.

- Milder insect allergies are limited to swelling and redness that may encompass an entire leg or arm. These may require medical attention and should be discussed with your doctor or allergist.

- Any symptoms extending to other areas of the body may indicate anaphylaxis. Other symptoms include wheezing, difficulty breathing, swelling in the throat or tongue, widespread hives, itching or swelling, feeling faint, or losing consciousness. Call 911. (For more information, see Anaphylaxis on page 211.)

- If you have an allergic reaction to an insect sting, discuss possible treatments, such as the EpiPen or VIT, with your doctor or allergist.

- If you are allergic, ask your doctor about wearing a MedicAlert bracelet. Applications are available in many doctors' offices and from the Internet at www.medicalert.org.

- If you are going to be far from a hospital, you may want to carry some antihistamine pills and prescription prednisone pills with you, in addition to an EpiPen.

- Replace unused EpiPens that are outdated or deteriorating. The solution may turn brown even before it becomes outdated and is then no longer effective.

- If you do need to use your EpiPen, call 911 and go to an emergency room immediately for follow-up care.

PART FIVE

Common Allergic Symptoms:
CAUSES & TREATMENTS

Symptom
SOLVERS

ARE SNEEZING and wheezing keeping you up at night? Just can't stop scratching that itchy patch of skin? Wonder why the whites of your eyes look a little pink?

You may have an allergy, but finding out what kind and what is triggering your symptoms can take some detective work. If you follow the clues in the following Symptom Solver charts, you'll find lots of evidence to help you determine the origin of your problem.

The following charts will help take the mystery out of what kind of allergy is causing your runny nose; coughing and wheezing; red, watery eyes; rash; or ear in-fection and lead you to the most promising treatments. These symptoms are "equal of-fenders"—they're associated with an assort-ment of allergic conditions from food to pollen.

For convenience, we have listed the treat-ment plans for eye, ear, and skin problems in this section. To accommodate the more extensive information relating to runny nose and sneezing, and coughing and wheezing, treatment is listed under the Action Plans in part 4.

Pay attention to our danger signs, and if any of your symptoms persist for more than 1 week, be sure to consult your doctor.

Allergy Symptom Solver
RUNNY NOSE AND SNEEZING

Upper respiratory symptoms such as runny nose and sneezing
can occur with many different diseases. The chart below lists
those most commonly associated with allergy.

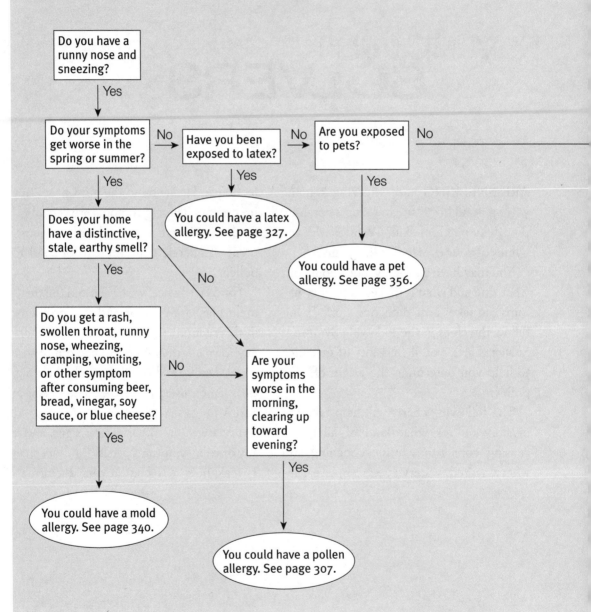

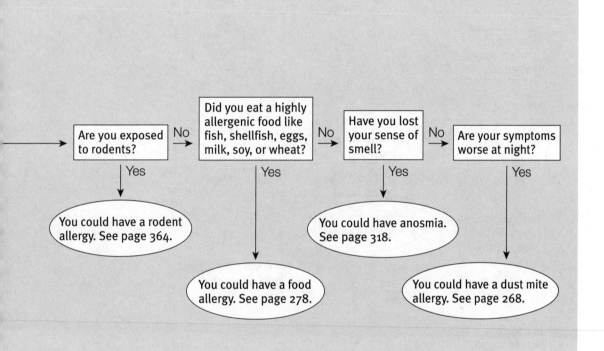

Allergy Symptom Solver
COUGHING AND WHEEZING

Coughing and wheezing can occur with many different diseases. The chart below lists those most commonly associated with allergy.

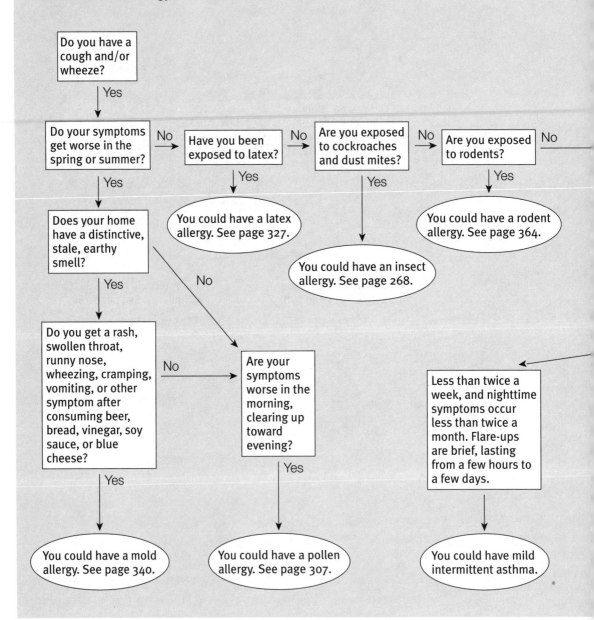

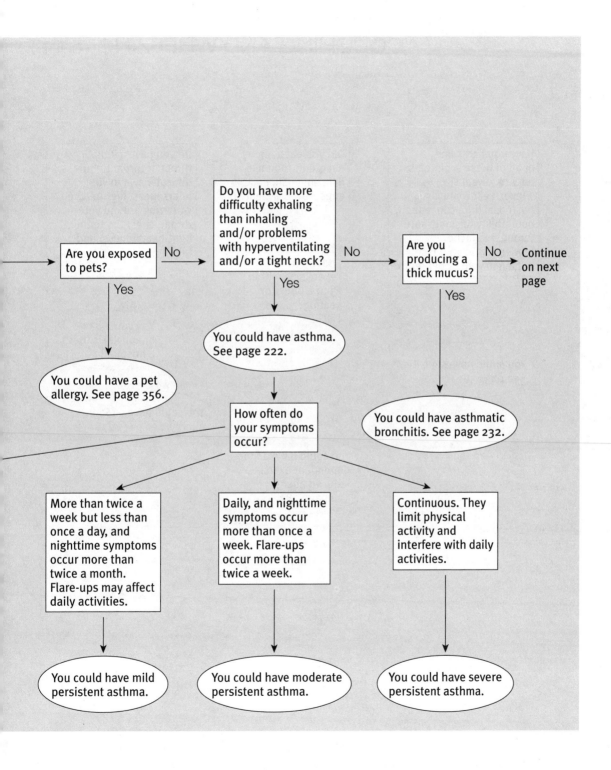

Are you exposed to pets?

No →

Do you have more difficulty exhaling than inhaling and/or problems with hyperventilating and/or a tight neck?

No →

Are you producing a thick mucus?

No → Continue on next page

Yes ↓

You could have a pet allergy. See page 356.

Yes ↓

You could have asthma. See page 222.

Yes ↓

You could have asthmatic bronchitis. See page 232.

How often do your symptoms occur?

More than twice a week but less than once a day, and nighttime symptoms occur more than twice a month. Flare-ups may affect daily activities.

Daily, and nighttime symptoms occur more than once a week. Flare-ups occur more than twice a week.

Continuous. They limit physical activity and interfere with daily activities.

You could have mild persistent asthma.

You could have moderate persistent asthma.

You could have severe persistent asthma.

Allergy Symptom Solver
COUGHING AND WHEEZING (cont.)

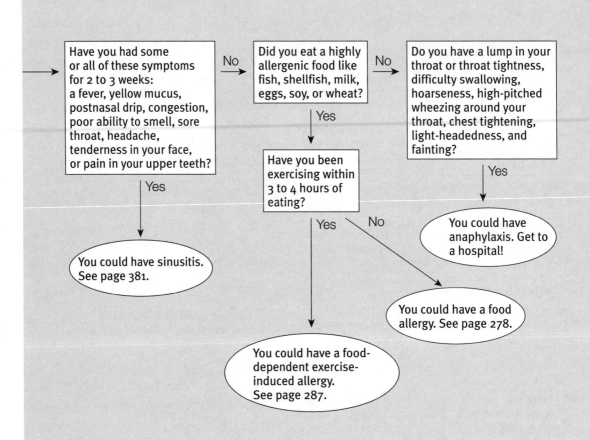

Symptom Solver:
SKIN PROBLEMS

YOUR SKIN IS the window of your body's immune system.

Although this certainly doesn't have the same poetic ring as the saying "the eyes are the windows of the soul," it's more medically accurate.

When you cross paths with the wrong foods, inhaled particles, drugs, animals, chemicals, or even items like latex and nickel, a variety of signs like itchy spots, red welts, and sore cracks can flare up on your 17 or so square feet of skin like warning lights on a dashboard.

Skin conditions that have an allergic link include hives and angioedema (swelling of the tissues beneath the skin), atopic dermatitis, and contact dermatitis. Fortunately, you may be able to eliminate these when they appear on the surface of your skin. Better yet, it may be possible for you to avoid them in the first place.

The Allergic Process in the Flesh

Hives and angioedema are essentially the same condition and are the component of anaphylaxis that affects only your skin and underlying tissues. (For more information, see Anaphylaxis on page 211.)

They occur when an allergen—say, pollen or a bit of peanut protein—causes the mast cells in your body to send out inflammatory chemicals, including histamine.

About half of the people who have these reactions will have hives and angioedema at the same time. Forty percent will have only the hives, and another 10 percent will have only angioedema.

While these conditions can pop up together or at different parts of your body, angioedema usually flares in places where the skin is soft or loose, like the eyes, mouth, genitals, and the backs of your hands and feet. More ominously, angioedema can cause the mucous membranes in your throat to swell, which may lead to breathing problems that must be treated as an emergency.

Why the Welts Are Dealt

Hives can come and go within 24 hours in an acute burst or can drag on in a chronic form.

Also, a type called physical urticaria can be caused by aspects of the environment like heat and pressure. Here's more on each type.

Acute. This is the most common kind. Often the cause of the attack is identifiable from a culprit, such as an allergy to a drug, a food, or latex. Nuts, eggs, shellfish, soy, wheat, and milk are the cause of 90 percent of proven food-induced hives, though chocolate, fish, tomatoes, and berries are also known triggers.

Frequently implicated drugs include aspirin, ibuprofen, angiotensin-converting enzyme (ACE) inhibitors for blood pressure, and codeine. Other triggers include bug bites, immunotherapy shots, viral or bacterial infections, and emotional stress.

Acute attacks of hives, by definition, last for fewer than 6 weeks.

Chronic. This is a more frustrating form of hives. By their definition, chronic hives last more than 6 weeks, and in many cases, doctors have no idea what's causing the outbreak.

They eventually just disappear on their own, with or without treatment. About half the time, the hives will vanish in 3 to 12 months. But a small number of people may have to cope with them for more than 20 years.

Cases may be caused by long-term use of a drug or a chemical, such as a food additive, or by infections or diseases like lupus, lymphoma, thyroid disease, vasculitis, or polycythemia vera, a blood disorder.

Physical. Triggers of these hives include pressure or rubbing on the skin, physical exertion, sunlight, water, and changes in temperature. For example, cholinergic urticaria, caused by increased heat due to exercise or a warm shower, will trigger tiny pinpricks of hives surrounded by redness.

With cold-induced urticaria, an ice cube placed against the arm will leave a square welt with a protruding line corresponding to the cube and the melted water running from it. One condition this danger poses is that while swimming in cold water, a person can go into a full-body reaction and drown.

Angioedema—Swell, but Not So Swell

Patients with angioedema can show an alarming amount of swelling—enough to make their eyes swell completely shut before turning back to normal with treatment. Because angioedema can swell the mucous membranes in the throat, it can cause a medical emergency, requiring prompt treatment to relieve breathing.

Atopic Dermatitis

Atopic dermatitis—also known as eczema— is a riddle wrapped up in an enigma, bundled into a layer of itchy, red skin.

It often strikes people who also have asthma or allergic rhinitis (hay fever) or have a family history of them; the three conditions are known as the atopic triad. (An atopic person is predisposed to being hypersensitive to environmental triggers.) In fact, about 80 percent of kids with atopic dermatitis go on to develop allergic rhinitis or asthma.

Allergists and dermatologists are still at odds, however, about exactly what role allergies play in atopic dermatitis. While allergens such as food, latex, and airborne particles can provoke symptoms in some people, the more pressing problem of people with atopic dermatitis is that their skin is easily insulted by a range of objects and conditions that the rest of the world can easily handle, such as wool sweaters, sunlight, detergents, fruit juices, stress, perfumes, high humidity, low humidity, and panty hose.

For more information about the symptoms of atopic dermatitis, see the Symptom Solver chart on page 423.

Managing Atopic Dermatitis

The mainstay of medical treatment for atopic dermatitis has been steroids, primarily rubbed on the skin as a cream. While

New Drug May Offer Hope for Atopic Dermatitis

Doctors seeking another weapon against atopic dermatitis found it in an unlikely candidate—a lowly fungus growing in the soil of Japan's Mount Tsukuba.

While corticosteroid creams have long been at the forefront of treating atopic dermatitis, their side effects—ranging from thinning the skin to affecting children's growth patterns—make them undesirable for long-term use.

That's why this fungus—*Streptomyces tsukabaensis*—was viewed with such promise. A drug made from it, tacrolimus, is used to suppress patients' immune systems to keep them from rejecting a transplanted kidney or liver.

Researchers recognized the potential the drug could have in inhibiting the inflammation that contributes to atopic dermatitis, but sadly, taking tacrolimus by mouth has a wide range of considerable side effects. Fortunately, a tacrolimus cream has been developed that would simply be rubbed on the skin and produces minimal side effects. Doctors are pleased at the possibilities it will offer in treating this condition over the long term without corticosteroids.

these are effective and come in varying strengths, they're not safe for long-term use, says John Hanifin, M.D., professor of dermatology at the Oregon Health Sciences University in Portland and an atopic dermatitis expert.

After about 3 weeks of daily use, they can damage the skin, thinning it and causing stretch marks. People who use it around their eyes for too long risk cataracts and glaucoma. In children, absorption of the drug may interfere with their growth.

Fortunately, the most important step that people can take to handle their atopic dermatitis—more important than steroids even, says Dr. Hanifin—is an all-natural, self-care approach.

First, keeping the skin moisturized so that it doesn't dry out and crack is absolutely essential. The trick to keeping your skin moisturized is to understand the riddle that water represents. It can both dry out and moisturize your skin, Dr. Hanifin points out.

A long soak followed by patting dry with a towel moisturizes—whereas wetting for

Could You Be Allergic to Your Own Hormones?

It is generally accepted that hormones can influence the severity of certain skin conditions. For example, young women tend to have acne flare-ups that coincide with the hormonal changes that come with their menstrual cycles. Some doctors believe, however, that people may actually develop skin conditions or other symptoms as a result of an allergy to their own hormones.

One of these doctors, Walter Shelley, M.D., Ph.D., professor emeritus of dermatology at the Medical College of Ohio in Toledo, says that he has treated a number of women who developed skin outbreaks from their own hormones, primarily progesterone and estrogen. Still, they were few and far between.

These women typically show up with welts, rashes, acne, or other skin problems that appear or get worse a few days before their periods begin. The timing of these outbreaks is a key sign, Dr. Shelley says, since that's the point in the month when a woman's progesterone and estrogen levels are running high to help prepare her uterus in case it needs to start carrying an embryo.

Symptoms of hormone allergy aren't limited to the skin, though. It may also create problems in fertility, like miscarriages or difficulty getting pregnant, says Alan Beer, M.D., founder of the reproductive medicine program at the Finch University of Health Sciences at the Chicago Medical School.

short periods of time and then rubbing yourself with a towel to dry off has a drying effect.

In addition, avoid wool sweaters, sunlight, and perfumes. The specific triggers will be different for everyone. Also watch out for tight or heavy clothing or heavy sheets and blankets that trigger sweating. Sweaty skin, at least as far as people with atopic dermatitis are concerned, equals itchy skin, Dr. Hanifin says. "You want to always keep things kind of cool." Finally, treat infections quickly.

While doctors are still debating the exact role of allergies in atopic dermatitis, it's certainly worth investigating with a physician whether an allergy may be contributing to your problems. Food allergy could be a possibility, though it's most common in kids younger than age 2. Since skin-prick tests and radioallergosorbent tests (RAST) falsely report that many foods are allergenic, the best way to test for food allergy is by controlled, double-blind food challenges at the doctor's office.

A fertility specialist, Dr. Beer regularly tests his patients for allergies to their hormones or neurotransmitters, which are chemicals in the body that nerve cells use to communicate and that play a role in the uterus during pregnancy.

Other hormones a woman may be allergic to include human chorionic gonadotropin (HCG), which is produced by the placenta during pregnancy and is given as a chemical to produce ovulation, and thyroid hormones, Dr. Beer says.

Along with skin conditions and pregnancy complications, hormone allergies can also trigger symptoms such as worsening PMS, spotting a few days before a period, and weak bones, Dr. Beer says.

If you have a potential hormone allergy, Dr. Beer recommends that you visit an allergist or immunologist who is familiar with this problem. The doctor can pinpoint which hormone, if any, is causing your problems through skin-prick tests or by checking your blood for antibodies to the hormones.

Antihistamines may solve your problem, Dr. Shelley says, though he found even better success with the medication tamoxifen (Nolvadex). This drug, commonly used to reduce the risk of breast cancer, may help by blocking the effects of estrogen inside the body, he says.

A more serious option that doctors have used to cure the allergy is oophorectomy, or surgery to remove the ovaries.

Tame Your Skin with Herbs

When London-based herbalist Douglas Schar, who holds a diploma in phytotherapy and is a member of the National Institute of Medical Herbalists, advises people with skin conditions at his herbal practice, he takes a two-pronged approach to helping them clear up their patchy, itchy problems. He treats the inflammation and treats the underlying immune system failure.

The following are some of his favorite herbs for treating allergic skin conditions. They don't work equally well for everyone, so you may have to experiment to find what helps you. Also, keep in mind that herbs won't necessarily offer overnight success.

Herbs for Symptom Relief

Aloe. The same clear gel from the aloe plant that many people use for minor kitchen burns is also useful for dermatitis because of its anti-inflammatory properties.

Simply snip off a leaf from an aloe plant, remove any spines, split it lengthwise, scrape out the gel, and smear it onto the affected area three times a day. Or buy a container of aloe gel and use that. (Be sure to get pure gel, not another type of product with aloe as an ingredient).

Marshmallow. This isn't the same sort of marshmallow that makes s'mores so tasty. Instead, the root of this plant is useful for soothing irritated, angry skin.

Simply mix ½ teaspoon of powdered marshmallow root into ½ cup of cold water and apply it to affected areas three times a day.

Calendula. The flowers of this relative to burdock and chamomile contain chemicals that reduce inflammation, speed healing, and fight infection from bacteria, fungi, and viruses.

To make your own calendula cream, mix a 4-ounce bottle of 1:5 calendula tincture with 4 ounces of cold cream. Apply it three times a day to affected areas and store in a sealed container.

Herbs for the Bigger Picture

Oregon grape. "The real star in my book, in the constitutional department, is Oregon grape. That's the one I've seen perform time and time again," Schar says.

This isn't the same kind of grape that we use for jelly and wine, though the plant does produce grapelike berries. The part used medicinally is the root, which contains the chemical berbamine. This chemical has anti-inflammatory properties that are helpful for treating atopic dermatitis.

In addition, Schar says, the plant works to stop tiny blood vessels from leaking fluid into your skin, which is the process that leads to hives and angioedema.

Take Oregon grape orally. Three times a day either take 1 teaspoon of 1:5 tincture or 20 drops of 1:1 tincture. You should try this treatment daily for 3 months before deciding if it's working for you. Pregnant women and nursing mothers should avoid using this herb.

Burdock. Herbalists use the roots of this widespread weed to regulate immune function—boosting it when it lags and quieting it when it overreacts. One of its many uses is to soothe dermatitis.

Burdock takes a minimum of 2 weeks to work and may require 3 months to take effect. Take it three times a day. One dose would be a cup of tea made with a gram of dried root boiled in a cup of water; two 500-milligram tablets of dried root; or 1 teaspoon of 1:5 tincture or 20 drops of 1:1 tincture.

Nettle. Ironically, the nettle plant, which will leave you with a red, painful sting if you brush against it, can also help clear up your hives or dermatitis.

You may need to use it for weeks or months to see an effect. Three times a day, drink a tea of 3 grams of dried herb boiled in water and strained; take a teaspoon of 1:5 tincture or 20 drops of 1:1 tincture; or drink 10 milliliters of fresh nettle juice. Take only one dose a day for the first few days to ensure that the nettle doesn't spark an allergic reaction.

In addition to these herbs, you can also try one of the following sources of an essential fatty acid called gamma-linolenic acid (GLA): evening primrose oil, black currant oil, or borage oil. GLA has anti-inflammatory properties and promotes healthy skin. Follow the instructions on the label for dosage information.

Contact Dermatitis

Here's some good and bad news about contact dermatitis: Of the more than six million chemicals that your skin can encounter in the environment, only 3,000 have been implicated in allergic contact dermatitis. That's the good news.

The not-so-good news is this: Virtually any chemical can still cause contact dermatitis under the right circumstances. That's because contact dermatitis—which happens when your skin breaks out because you've touched the wrong substance—takes two forms.

Allergic contact dermatitis. This type occurs when you touch a substance that provokes an allergic reaction in your skin, causing an itchy, red rash that may contain fluid-filled blisters. Only people who are allergic to the substance will get a reaction from it, and a day or two may pass between touching the item and developing the symptoms. Poison ivy is one of the better-known causes of this, but other common triggers include latex, adhesive tape, and hair dye. Only about 20 percent of contact reactions are allergic in nature.

Irritant contact dermatitis. This form occurs when you touch a substance that directly damages your skin. The longer you're touching the substance—or the more concentrated it is—the worse the damage will be. Bleach and acid are examples of irritants, but more common ones include soaps, detergents, and plain old water.

Dermatitis caused by irritants tends to hurt or burn—in fact, the wound can look like an actual burn—as opposed to the itch of allergic causes. Irritants make up 80 percent of contact dermatitis cases.

Trouble can strike in the comfort of home—from household cleaners to perfumed personal-care products to a kitchen sink full of soapy water. At work, depending on your occupation, you can run into a spectrum of dermatitis triggers like latex gloves (health care workers), potassium dichromate (cement workers), and photography chemicals (photographers). In fact, of all the diseases that are caused by work, contact dermatitis is the most common. (For more information, see The Allergy-Free Workplace on page 111.)

The best way to avoid contact dermatitis is very straightforward, if not always easy to follow: Don't touch the things that make you break out. If your dermatitis chronically bothers you, you may need to visit a dermatologist for skin testing to find what's causing the problem. Using a patch test, the doctor can place small amounts of allergens on your skin and cover them with patches of tape, along with plain tape with no allergen that serves as a control.

If your skin turns red and swollen under an allergen but not under the plain patch, you're most likely allergic to that substance. (For more information on signs and symptoms, see the Symptom Solver chart on page 423.)

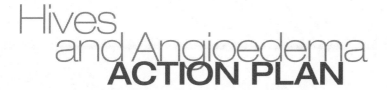

Hives and Angioedema
ACTION PLAN

🌿 *indicates a natural remedy*

🌿 Eliminate anything that you know will trigger hives or angioedema. This includes foods and drugs as well as physical triggers like cold water and objects that rub your skin.

🌿 Apply cool, moist compresses to the hives to cut down on itching.

🌿 Also to soothe the itch of hives, soak in a tub of lukewarm water with an added oatmeal bathing product, such as Aveeno Soothing Bath Treatment.

• You may need an epinephrine injection from your health care provider to treat acute hives or angioedema, particularly when it involves the throat.

• Your doctor may prescribe antihistamines, which reduce itching and minimize the welts. They're more useful, however, when you take them to prevent problems, rather than waiting until after problems appear.

🌿 If your problems are caused by aspirin, you may also need to avoid non-steroidal anti-inflammatory drugs and tartrazine since they may also trigger symptoms. Tartrazine, also known as yellow dye no. 5, is a coloring ingredient used in drugs, cake mixes, and lemon-lime sodas.

🌿 Don't let stress get the best of you. By staying calm, you can cut down on your episodes of hives and swelling. (See Allergy-Free Stress Busters on page 173.)

Atopic Dermatitis
ACTION PLAN

🌿 *indicates a natural remedy*

🌿 During outbreaks, soak in the tub in lukewarm water twice a day for 15 to 20 minutes or until your fingertips wrinkle. Jumping in and out of the shower will dry your skin. When your skin is under good control, a lukewarm shower is fine. Don't use washcloths or scrub your skin.

🌿 Use a mild soap or cleanser or Oil of Olay Sensitive Skin Bar.

🌿 After you get out of the tub, pat yourself dry with a towel. (Do not rub.) Within 3 minutes, apply an ointment or cream to your skin to keep the moisture in. Inexpensive options include petroleum jelly and vegetable shortening (avoid the shortening if you're allergic to soy). Follow the same advice when you get your hands wet.

🌿 Stay away from lotions. Because of their water content, they're more drying.

🌿 Keep away from things that irritate your skin, and avoid food and inhalant allergens that have been proven to affect you.

• If you're going to use steroids, whether rubbed on your skin or taken orally, use them no more than is absolutely necessary.

• Ask your doctor if you're a good candidate for a form of the drug tacrolimus (Protopic) that you rub on your skin. The drug can quell symptoms without the dangers of steroids.

🌿 If you have a history of atopic disease (asthma, allergic rhinitis, dermatitis), consider avoiding occupations in which you'll get your hands wet and encounter irritants like detergents and solvents.

🌿 To keep your skin moist and cool during severe outbreaks, wear a pair of damp pajamas to bed under a dry pair.

🌿 To ease the itching, take a cool bath with an oatmeal product such as Aveeno Soothing Bath Treatment.

• Consider trying products containing tar, which have long been used to ease itching as well as to disinfect and exfoliate your skin and bring down inflammation. Although these products are available over the counter, check with your doctor before using them. Keep in mind, however, that these can stain your tub, clothing, and, temporarily, your skin. Since they can be irritating, don't put them on extremely inflamed skin.

• Keep an eye out for the warning signs of infections, and treat them quickly when they appear. Watch for signs like extensive clear fluid oozing out, honey-colored crusting, and pus.

🌿 Keep your stress level under control, which may also help keep skin outbreaks in check. (See page 173 for specific stress relievers.)

• If your symptoms are severe, consider getting tested for allergies. The physician may conduct a skin-prick test or a radioallergosorbent test—which detects allergies by exposing a sample of blood serum to a disk bearing the suspected allergen—and food challenges to uncover allergens.

🌿 If tests show that you're allergic to dust mites, consult the tips for ridding your home of them on page 275. Start with a mite-proof mattress cover and pillowcases. Avoid vinyl covers, since these can make you sweaty.

🌿 Avoid skin products with alcohol or astringents, as they can be drying.

🌿 If you don't have a dishwasher, have a family member wash the dishes.

• Use sunscreens that don't contain PABA, which can irritate your skin.

🌿 A little sunshine can be beneficial to your skin, but avoid staying out in the sun so long that you sweat or get a sunburn. Also, some doctors use special ultraviolet lights in the office to ease dermatitis.

🌿 Use cotton bedding instead of synthetic or wool fabrics.

🌿 Avoid clothing that's tight or doesn't breathe.

🌿 When cutting meat, fruit, or vegetables—especially onions and garlic—be sure to keep the juices off your hands.

🌿 Use air-conditioning to keep cool and avoid sweating.

🌿 Avoid foods that increase bloodflow to your skin, like hot and spicy foods, red wine, and other alcohol. These can make you itch more.

🌿 If the sweating from exercise irritates you, consider swimming. Just be sure to rinse off the chlorinated water immediately afterward.

🌿 Keep your fingernails clipped short to minimize damage to your skin from scratching. Wear gloves or socks over your hands when you sleep.

🌿 Wash new clothes before wearing them to reduce chemical irritants.

• Because laundry detergent that lingers in clothing can irritate your skin, use a liquid detergent and put the clothes through an extra rinse cycle in the washer.

🌿 Give infants with atopic dermatitis sponge baths in tepid water.

Contact Dermatitis
ACTION PLAN

🌿 *indicates a natural remedy*

🌿 Minimize—or better yet, avoid—touching the allergens and irritants that will trigger an outbreak.

• Depending on your symptoms, your doctor may want to prescribe oral or topical corticosteroids. Use these only if they're absolutely necessary, and carefully follow the doctor's instructions on the proper use.

• Consider antihistamines, which can relieve itching and, at least in the older, sedating forms, help you sleep.

• Buy calamine lotion, which you may find soothing, but avoid using brands containing diphenhydramine, since it can trigger sensitization.

🌿 If you get an irritant or allergen on your hands or clothing, be sure to wash the substance off, as you can transfer it to other parts of your body, where it can spark more dermatitis.

🌿 To soothe itching, apply to the outbreak a compress of cloth soaked in cool water. You may also find Domeboro, an over-the-counter astringent that you mix in water, effective at relieving itch and inflammation.

🌿 Also, try soaking in a bath with a special oatmeal bathing product to soothe inflamed skin.

🌿 Wear cotton-lined gloves to help protect your hands from items you can't avoid.

Allergy Symptom Solver
SKIN PROBLEMS

Skin problems can occur with many different diseases. The chart below lists those most commonly associated with allergy.

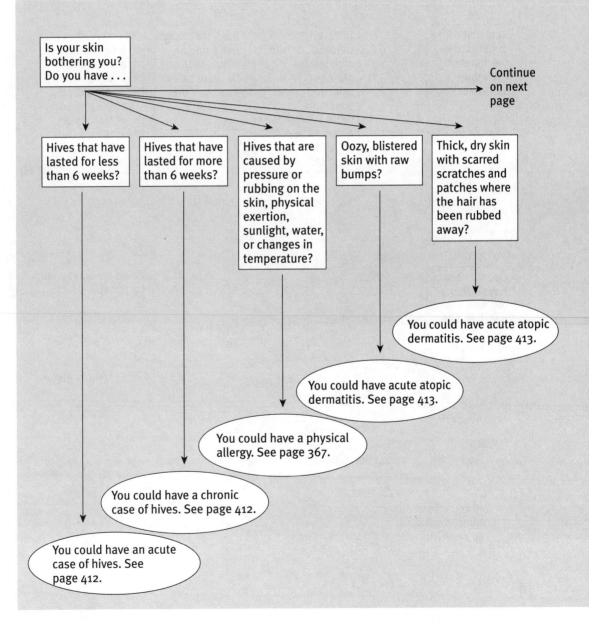

Continue on next page

Is your skin bothering you? Do you have . . .

- Hives that have lasted for less than 6 weeks?
- Hives that have lasted for more than 6 weeks?
- Hives that are caused by pressure or rubbing on the skin, physical exertion, sunlight, water, or changes in temperature?
- Oozy, blistered skin with raw bumps?
- Thick, dry skin with scarred scratches and patches where the hair has been rubbed away?

You could have acute atopic dermatitis. See page 413.

You could have acute atopic dermatitis. See page 413.

You could have a physical allergy. See page 367.

You could have a chronic case of hives. See page 412.

You could have an acute case of hives. See page 412.

Allergy Symptom Solver
SKIN PROBLEMS (cont.)

Skin that broke out because you touched the wrong substance?

Itchy, bright red patches covered with silvery scales on your skin, and possibly your nails are dotted with pits and may be separated from the bed?

Rash that looks like a line or streak that broke out 6 to 72 hours after touching a plant?

Widespread itching, welts and hives on your skin, and possibly a drop in blood pressure, swelling of skin, fluid in lungs, and difficulty breathing?

Does your skin have an itchy red rash possibly with fluid-filled blisters?

You could have anaphylaxis. Get to a hospital!

You could have a poison plant rash. See page 373.

Yes   No

You could have psoriasis. See your doctor.

You could have irritant contact dermatitis. See page 418.

You could have allergic contact dermatitis. See page 418.

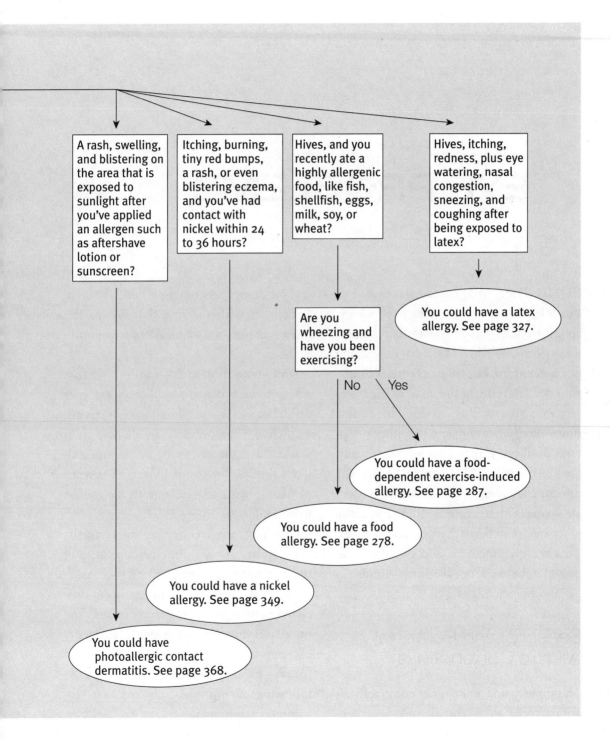

A rash, swelling, and blistering on the area that is exposed to sunlight after you've applied an allergen such as aftershave lotion or sunscreen?

Itching, burning, tiny red bumps, a rash, or even blistering eczema, and you've had contact with nickel within 24 to 36 hours?

Hives, and you recently ate a highly allergenic food, like fish, shellfish, eggs, milk, soy, or wheat?

Hives, itching, redness, plus eye watering, nasal congestion, sneezing, and coughing after being exposed to latex?

You could have a latex allergy. See page 327.

Are you wheezing and have you been exercising?

No   Yes

You could have a food-dependent exercise-induced allergy. See page 287.

You could have a food allergy. See page 278.

You could have a nickel allergy. See page 349.

You could have photoallergic contact dermatitis. See page 368.

Symptom Solver:
EYE PROBLEMS

COMPUTERS AND contact lenses are just a couple of factors contributing to an allergic condition that affects 40 million Americans—conjunctivitis. The word may sound like a mouthful, but conjunctivitis is simply your doctor's term for the itchy, red, and watery eyes you tend to develop alongside a runny nose, wheezing, and the other symptoms of allergic rhinitis (hay fever). Actually, conjunctivitis isn't that simple. In fact, the disease takes about as many forms as there are irritants that cause it. Remember the nasty case of pinkeye that you had as a kid? That was conjunctivitis, too, only that was caused by bacteria, not allergens. Viruses can cause conjunctivitis as well.

Seasonal and Perennial Allergic Conjunctivitis

The three major branches of conjunctivitis are bacterial, viral, and allergic, with several outcroppings coming off each branch. Let's start with the one that affects the most people—seasonal allergic conjunctivitis.

You know those itchy, watery eyes that you get every time the pollen count goes up? That's seasonal allergic conjunctivitis, and while it can occur alone, chances are it will attack at the same time as your other allergic rhinitis symptoms. In fact, 56 percent of people with allergic rhinitis also suffer from conjunctivitis.

While seasonal conjunctivitis torments your eyeballs only during certain times of the year, perennial conjunctivitis never takes a season off. Seasonal conjunctivitis is associated with exposure to natural pollens and mold, but dust mites and animal dander—allergens that don't go away after the pollen season—provoke the perennial kind. See the following Symptom Solver chart for common symptoms.

About 3 percent of the population has a skin allergy that is much more severe than ordinary allergic rhinitis—atopic dermatitis. If you have it, your skin allergies have the potential to migrate to your eyes and cause atopic keratoconjunctivitis. This condition is usually triggered by the same allergens as seasonal or perennial conjunctivitis, but the symptoms are even stronger. You may need to see an allergist or a dermatologist in addition to an ophthalmologist.

Vernal Keratoconjunctivitis

Much less common than seasonal allergic conjunctivitis, vernal keratoconjunctivitis used to be referred to as cobblestone conjunctivitis because of the pattern of bumps it causes on the inside of the eyelids. According to Edward Paul, O.D., director of Atlantic Eye Associates in Hampstead, North Carolina, "Vernal keratoconjunctivitis is symptomized by intense itching, caused by the histamine release involved." The upper eyelid displays cobblestone-like bumps. Vernal keratoconjunctivitis is very rare—it accounts for only 0.1 to 0.5 percent of ocular disease worldwide, most frequently in regions with a warm, dry climate like northern Africa and the Mediterranean. It is primarily a disease that affects children and young adults, with the majority of them being males between the ages of 3 and 20.

Like seasonal allergic conjunctivitis, vernal keratoconjunctivitis usually strikes in the spring, summer, and fall.

Allergies . . . Or Just Dry Eyes?

Sometimes, your red and irritated eyes may not be a case of allergic conjunctivitis at all. Instead, you may just have a case of dry-eye syndrome. People often spend a good amount of their workday in a room with fluorescent lights, air-conditioning, and a computer screen—all of which have the potential to dry out your eyes.

Studies have shown that people working intensely on a computer blink about half as much as they normally would. As a result, their eyes aren't getting enough moisture. One of the best solutions to dry-eye syndrome is to get plenty of water. Drinking eight glasses a day will ensure that your body is getting an adequate intake of moisture. Edward Paul, O.D., director of Atlantic Eye Associates in Hampstead, North Carolina, also recommends an oral supplement of flaxseed oil to relieve your irritated eyes. Finally, remember to take numerous mini-breaks to look away from the computer.

Giant Papillary Conjunctivitis

Unlike the previously discussed forms of conjunctivitis, giant papillary conjunctivitis (GPC) has no relationship at all to allergic rhinitis, yet this condition affects a group that has more than 25 million members in the United States alone—people who wear contact lenses.

Although it is rare for well-maintained contact lenses to present any problems to their wearers, certain factors can cause GPC, a particularly nasty eye problem that results from irritants on contact lenses. Nobody is exactly certain what irritants cause GPC. Some popular candidates are mucus, calcium, and the wearer's own protein. However, the reason the condition occurs is not as important as who gets it: individuals who don't spend enough time cleaning their contacts.

The symptoms of GPC are quite similar to the symptoms of vernal keratoconjunctivitis. "The way you make the difference in diagnosis is if they wear contact lenses, you call it GPC, and if they don't, you call it vernal," says Dr. Paul. Luckily, GPC can be avoided altogether by being more hygienic about wearing and cleaning your contacts.

Contact Dermatitis

The last type of eye allergy is not a form of conjunctivitis. Without question, though, it can be just as irritating as any of the others. A host of irritants can trigger an eye allergy, even if the particular irritant doesn't come in close contact with your eyes. Some common culprits are cosmetics, hair dye, nail polish, and even some medications. "People can have reactions to a product not normally used around the eyes, such as nail polish, when they rub their eyes while wearing the product," notes Michael B. Raizman, M.D., associate professor of ophthalmology at Tufts University School of Medicine in Boston.

Most of the time, the best solution is to identify and remove the irritant, but sometimes applying cold compresses, made by soaking a clean washcloth in cold water, or using an over-the-counter 1 percent hydrocortisone topical cream around the eye, may be a helpful relief. "Just be careful not to get the cream in your eyes," notes Dr. Paul. (See the Action Plan.)

Nonallergic Conjunctivitis

If your eye problem isn't caused by an allergy, the culprit could be a bacterium or virus. The bacterial and viral forms of conjunctivitis are generally nastier than their allergic counterparts. Plus, they're contagious.

If you're concerned that you might have a bacterial or viral eye infection, see your doctor.

Eye Problem
ACTION PLAN

If you're experiencing problems with your vision, always see a qualified doctor for an evaluation. In addition, check out the following strategies for relieving the itchy, watery eyes associated with such conditions as seasonal and perennial conjunctivitis.

Relieving Seasonal and Perennial Conjunctivitis

indicates a natural remedy

- Wear wraparound glasses if you work outside, keep windows closed and the air conditioner on during high-pollen seasons, and change clothes and shower after coming in from outdoors. Most of all, just be aware of what is irritating your eyes and avoid it.
- Don't rub your itchy eyes. "You release a lot of inflammation in the eyes just from the mechanical force of rubbing," says Dr. Raizman.
- Consider supplements. Two 500-milligram doses of vitamin C taken daily with 2,500 milligrams of quercetin have been an effective natural weapon against eye allergies for some, Dr. Paul reports. Both have natural antihistaminic activity.
- Relieve symptoms by applying cold compresses to your eyes. Soak a clean washcloth in cold water, wring out excess water, and apply to eye area. Or, for an extra bit of relief, soak your cold compresses in calendula lotion before applying them.
- Brew some ordinary tea, allow the bags to cool, and then apply the bags to your closed eyelids for 10 minutes.
- Try a natural alternative to your regular eyedrops. Nonprescription Viva-Drops and Similasan have brought relief to Dr. Paul's patients.
- Over-the-counter antihistamine eyedrops (like Visine-A and Vasocon-A) may be effective for minor irritation, but the antihistamine in these products is often far too weak to be useful in more serious situations.

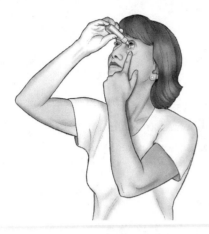

To administer eyedrops, tilt your head back or lie down on a couch. Pull your lower lid away from your eye so that it forms a little pocket. Then, squeeze the eyedrop into the pocket. Do not let the dropper touch your eye or eyelid. Bacteria can contaminate the eyedropper if it touches you. Contact with the dropper can also scratch your cornea.

- Sometimes, the prescription oral antihistamines taken for other allergic rhinitis symptoms can be quite helpful for allergic conjunctivitis symptoms. The nondrowsy forms such as fexofenadine (Allegra), loratadine (Claritin), and cetirizine (Zyrtec) are good choices.
- If you've tried everything but your eyes are still driving you crazy, see your doctor about prescription eyedrops. Dr. Raizman recommends ketotifen (Zaditor) and olopatadine (Patanol) as two extremely effective antihistamine eyedrops, and Dr. Paul names Crolom (sodium cromolyn) as an effective mast cell stabilizer for more severe conditions.
- For serious cases, your doctor may prescribe corticosteroid eyedrops such as loteprednol (Alrex). These are stronger, but they hold the potential for side effects, such as increased eye pressure and cataracts.

Relieving Vernal Keratoconjunctivitis

- The symptoms of vernal keratoconjunctivitis are usually severe and can cause permanent eye damage, so your doctor may start you out on strong corticosteroid eyedrops like Alrex.
- Be patient. Vernal keratoconjunctivitis usually takes months to treat. To overcome it, you'll need to be vigilant about taking your medication.

Relieving Giant Papillary Conjunctivitis

- Always take your contacts out overnight. Leaving them in is like begging for eye irritation.

🌿 Choose disposable contact lenses over reusable ones so that the allergen-causing protein never gets a chance to build up on the lenses.

• If you have reusable contacts, use a protein remover once a week as a complement to your regular saline solution. Dr. Paul recommends enzymatic cleaner tablets as an effective protein remover.

Relieving Contact Dermatitis

🌿 The cause of your allergy may be cosmetics, soaps, lotions, nail polish, perfumes, dyes, or even medication. Take stock of any of these items you come in contact with on a daily basis and avoid the potential allergen. In addition, try to find allergy-free alternatives to the items you're sensitive to.

• You may need a topical cream to treat the eyelid and the skin around the eye. Dr. Paul recommends a 1 percent hydrocortisone cream, which is available without a prescription. Use for no longer than 2 weeks, and do not allow the cream to get into your eyes, Dr. Raizman notes.

Allergy Symptom Solver
EYE PROBLEMS

Eye problems can occur with many different diseases. The chart below lists those most commonly associated with allergy.

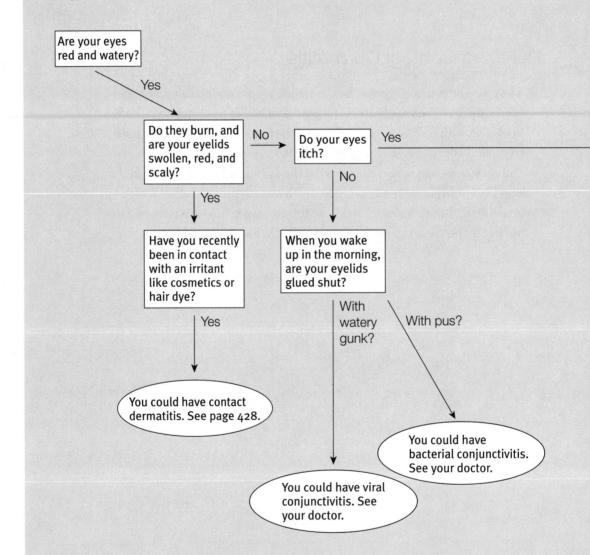

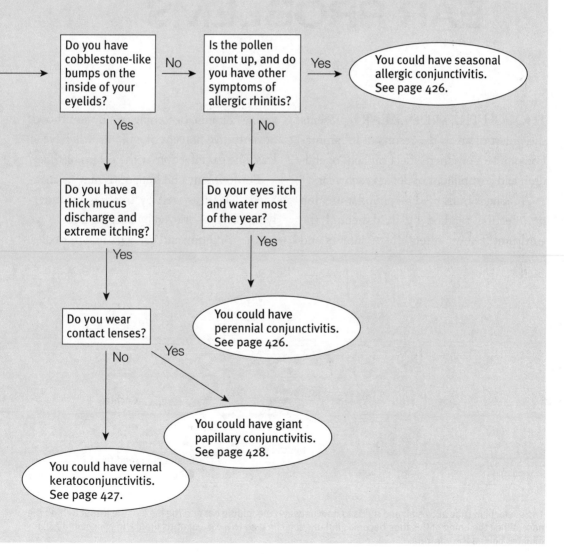

Symptom Solver:
EAR PROBLEMS

THOUGH THE MIDDLE EAR represents the tiniest of areas, the results of inflammation or infections there affect millions of children and cost billions of dollars each year.

At issue is otitis media—an inflammation or infection marked by fluid behind the eardrum. It most often affects infants and young children, becoming rare by adulthood. Seventy-five percent of children will have at least one ear infection by their third birthday.

But for many children, otitis may be managed at least as well by treating an underlying allergy—or even by keeping a close eye on the condition and using natural remedies.

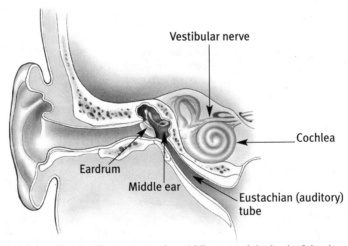

The eustachian tube allows air and fluids to flow between the middle ear and the back of the throat behind the nose. When the lining of this tube becomes inflamed, it can lead to a case of otitis media, in which fluid accumulates behind the eardrum.

The Culprit: A Blocked Eustachian Tube

An episode of otitis media begins in the eustachian tube. This is the tunnel that allows air and fluids to flow between the space behind the eardrum, known as the middle ear, and the back of the throat behind the nose.

When the lining of this tube becomes inflamed, as it can by a cold or other virus, the tube can swell shut and pinch off the middle ear, says Joel M. Bernstein, M.D., Ph.D., clinical professor of otolaryngology and pediatrics at the State University of New York at Buffalo.

Dr. Bernstein thinks that about 40 percent of kids may have allergies like allergic rhinitis (hay fever), which contribute to otitis by increasing mucus and swelling and by creating favorable conditions for a bacterial infection in the middle ear. Common symptoms are earache, fever, and muffled hearing. Eventually, the eardrum may rupture under the pressure exerted by the fluids in the middle ear, releasing the fluid into the outer ear.

Another form of otitis in which allergy may play a role—otitis media with effusion—doesn't necessarily involve a viral or bacterial infection or cause fever and pain, but it can result in decreased hearing.

Ménière's Disease

Deep within your inner ear, lodged behind the eardrum, is a complex structure called the vestibular labyrinth, which teams up with your eyes, neck, and feet to give you a sense of balance.

Ménière's disease can knock this structure for a loop. The disorder is primarily known for the vertigo it brings—a nausea-inducing feeling that the room is spinning.

Doctors still aren't sure what leads to Ménière's symptoms, says Jennifer Derebery, M.D., associate clinical professor of otolaryngology at the University of Southern California and an associate at the House Ear Clinic and Institute, both in Los Angeles. But her research indicates that allergies may play a role for some patients. She found that about twice as many people with Ménière's disease had allergies to foods like milk or wheat or to airborne particles like pollen and mold than the general population.

If you have Ménière's, your doctor should consider testing for an allergic link if:

• Your symptoms get worse in the spring and summer, implying pollen or mold allergies.
• Your symptoms get worse after you eat a specific food.
• You've ever had other allergic conditions, such as allergic rhinitis, asthma, or eczema.
• You have a parent or sibling with allergies.

Two Approaches to Treatment

If otitis is left unattended, complications can develop, ranging from ruptured eardrums and hampered hearing that can lead to speech impediments to rare but life-threatening cases of brain abscess and meningitis. That's why it's important to take children to the doctor when they show symptoms.

American doctors have commonly treated otitis with antibiotics to try to shut down any possible bacterial infection. If the otitis is caused by a viral infection, however, antibiotics will be useless, since they kill only bacteria. Doctors in the United States also often install tubes in the eardrums to allow fluid to escape and air to enter.

In contrast, doctors in the Netherlands are much less quick to prescribe antibiotics, preferring instead to monitor their patients for a few days first. They've found that about 80 percent of the children recover from their otitis without antibiotics and their common side effects, says Dr. Bernstein.

To investigate a possible allergy link, consult an allergist or pediatric allergist who can use skin-prick tests to check to see if your child is sensitive to allergens like pollen or molds or to foods like milk, wheat, eggs, peanuts, or soy, suggests Talal Nsouli, M.D., associate professor of pediatrics and allergy/immunology at Georgetown University Medical Center in Washington, D.C.

If children indeed have allergic conditions that are contributing to their otitis, they may be helped by such measures as learning to avoid the allergen, using medications such as antihistamines and intranasal corticosteroids, and getting allergy shots to build up a tolerance to the allergen. An elimination diet can help with food allergies.

When Surgery Is the Answer

If otitis media continues to be a problem for 4 to 6 months or more, a second opinion or review of all treatment options is advisable, according to Talal Nsouli, M.D., associate professor of pediatrics and allergy/immunology at Georgetown University Medical Center in Washington, D.C. If all other forms of treatment fail, an operation called a tympanostomy with tube placement is a last resort for children who suffer from persistent otitis media. In this procedure, the doctor will cut a tiny hole into the eardrum and insert a tube into it to let it drain air and fluids.

Typically, tubes should be reserved for patients who've had otitis media with effusion in both ears for at least 4 months or in one ear for at least 6 months, or who have had a hearing loss of more than 25 decibels. Tubes are warranted for people with acute otitis media if it has flared up more than two or three times during medication.

Ear Problem
ACTION PLAN

Symptoms of otitis media should always be monitored closely, since they could lead to hearing loss or develop into more serious conditions if left unattended.

Addressing Acute Flare-Ups of Otitis Media

indicates a natural remedy

- See the doctor if your child is showing signs of an ear infection, including tugging or pulling at one or both ears, fever, fluid draining from the ear, irritability, difficulty sleeping, or difficulty hearing.
- The decision to use antibiotics versus watchful waiting should be made by a doctor and will depend a lot on the age of your child and how severe the symptoms are. The doctor will be more likely to want to use antibiotics if the child is under 2 years old or has a red, bulging eardrum.
- Pain relievers containing acetaminophen and ibuprofen can be helpful for treating otitis pain.
- Consider giving your child products with xylitol. A Finnish study found that kids who chewed gum with this natural sweetener had 40 percent fewer occurrences of acute otitis. Gum with xylitol is available in health food stores and some drugstores in the United States, along with toothpastes with xylitol. (The Finnish study didn't look at the effectiveness of xylitol toothpaste, though xylitol gum can help suppress the bacteria that cause cavities.)
- If the child is older and the symptoms aren't as severe, the doctor may want you to monitor the situation for a few days to see if it improves on its own before trying antibiotics.
- Mullein oil or infused garlic oil may be helpful if the eardrum hasn't recently ruptured. These oils can be used simultaneously with antibiotics prescribed by your doctor. You can find a preparation containing either mullein oil or infused garlic oil (do not use pure essential garlic oil in the ear) at most health food stores.

The oil may be warmed in a glass dropper bottle by dipping it briefly into a pot of hot water on the stovetop. The oil should be warm to the touch, not boiling, of course. Place 3 to 5 drops of mullein or infused garlic oil into the child's ear every few hours as needed. The oils soak through the eardrum to fight infection with their antimicrobial properties. "If the eardrum has recently ruptured, symptomized by intense pain followed by a sudden relief along with acute drainage of pus or blood from the ear canal, this treatment is not advised," says Robert Rountree, M.D., a holistic physician in Boulder, Colorado, and coauthor of *Immunotics*.

🌿 To effectively treat the pain, warm a few drops of olive oil, using the water method mentioned above, until it's just slightly warm to the touch, and place a few drops into the child's painful ear. Be sure the oil is neither cold nor hot. Again, it is not advisable to use oils in the ear if the eardrum has recently ruptured, Dr. Rountree notes.

🌿 The fluid left behind after a flare-up may need up to 6 weeks to drain away. If your child has no other symptoms, there's no need to treat this fluid.

Combating Chronic Otitis the Natural Way

There are a number of relatively simple steps that you can take to minimize your child's chances of developing chronic otitis.

- Consult with an allergist to see if your child may have allergies to food or airborne allergens like pollen.
- Don't smoke or let others do so around your child. Studies show that kids who live with adults who smoke have more ear infections.
- Refrain from putting your baby to bed with a bottle. Drinking in a reclined position makes infants more likely to get acute otitis, perhaps because the fluid is prone to backing up into the eustachian tube. Better yet, breast-feed.
- Minimize the time your child spends with a pacifier. A study in Finland found that infants who used a pacifier only occasionally, such as while going to sleep, had fewer cases of acute otitis.

Allergy Symptom Solver
EAR PROBLEMS

Ear problems can occur with many different diseases. The chart below lists those most commonly associated with allergy.

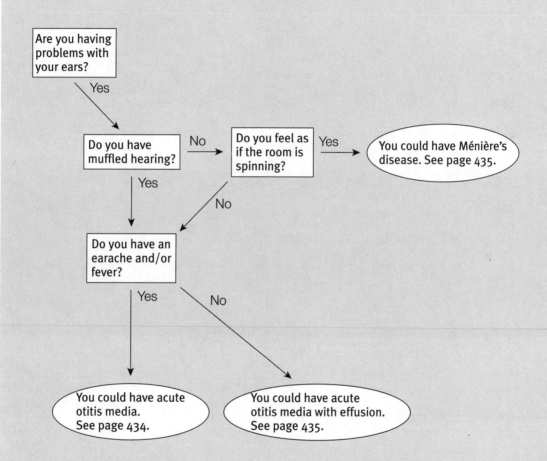

PART SIX

The Hidden Allergy
CONNECTION

Unearth the Causes of Some Mysterious CONDITIONS

ALLERGIES DON'T ALWAYS announce themselves with symptoms as obvious as the sneezing of allergic rhinitis (hay fever) or the anaphylaxis of peanut allergy. But sometimes they produce symptoms like fatigue, headaches, and depression. And the trigger that sets them off can be much harder to discover than ordinary pollen. We say that these symptoms or conditions have hidden allergy connections.

The topics covered in this section are not the ones most people think of when they consider allergies. And these "hidden allergy connections" can be controversial, tenuous, or still in the realm of scientific speculation. They sometimes go beyond the strict definition of allergies to include "sensitivities" and other reactions resembling allergies.

Here's a summary of what you'll find in this section.

Attention-deficit hyperactivity disorder (ADHD). Taking behavior-controlling drugs like Ritalin may not be the only solution to ADHD—not if food sensitivities are contributing to the problem. While this may occur less than 10 percent of the time, for these children, avoiding the allergen triggers may lead to some improvement. We will show you how to experiment with a food elimination diet to spot the culinary culprits.

Candidiasis. Some alternative and environmental-medicine doctors believe that an overgrowth of the yeast *Candida albicans* in the intestines can also contribute to chronic fatigue, fibromyalgia, and related symptoms like depression, anxiety, and muscle and joint pain. In this chapter, we will explain how candida may penetrate the intestinal wall, pumping allergens and toxins into the bloodstream. And we will, of course, offer some natural solutions.

Chronic fatigue syndrome. You may have already read about intestinal permeability in

443

earlier chapters. In the Chronic Fatigue Syndrome chapter, we will show you how some experts believe that excessive permeability and other allergy-related problems can fill the immune system's "rain barrel" to overflowing, leading to more allergies and to problems like chronic fatigue and fibromyalgia.

Depression. Allergies seem to increase irritability and mood swings in adults. While they are unlikely to be the only cause of major depression, statistical studies show that allergies can sometimes make a bad situation worse. In this chapter, we will explore the theory that inflammation from allergies can increase the production of cytokines, a chemical that may trigger depression. Cytokines also show up as a link between allergies and fatigue in the Chronic Fatigue Syndrome chapter.

Headache. Allergies may cause no more than 15 percent of headaches. But if eliminating, say, milk, chocolate, or pickled herring from your diet cures you of headaches, that's nothing to sneeze at. We will explain how some experts believe that a chemical in these foods can cause swelling—or what is sometimes called a "brain allergy"—which can lead to a migraine. And a simple change of diet may eliminate the need for frequent use of nonsteroidal anti-inflammatory drugs (NSAIDs).

Inflammatory bowel disease. Speaking of the intestines, we will explore how alternative practitioners believe that a component in dietary fats called essential fatty acids can contribute to intestinal inflammation that may aggravate inflammatory bowel disease and Crohn's disease. And we will show how adding omega-3 fatty acids from fish oil and reducing omega-6 fatty acids from beef can help reduce this inflammation. The inflammatory mechanism here, while not a true allergy, is similar to allergic inflammation, and some doctors believe that modifying the intake of fatty acids can reduce problems such as inflammation from rheumatoid arthritis. (See The Allergy-Free Supplementation Schedule on page 149.)

Multiple chemical sensitivity. And finally, there is multiple chemical sensitivity, a sort of allergy nightmare where everything from perfumes to pesticides to fresh paint can unleash problems ranging from headaches to hyperactivity. In this chapter, you will see that professional theories struggle to define this mysterious condition and determine how to treat it.

Attention-Deficit Hyperactivity DISORDER

DOCTORS HAVE A LOT OF fancy names for it. Over the years, it has been known as minimal brain dysfunction, hyperkinetic reaction to childhood, attention-deficit disorder, and the one that has stuck (at least for now): attention-deficit hyperactivity disorder (ADHD). But what most parents call it is probably unprintable.

The truth is that ADHD has many faces, many names. It afflicts the poor, the rich, and the famous alike. Leonardo da Vinci, Ludwig van Beethoven, Thomas Edison, and Albert Einstein all may have had it. Further, up to 15 percent of school-age children may have ADHD, a cluster of behavior problems first described in 1902.

For yet undetermined reasons, boys are more than twice as likely to have ADHD than girls. Many parents of children who have this disorder can't recall a time when their child wasn't constantly fidgeting, wasn't always "on the go," wasn't talking too much, wasn't "hell on wheels."

Children with ADHD may exhibit most, if not all, of these signs. Most of these children are both hyperactive and unusually inattentive. Others may only have problems concentrating—a condition that was once called attention-deficit disorder without hyperactivity but is now considered a milder form of ADHD. Yet whatever you call it, and no matter how it manifests itself, the parents of these children—and often the children themselves—search desperately for ways to control it. In some cases, children attempt to self-medicate with alcohol, tobacco, and other addictive substances.

Treatment: The Reign of Ritalin

According to most doctors, the answer is drugs such as methylphenidate (Ritalin), a potent stimulant that helps children with ADHD symptoms focus their attention and regulate their behavior. But a growing number of physicians have a different idea. They feel that the underlying causes of ADHD symptoms should be searched for.

One of the possible causes being looked at is allergies, including sensitivities to foods, pollen, cosmetics, perfume, glues, pesticides, environmental chemicals, animal dander, molds, and even household dust.

"Using drugs to treat ADHD symptoms

The Ritalin Riddle: Is It the Best Choice?

To Mary Ann Block, D.O., medical director at the Block Center near Dallas, ADHD, or attention-deficit hyperactivity disorder, has a totally different meaning. To her, it stands for "Another Devalued, Helplessly Drugged child." "To many physicians, ADHD seems to mean 'let me write this prescription for you.' And nothing more is done," says Dr. Block. "I'm not antidrug by any means, but drugs treat only the symptoms of ADHD; they don't fix the underlying cause."

Up to 30 percent of children who have ADHD symptoms are treated with medications such as Prozac, Dexedrine, and Tofranil. But methylphenidate (Ritalin), which is taken by at least two million children daily, is by far the most commonly prescribed drug for ADHD symptoms, Dr. Block says. More than 10 tons of the drug are produced annually, and the number of children taking it has quadrupled in the past decade. Despite its popularity and its long track record of being a "short-term quick fix," it may not be the best treatment for your child, Dr. Block warns.

"In my mind, Ritalin is just 'pediatric cocaine.' Both drugs use the same receptor site in the brain, give the same 'high,' and in medical research, they're used interchangeably," Dr. Block says. "It's no surprise to me that we have a drug problem in this country when we prescribe potentially addictive drugs such as Ritalin to children as young as 3 years old."

Ritalin, even when used for just a few weeks, can have serious side effects, including irritability, insomnia, tics, decreased growth, and psychotic-like symptoms, according to Dr. Block. The long-term effects—and many children do take this drug for years or even decades—are not well-known. So before your physician hands you a prescription for this potent drug, ask for a second opinion and explore all other options first, she suggests. You might be surprised how quickly nondrug treatments can give a whole new meaning to ADHD and transform your child into an "Adorable, Dynamic, Huggable, Delightful" person.

merely covers up the symptoms. The drugs don't fix the underlying cause," says Mary Ann Block, D.O., medical director at the Block Center near Dallas and author of *No More Ritalin: Treating ADHD without Drugs*. "Doctors should be searching for the underlying cause of the symptoms, and allergies do seem to be one of the dominant underlying causes."

Meanwhile, some doctors and organizations, including the National Institute of Mental Health, contend that allergies rarely, if ever, cause ADHD. It is a controversy that likely won't be resolved soon.

"The whole issue of ADHD is emotionally charged. It almost seems like a political campaign. To listen to people on one side, you can't believe they exist in the same world as people on the other side. There is as much opinion as there is fact involved in much that is written or said about this condition," says L. Eugene Arnold, M.D., psychiatry professor emeritus at Ohio State University in Columbus, member of a National Institute of Mental Health steering committee for a treatment study of children with ADHD, and author of a textbook on ADHD diagnosis and treatment.

Treatment: The Dietary Directive

The truth is that an increased chance of ADHD symptoms is probably caused by a number of underlying factors, including genetic abnormalities and birth injuries due to lack of oxygen from chord trauma during labor or use of forceps or suction during delivery. Other factors may be biochemical disturbances and toxins, according to Dr. Arnold. Allergies or other hypersensitivities may aggravate ADHD symptoms in a small proportion—possibly less than 10 percent of children who have the disorder—though the exact percentage is not known, he says.

Notably, however, of those children with ADHD who are affected by allergies, perhaps as many as 7 out of 10 improve when the troublemakers are eliminated from their diets or surrounding environments, says William G. Crook, M.D., of his experience treating ADHD patients as a pediatrician in Jackson, Tennessee.

In many cases, the culprit is a food or beverage. "It's usually the foods the child likes the best and is eating all of the time that are causing the problems," Dr. Block notes. "So ask yourself what foods your child eats every day. Then ask yourself if your child would be extremely unhappy if you said, 'No, you can't have that.' Take all of these foods out of your child's diet and see what happens."

The notion that allergens can affect behavior and not just cause rashes and wheezing isn't a new one. In the 1970s, California allergist Benjamin Feingold, M.D., claimed that artificial colorings and flavorings as well as salicylates, natural chemicals found in foods such as tomatoes, apricots, and berries, could trigger ADHD. From this finding, he developed what became known as the Feingold diet, which eliminated troublesome ingredients from the child's diet. Up to 50 percent of the children placed on this diet, according to Dr. Feingold, exhibited fewer symptoms of ADHD.

Despite the conventional viewpoint that food allergies can cause hives or make your throat close up but not affect how you feel, think, or act, Dr. Feingold's diet is still used by many parents. But some physicians, including Dr. Block, believe it doesn't go far enough in all cases. Almost any food or beverage can trigger ADHD symptoms in any

The Natural ADHD Treatment Program

Drugs such as methylphenidate (Ritalin), when used in combination with counseling, may improve the behavior of some, but not all, children with attention-deficit hyperactivity disorder (ADHD), says William G. Crook, M.D., a pediatrician in Jackson, Tennessee, and author of *Help for the Hyperactive Child*. So before you subject your child to drugs or counseling, you might want to ask a nutritionist or other health professional to supervise the following nondrug treatment program designed by Dr. Crook.

Clean up your child's diet. Many children with ADHD improve substantially when chemically enhanced foods are stricken from their diets. So curtail or sharply limit your child's consumption of processed foods and beverages, particularly those that contain processed sugars, artificial sweeteners, saturated oils, food colorings, caffeine, phosphates, and other additives. Instead, serve your child a balanced diet that contains more fruits, vegetables, whole grains, and natural sweeteners such as honey or maple syrup. Ideally, buy organic foods and products produced on nearby farms and gardens.

Clean up your child's environment. Tobacco smoke, pesticides, perfumes, colognes, glues, deodorants, and other odorous or toxic substances can shrivel your child's attention span and trigger behavioral problems. Eliminate as many of these substances from your home as possible. Ask your child's teacher or principal to make accommodations for your child so that exposure at school is minimized. If your child usually rides a bus to school, consider driving him there yourself instead since some children are sensitive to diesel fumes.

Try an elimination diet. Put your child on a 5- to 10-day elimination diet to identify ingredients that seem to aggravate his behavior. Common culprits include food coloring, milk, wheat, sugar, citrus, and yeast.

given child, she says. Instead, Dr. Block and others advocate a more comprehensive elimination diet that temporarily excludes certain foods from the child's menu, such as:

- Chocolate
- Citrus
- Corn
- Milk and other dairy products
- Processed meats and other processed or packaged foods
- Soft drinks and artificial juices
- Sugar
- Wheat
- Yeast

If you discover dietary ingredients that adversely affect your child's behavior, you can make permanent adjustments. (For more on elimination diets, see Food Allergies and Intolerances on page 278.) But it still might be wise to consider supplementing this approach with other treatments, Dr. Arnold says.

"It doesn't have to be an either-or proposition. Dietary modification can be used in conjunction with behavioral treatment or medication," Dr. Arnold says. "In some cases, at least it is claimed, you can reduce the amount of medication needed if you place the child on a proper elimination diet."

While proponents and critics of the allergy-ADHD connection may disagree about much, they do agree on one thing: keeping the best interests of your child in mind. If necessary, seek out second or even third opinions. You can get information about ADHD causes and possible solutions by sending $3 and a stamped, self-addressed envelope to The International Health Foundation, PO Box 3494, Jackson, TN 38303. You can also find out more about children's nutrition and learning by writing to the Block Center, 1721 Cimarron Trail, Suite 4, Hurst, TX 76054. Include a stamped, self-addressed envelope.

"Parents who have children with ADHD symptoms and suspect that allergies may be the cause of the problem need to be advocates for their children. They need to take the situation into their own hands," Dr. Block says. "If you were buying a car, you wouldn't just go to one dealership and fork over your money without shopping around first. Give your child with ADHD symptoms at least that much time and energy."

CANDIDIASIS

FOR MORE THAN 150 YEARS, we have known that we are not alone in our bodies. Four hundred different types of organisms, most of them harmless, reside in the dark recesses of the digestive tract alone. But what happens when these little creatures beneath turn against us?

In 1978, that's exactly what Dr. C. Orian Truss of Birmingham, Alabama, decided to find out. In particular, he was interested in *Candida albicans*, a yeast that naturally occurs in the human body. Before Dr. Truss presented his theories, *Candida albicans* was known to cause yeast infections in women—and not known for much else. But Dr. Truss believed that the yeast was the source of more misery than it was given credit for. He saw the overgrowth of intestinal candida (rhymes with *Canada*) as the cause of fatigue, lethargy, depression, difficulty in concentrating, and a host of other problems. The condition soon came to be known as candidiasis hypersensitivity.

The Quarrel over Candidiasis

Dr. Truss's ideas have been the source of controversy ever since he first presented them, and the medical community is divided on whether or not candidiasis (pronounced "can-duh-DIE-uh-sis") hypersensitivity even exists. Several respected physicians not only see it as a dangerous disease but also consider the *Candida albicans* yeast a potentially harmful allergen. Others are not so certain. The American Academy of Allergy, Asthma, and Immunology dismisses the disease entirely. In their position statement, they conclude: "The concept of candidiasis hypersensitivity is speculative and unproven."

The only thing about candidiasis hypersensitivity that doctors do seem to agree on is that the yeast *Candida albicans* does exist. In a healthy person, candida resides in the mouth, skin, intestinal tract, and, in women, the vagina. A healthy immune system and "good" bacteria prevent the yeast from growing out of hand.

Causes of Candidiasis

How does this natural and seemingly harmless yeast cause so much trouble? A whole host of factors can cause candida to grow beyond its normal levels. Everything from hormonal changes (such as those that go along with monthly periods, pregnancies, or the use of birth control pills) to a diet high in sugar and carbohydrates can trigger candida growth. Other common causes of growth include stress and the use of antibiotics. "Any antibiotic can make you more prone to yeast infections," says Elson Haas, M.D., medical director and founder of the Preventive Medical Center of Marin in San Rafael, California. "This usually occurs with vaginal yeast, but it can cause growth of intestinal yeast as well."

Candida is also associated with a host of other diseases, ranging from autism to cancer. Healthy newborns often develop candida infections in the mouth and throat (known as thrush), and the yeast is also a well-known cause of diaper rash. People with suppressed immune systems, such as AIDS patients, also are common victims of yeast overgrowth.

This much is scientifically well-documented. What happens next is where medical experts disagree.

Believers in the candida-allergy connection theorize that once *Candida albicans* starts multiplying, the yeast changes shape into its mycelial fungal form. In this form, candida grows long, rootlike structures known as rhizoids that dig into the intestinal walls like tree roots into soil. Once in place, these rhizoids act as pipelines for candida, pumping toxins and allergens generated by the fungus into the bloodstream. And just like that, the normally harmless yeast can become the source of your problems.

Symptoms of the Syndrome

In particular, it is at the point when the rhizoids are pumping toxins and allergens into the bloodstream that a person with a yeast allergy will feel the effects the most. Candidiasis may just mean overgrowth of yeast in the intestinal tract, says Dr. Haas. "Just like people have hay fever (allergic rhinitis), you can become allergic to particular molds and yeasts."

Whether candidiasis hypersensitivity truly exists—and whether it is the real cause of the following symptoms—may be controversial, but the symptoms themselves are real and can make your life miserable. Among patients diagnosed with the disease, doctors have seen these symptoms.

- Chronic yeast infections
- Coated tongue
- Toenail fungus
- Abdominal bloating
- Muscle and joint pain
- Chronic fatigue
- Irritability
- Mood swings
- Depression
- Anxiety
- Difficulty in concentrating

Talking to Your Doctor

Because the diagnosis covers such a multitude of symptoms, many doctors think that candidiasis is more of an emotional or psychological problem than a physical one. Moreover, the yeast is always present, even in the body of a healthy person. This makes it difficult for doctors to prove that the yeast is the actual cause of any health problems. Sure, candida might show up in a patient's stool sample, but the naturally occurring yeast would probably show up there even if the patient were not sick. This simple fact would seem to make it impossible to pin any specific symptoms on candida.

Believers have another explanation, how-

ever. "Candida can masquerade as just about anything," says Sherry A. Rogers, M.D., a fellow of the American College of Allergy, Asthma, and Immunology and a board-certified specialist in environmental medicine. While doctors argue about whether or not candidiasis hypersensitivity actually exists, for many people who experience the symptoms, nothing except candidiasis treatment seems to help.

Dr. Rogers has seen it time and time again: Patients show strong symptoms of candidiasis, yet their previous physicians don't make the proper diagnosis. "I just saw a 45-year-old man for a 1-year follow-up last week. He came to my office a year ago with a 4-year history of being disabled from work because he had been diagnosed with fibromyalgia," she says. "We tested his intestinal contents, because I was suspicious from his history that he had high levels of candida. Sure enough, he did, we treated it, and in 3 weeks his symptoms of 4 years were gone, and they've been gone ever since then."

If you exhibit any or all of the symptoms listed above and you can't seem to pinpoint the cause of your misery, talk to your doctor.

Keep in mind, though, that even inquiring about this disease may not be easy. Since candidiasis hypersensitivity is so controversial, Richard Layton, M.D., a physician in specialized pediatrics and allergy and integrated medicine in Towson, Maryland, recommends that you inform your doctor that you think you might have a "yeast or mold problem."

While the existence of candidiasis hypersensitivity is questioned by many physicians, some, like Dr. Layton, will listen to your symptoms, look into your medical history, and consider the possibility that candidiasis might be your problem. "The key is to take a full history and try to break it down," he says. "Rather than getting pigeonholed into candidiasis, I try to look at all the connections."

The Common Yeast Problem

Probably the most common form of candidiasis—and the one that all doctors agree is legitimate—is vaginitis, more commonly known as a yeast infection. The characteristic symptoms are vaginal itching, burning, and swelling, and white or yellow discharge. Yeast infections usually can be self-treated; numerous conventional and natural treatments can alleviate the symptoms. (For specific information on treating this condition, see "Attack the Common Yeast Infection" on page 454.)

A yeast infection is irritating, but it's nothing to be overly concerned about. Seventy-five percent of women will experience at least one during their lifetimes. But if your infections become recurrent and are accompanied by some of the symptoms listed above, your problem may be bigger than a simple yeast infection. In this case, you may want to try some of the treatments used for candidiasis hypersensitivity, such as a diet low in sugar, supplements of "good" bacteria, and, when necessary, over-the-counter and prescription antifungals.

Vaginitis is primarily a "women-only" condition, but other problems associated with yeast can affect both genders equally. Dr. Layton does treat more women than men for gut-related yeast problems, but that doesn't necessarily mean candidiasis affects women only. "Women tend to be more aware of what's wrong, while too many men, including myself, don't pay attention to details," he explains.

The Battle Plan for Beating Candidiasis

Whether you're a woman or a man, candidiasis hypersensitivity usually can be treated without antibiotics. In fact, the first thing that Dr. Layton does when he sees a potential case of candidiasis isn't fill out prescriptions; instead, he gets that person back on a healthy diet.

• The candida yeast thrives on sugar, so the best way to kill it off is to quit eating the sweet stuff. When Dr. Layton sees children with what may be a candidiasis problem, he immediately suggests cutting back on junk food.

• If you're sensitive to the candida yeast, it's likely that you will be sensitive to other molds as well. So yeasty foods (bread, beer, cheese, and mushrooms) are definitely a good thing to avoid.

• One food that actually curbs the growth of *Candida albicans* is good old-fashioned yogurt. Live-culture yogurt contains *Lactobacillus acidophilus*, a type of "good" bacteria in the body. Since an adequate amount of this bacteria maintains yeast at a normal level, adding a little more plain, unsweetened yogurt to your diet certainly will not hurt.

• Meats and fresh vegetables are also part of the anticandidiasis diet, as well as whole

Attack the Common Yeast Infection

Yeast infections are common, generally harmless—and irritating. To knock them out, follow the steps below.

• Try a natural alternative. Take 600 milligrams of garlic concentrate tablets three times daily for 1 month, says Robert Rountree, M.D., a holistic physician in Boulder, Colorado, and coauthor of *Immunotics*.

• If garlic supplements are ineffective, try an over-the-counter treatment, says Richard Layton, M.D., a physician in specialized pediatrics and allergy and integrated medicine in Towson, Maryland. (The best known are Gyne-Lotrimin and Monistat 7.)

• If that still doesn't do the trick, see your doctor. Generally, Dr. Layton recommends 150 milligrams of fluconazole (Diflucan) for a serious acute infection. For a chronic yeast infection, dosage and duration will depend on the individual patient's history.

• To prevent recurrent vaginitis, wear loose, all-cotton underwear, and avoid irritants such as scented toilet paper and perfumed bubble bath, says Shari Brasner, M.D., an obstetrician and gynecologist at Mount Sinai School of Medicine in New York City.

• Certain antibiotics like penicillin can trigger a yeast overgrowth by killing off *Lactobacillus acidophilus* and other "good" bacteria. To prevent this from occurring, take an acidophilus supplement along with the antibiotic to maintain your levels of these bacteria. Dr. Brasner recommends two acidophilus tablets three times a day, with meals, as a preventive measure against yeast infections.

grains and nuts, Dr. Rogers says. None of these foods feed the candida yeast, so, in essence, they can "starve" the yeast down to a healthy level.

• Complement your yeast-free diet with supplements that contain *Lactobacillus acidophilus*, *L. bifidus*, and other "good" bacteria. A product with garlic or biotin also helps fight yeast overgrowth, says Dr. Layton.

• If this regimen yields no results after a few weeks, talk to your doctor about antifungals.

Taking Your Body Back

Candidiasis hypersensitivity differs from many conventional diseases because it's not caused by harmful bacteria or viruses. Instead, the body of a person with candidiasis has been weakened in such a manner that a normally harmless organism can wreak havoc. The most common causes of this wearing down of the immune system are antibiotics, sodas, processed foods, sugars, and a leaky gut, says Dr. Rogers, who calls the disease a product of our drug culture. "The person has a weakened immune system, so harmless bugs become harmful," she explains. "So we make the person stronger."

A lot of times, that strength can come from an act as simple as cutting sugar and yeast out of your diet. If you're suffering and your doctor can't find the solution, the culprit could be *Candida albicans*. And with 400 other forms of bacteria living harmlessly within your digestive tract, there's no reason that *Candida albicans* should get to act so wild. It's time to make that yeast behave.

Chronic Fatigue SYNDROME

FEELING LIKE A SLUG in the mud and wondering why?

If you've been experiencing extreme exhaustion for 6 months or more and your doctor hasn't been able to identify the cause, you might have chronic fatigue syndrome (CFS). And if you do have CFS, allergies could be playing an important role, says Leo Galland, M.D., director of the Foundation for Integrated Medicine in New York City and author of *Power Healing*.

Scientists are still trying to uncover the source of CFS, which was once known as the yuppie flu. According to the Centers for Disease Control and Prevention, you may have chronic fatigue syndrome if you have severe chronic fatigue for 6 months or more, with no other medical explanation, and you have four or more of the following symptoms.

• Substantial impairment of short-term memory or concentration

• Sore throat
• Tender lymph nodes
• Muscle pain
• Multijoint pain without swelling or redness
• Headaches of a new type, pattern, or severity
• Unrefreshing sleep
• A post-exertion feeling of general discomfort or uneasiness lasting more than 24 hours

Despite these criteria, some doctors question whether CFS truly exists, since a specific cause has not been identified. Some of these doctors believe the source of the condition may have more to do with psychological, rather than physical, symptoms. If you have the symptoms listed above, be sure to discuss them with your doctor, and—since many of the symptoms are common to other conditions—make sure that the two of you explore all possible explanations.

Fibromyalgia: A Common Companion

Although chronic fatigue syndrome and fibromyalgia have distinct definitions, many people who have CFS also have fibromyalgia. And fibromyalgia occurs seven times more frequently in women than men.

According to the American College of Rheumatology, you may have fibromyalgia if you meet the following guidelines.

• You have widespread aching, stiffness, and fatigue originating in the muscles and soft tissues for at least 3 months.

• You also have pain when pressure is applied to 11 or more of 18 tender points around the body.

Anyone who believes that they have CFS or fibromyalgia should see a doctor with expertise in treating these conditions. There is no single cure for either condition, though doctors say that many people can reach a point where they feel substantially better most of the time. National organizations and local support groups can help you find a qualified doctor. The CFIDS Association of America posts a wide range of information. Go to www.cfids.org on the Internet or write to them at PO Box 220398, Charlotte, NC 28222-0398.

The Allergy Link

Though no one knows exactly what causes CFS, researchers have found that more than half of the people with CFS they've studied also have allergies. "I believe that being an allergic individual predisposes you to chronic fatigue syndrome," says Dr. Galland. "Chronic fatigue syndrome seems to be associated with an overreactivity of certain parts of the immune system, which is similar to what we see in people with allergies."

And when allergies are part of the cause, treating the allergies can be a part of the cure. "I've found that close to three-fourths of my patients will find their fatigue improves when their allergies improve," Dr. Galland notes. This improvement varies widely, but sometimes it can be dramatic. "There have been some patients in whom disabling chronic fatigue totally goes away when their food allergies were treated," he reports.

Finding and treating the culprits, however, is not always easy. With chronic fatigue, if there is one food allergy, there are probably many. Further, even nickel allergy could play a role in this condition. A study found that nickel allergy occurred in more than one-third of all CFS patients, rising to more than half of female CFS patients. These are about double the normal rates. The researchers speculate that nickel could be one factor causing chronic overstimulation of the immune system, triggering chronic fatigue.

Environmental allergens and irritants can also compound your fatigue. "Mold allergy is an important cause of fatigue and muscle aches. A significant proportion of people with chronic fatigue syndrome and fibromyalgia have mold sensitivity," says Dr. Galland. In addition, environmental chemicals can be a big problem—people with chemical sensitivities are the hardest to treat.

If you have been diagnosed with CFS or fibromyalgia, you should see an allergist to get a thorough evaluation for allergies, says Dr. Galland. One clue, however, to whether your fatigue is caused by allergies is how it responds to exercise. "I've found that the kind of fatigue linked to allergy is lethargy or sluggishness. And about 90 percent of the time, the people who have allergic fatigue find that if they go out and engage in vigorous exercise, they feel better," he says.

On the other hand, some people with chronic fatigue feel miserable after vigorous exercise. Dr. Galland believes this may indicate a viral type of CFS. Exercise is still an

Practical Strategies for Taking Control of Your Symptoms

If you have been diagnosed with chronic fatigue syndrome (CFS) or fibromyalgia, you may begin to feel powerless since these conditions are not thoroughly understood and the symptoms often leave you feeling worn out. Having a practical plan of action can help you regain a sense of control over your health. First, you should get a thorough evaluation for allergies, advises Leo Galland, M.D., director of the Foundation for Integrated Medicine in New York City and author of *Power Healing*. You should also ask yourself whether your fatigue corresponds to possible exposure to allergens. For example, does it vary with the pollen season or get worse when you spend time in a possibly moldy building? Be sure to mention any patterns you notice to your doctor, and do your best to avoid any allergens the two of you have identified. In addition, follow the tips below to help ease your symptoms and gain some relief.

- Rinse out your nostrils with a saline spray twice a day to remove allergens and histamine. Options include a neti pot or bulb syringe, using 4 ounces of warm water, ¼ teaspoon of salt, and ⅛ teaspoon of baking soda.
- Try sleeping in a recliner. Nasal congestion often is worse when you lie down, so sleeping with your head elevated may help.
- Consider trying nasal strips such as Breathe Right, which are used to hold the nostrils open. Some patients have found these to be helpful.
- Prescription nasal steroids such as fluticasone (Flonase) and mometasone (Nasonex) may be your best bet for both allergic and nonallergic rhinitis.

important part of treatment, but in this case you probably need to begin slowly, with small doses of an aerobic exercise that is gentle on your muscles, he says.

It's All in Your Nose

The benefits of exercise also were noted by Crawford Cleveland, M.D., an allergist in Pensacola, Florida, who studied the relationship of chronic rhinitis (hay fever–like symptoms) to fibromyalgia.

Dr. Cleveland and his colleagues looked at 47 consecutive patients who visited an allergy clinic with persistent rhinitis symptoms, such as sneezing, congestion, itchy eyes, postnasal drip, and sore throat. Then they looked for symptoms of fibromyalgia. Although less than 5 percent of the general

- Azelastine (Astelin), a prescription nasal antihistamine, may help. Be careful when using both over-the-counter and prescription antihistamines, however, since both could potentially make CFS symptoms worse.
- Discuss the benefits and drawbacks of immunotherapy with your doctor.
- Try taking 300 milligrams of feverfew, standardized to 0.3 to 0.7 percent parthenolides, three times daily. Or 300 milligrams of Siberian ginseng, standardized to 0.4 percent eleutherosides, two to three times a day. Although it's the least effective, you can try 300 milligrams of chamomile or one cup of fresh tea two to three times daily to reduce aches and fatigue.
- Small doses, typically 10 milligrams, of the prescription antidepressant doxepin at bedtime may improve sleep. Ask your doctor about this.
- Exercise. Begin slowly, with stretching exercises such as shoulder shrugs and side bends with arms outstretched. Gradually work up to an aerobic conditioning routine such as walking or bicycling for 20 to 30 minutes daily.
- Creatine may reduce after-exercise fatigue for people with CFS, says Dr. Lyon, but should not be used until you talk to your doctor to determine if you are ready for a more vigorous exercise program and the appropriate dosage. "We have patients load up with creatine at the same doses that bodybuilders use, initially, then have them stay on a maintenance dose," he says.
- Antibiotics may be necessary to treat sinus infections.
- When all else fails, surgery to correct deformities in the sinuses may be necessary.

Don't Discount Your Digestive Tract

One of the best ways to tackle allergies—and the fatigue they cause—may be to improve the health of your digestive tract, alternative and environmental doctors believe. Problems in the intestine can aggravate the immune system and increase your sensitivity to allergies, according to both Leo Galland, M.D., director or the Foundation for Integrated Medicine in New York City and author of *Power Healing*, and Michael Lyon, M.D., director of research at Oceanside Functional Medicine Research Institute in Nanaimo, British Columbia, Canada.

According to these doctors, even allergies like allergic rhinitis (hay fever) can get worse when problems in your gut overtax your immune system. "In anybody with chronic fatigue and in anybody with multiple food allergies, I always look at intestinal function. I find it very important to test for parasites, leaky-gut syndrome, and yeast overgrowth. That's usually the first area I look at," says Dr. Galland.

Though many conventional doctors question the validity of theories such as leaky-gut syndrome and any possible connection to allergies they might have, alternative doctors report some intriguing case studies. One of Dr. Galland's patients developed a debilitating case of fibromyalgia a year after she had been in Mexico on assignment and had gotten sick with diarrhea. Afterward, she had chronic constipation. She also had allergies to a half-dozen foods.

Dr. Galland became suspicious, and testing revealed the amoebic parasite *Entamoeba histolytica*. Soon after the parasite was eradicated and she cleaned up her diet, she began a dramatic recovery. "She is now even healthier than before she became ill," says Dr. Galland.

If you're having chronic digestive tract problems, get evaluated by a doctor for intestinal parasites, including *Giardia* and *Cryptosporidium*, says Dr. Galland.

Artemisia annua, or sweet wormwood, is a safe nonprescription alternative treatment for parasites such as giardia, says Dr. Galland. Be aware, though, that symptoms can become worse temporarily during treatment, and don't use it if you're pregnant.

You might also try adding yogurt or *Lactobacillus acidophilus* capsules to your diet to counter bad bacteria and reduce intestinal inflammation. Adding fiber to your diet can also help to support the friendly bacteria. Finally, avoid things that, according to alternative-minded doctors, can increase intestinal permeability. This means reducing or eliminating nonsteroidal anti-inflammatory drugs, drinking no more than one glass of wine or beer a day, and eliminating deep-fried foods and hydrogenated fats from your diet.

public has fibromyalgia, they found that among the patients they studied:

• Half had widespread but diffuse aching pain and fatigue lasting at least 3 months.

• Half had pain in 11 or more tender points on their bodies.

• Thirty-eight percent had both of these problems, thus meeting the full criteria for fibromyalgia.

Another study looked at rhinitis from the other statistical direction, first finding people with chronic fatigue syndrome, then checking for rhinitis. Seventy percent had it, including postnasal drip and nasal, sinus, and ear congestion.

Why You're Feeling Sleepy

The frequency of fibromyalgia among people with rhinitis was not entirely a surprise to allergists, who have long noted a syndrome of tiredness and generalized aching associated with food hypersensitivity and seasonal allergies. The real surprise was that one-quarter of the rhinitis patients did not have allergies. Yet they had fibromyalgia symptoms about as often as those with allergies. "We went into it thinking it was strictly caused by allergic rhinitis (hay fever)," says Dr. Cleveland.

This finding points to the rhinitis itself, rather than allergies, as a trigger of fibromyalgia and CFS, perhaps because the congestion causes a sort of sleep apnea that interferes with breathing during sleep, says Dr. Cleveland. He found that fatigue and sleep disturbances occurred at about the

same rate in the allergic and nonallergic subjects: 60 percent.

One theory of fibromyalgia is that it is caused by a lack of deep sleep, which is characterized by slow, delta brain waves. During delta-wave sleep, key hormones needed to repair the body, such as growth hormone, are produced. When a pioneering researcher in fibromyalgia, Harvey Moldofsky, M.D., professor emeritus of psychiatry and medicine at University of Toronto in Ontario, Canada, disrupted delta-wave sleep for several days in subjects of average physical fitness, they soon had the fatigue and aching muscles characteristic of fibromyalgia.

When Dr. Moldofsky tried this same experiment using college athletes, however, they did not develop the symptoms of fibromyalgia. Apparently, people who exercise regularly sleep better, says Dr. Cleveland, who notes that trained athletes are fairly resistant to any type of fatigue from chronic rhinitis, too. Although more research needs to be done, this suggests that getting more exercise may help anyone with fibromyalgia.

A Congestion Connection?

There may be an even closer link between nasal congestion and fatigue.

"Fatigue can come on virtually simultaneously with congestion, whether it's caused by hay fever or sick building syndrome," says Alexander Chester, M.D., clinical professor of medicine in the department of medicine at Georgetown University Medical Center in Washington, D.C. "I noticed it when I was quite young. Nasal stuffiness would produce a disproportionate level of fatigue. Many people with allergies feel run-down."

Dr. Chester theorizes that because of evolutionary reasons, irritation in the nose gives a trigger, neurologically, to create the fatigue. He believes the chronic congestion of sinusitis may trigger chronic fatigue syndrome. Therefore, if you clear up the congestion, you may clear up the fatigue. He says studies show that, when all else fails, surgery to correct deformities in the sinuses can be quite effective at restoring energy.

While he finds it intriguing, Dr. Galland has a problem with Dr. Chester's hypothesis: "There are people who have rhinitis and have no fatigue at all. But then people vary very much in the way they respond to allergies."

Could Biochemistry Be at Fault?

A more central cause of fatigue and achiness may lie in the chemicals released during the allergic response, including histamine and cytokines, says Dr. Galland.

Cytokines also cause much of the achiness and fatigue during the flu, so it's not

Cytokines: The Smoking Gun

Cytokines may be a key to understanding chronic fatigue syndrome (CFS), some researchers believe. Cytokines are chemicals that make you feel sick by triggering inflammation, fever, and lethargy, both as the result of illnesses and allergies.

Because allergies are the most consistent abnormality of the immune system in CFS, perhaps prolonged or excessive production of cytokines might be the problem.

Researchers from Denver and Seattle looked at the cytokines most associated with fever and lethargy and at one good cytokine that reduces inflammation. They found that in people with CFS, the levels of two of the harmful cytokines were more than three times higher than normal, and the good cytokine was almost undetectable.

These researchers think that allergies may be to blame because most of the people with CFS who had abnormal cytokine levels also had allergies. On top of that, cytokine levels increased during allergy season, and the test subjects with chronic fatigue also reported feeling worse during allergy season.

The participants who had allergies but no CFS also had abnormal—though less extreme—levels of cytokines, compared to the subjects who had neither chronic fatigue nor allergies.

The EPD Option

An alternative to immunotherapy that may work better to counter the fatigue of chronic fatigue syndrome (CFS) and fibromyalgia is enzyme-potentiated desensitization, or EPD, according to Michael Lyon, M.D., director of research at Oceanside Functional Medicine Research Institute in Nanaimo, British Columbia, Canada. A version of immunotherapy used by environmental-medicine doctors, EPD remains controversial in conventional-medicine circles.

"EPD appears to work by actually recreating tolerance. And loss of tolerance is really what allergy is," says Dr. Lyon.

In EPD, a fluid is injected that contains dozens of allergens along with an enzyme called beta-glucuronidase, which apparently reprograms immune cells to tolerate the allergens instead of mounting an allergic response, says Dr. Lyon. People undergoing EPD normally must be isolated from problem allergens during treatment, but studies that have skipped this step still have an 80 percent success rate, he adds.

EPD is just one part of the treatment that Dr. Lyon uses for people with CFS; it is not a cure by itself. "It does provide most people with CFS some degree of relief and improved quality of life," he says.

Other studies show that it is safer than conventional allergy shots because there seems to be no risk of anaphylactic reactions, says Dr. Lyon.

It is too early to say how much effect EPD has on reducing fatigue in CFS, says Dr. Lyon, but because the risk is minimal, it may be worth a try.

---

surprising that people with chronic fatigue syndrome feel like someone who is 5 days into the flu, notes Michael Lyon, M.D., director of research at Oceanside Functional Medicine Research Institute in Nanaimo, British Columbia, Canada.

Unfortunately, drugs to curb histamine and cytokine production may not always prove helpful. Over-the-counter antihistamines may cause daytime drowsiness—precisely what you don't want if you have chronic fatigue. And prescription antihista-mines, while generally nonsedating, can cause other problems. For example, prescription antihistamines such as fexofenadine (Allegra) and loratadine (Claritin) may make CFS symptoms worse in some people by inhibiting an enzyme in the liver and intestinal wall that helps the body detoxify drugs and chemicals from the environment and food, says Dr. Lyon. Some antidepressants, such as fluoxetine (Prozac), also inhibit this enzyme.

Another mainstay of allergy treatment—

immunotherapy—could be beneficial, though it is also not without its drawbacks. "Because immunotherapy is stimulating the immune system, it can also make the fatigue worse," says Dr. Galland. "There's no single answer to treating chronic fatigue." (A version of immunotherapy used by environmental-medicine doctors, known as enzyme-potentiated desensitization, may hold some promise for treating CFS. See "The EPD Option" on page 463 for more information on this treatment.)

Three herbs, however, may help reduce the aches and fatigue of allergies. The active ingredients from feverfew, Siberian ginseng, and chamomile reduced the production of inflammatory cytokines, at least in a test-tube study.

"That is probably part of the reason that they are helpful," says Mark Stengler, N.D., a naturopathic and homeopathic physician in La Jolla, California, adding that chamomile is probably the least effective of the trio.

DEPRESSION

IT WAS DUBBED the "Twinkie Defense," and it saved Dan White from a life sentence. In 1978, White, a former San Francisco city supervisor, shot and killed both Mayor George Moscone and supervisor Harvey Milk in their city hall offices. At his trial, White's attorneys argued that a junk-food diet had created a chemical imbalance in their client's brain and that as a result White had been depressed prior to the shooting.

White was convicted of in voluntary manslaughter—the least serious charge for homicide. In court, the defense was persuasive, but in scientific circles, the jury is still out. "It is unlikely that someone has major depression solely because of allergic reactions," says Paul S. Marshall, Ph.D., a psychologist at Hennepin County Medical Center in Minneapolis. "It would be extremely unusual for someone to have depression as the only symptom of an allergy.

In fact, I would be very surprised if that were the only symptom."

On the other hand, scientists acknowledge that allergens can contribute to mood alterations. In Dr. Marshall's 3-year study of 36 people with allergies, 69 percent reported feeling more irritable when their allergies flared up; 63 percent reported more fatigue; 41 percent said that they had difficulty staying awake; and 31 percent reported feeling "sad." So the idea that allergies might exacerbate mild depression in a few people who have other allergic symptoms isn't that far-fetched to some researchers.

"My guess is if there is a connection, it is not true for all people with allergies or all people with depression," says Marianne Wamboldt, M.D., associate professor of pediatrics at the National Jewish Medical and Research Center and associate professor of psychiatry at the University of Colorado

Health Sciences Center, both in Denver. "But for a small subset of individuals, it does appear that these conditions do seem to exacerbate each other."

Testing the Link

In her analysis of the incidence of allergies and depression among more than 7,000 Finnish twins, Dr. Wamboldt found that genetics may explain 10 percent of the connection between allergic disorders and depression. Other studies have suggested that people who have undergone allergy testing or received allergy shots are two to three times more likely to be diagnosed with major depression at some point in their lives, Dr. Marshall reports.

"Traditionally, allergists have said that depression is the result of the allergic symptoms—you're not sleeping well or not breathing well because your nose is stuffed up. Now we have a good deal of evidence that suggests there is a direct biochemical process going on in at least a few people," Dr. Marshall says.

Major Depression: A Serious Condition No Matter What the Cause

In most instances, allergies do not trigger major depression. But if you have any suicidal thoughts, seek immediate help from your doctor or qualified therapist, urges Marianne Wamboldt, M.D., associate professor of pediatrics at the National Jewish Medical and Research Center and associate professor of psychiatry at the University of Colorado Health Sciences Center, both in Denver.

In addition, if you have more than one of the following symptoms that persist for more than 2 weeks, seek professional care.

- You feel persistently sad, anxious, or empty, and you have lost interest in pleasurable activities, including sex.
- You feel tired or lack energy to do day-to-day chores.
- You feel restless and irritable, and you can't sit still.
- You have insomnia, early morning awakening, or a need to sleep more than usual.
- You have difficulty concentrating, remembering, or making decisions.
- You have fluctuations in your appetite or weight.
- You feel hopeless, worthless, pessimistic, helpless, and guilty.
- You're feeling down, and you're drinking more alcohol than usual.
- You're experiencing persistent crying spells.

THE HIDDEN CONNECTION

Depression and Allergies

Though researchers have investigated a possible link between allergies and depression, they have as yet been unable to determine the exact biochemical connection between the two. Some scientists speculate, however, that the same neurochemical pathways that trigger allergic reactions in the autonomic nervous system—the system that controls such automatic functions as breathing, heartbeat, and blood pressure—also may influence the central nervous system, which controls higher mental functions, including mood. There is also some research indicating that allergic reactions, thanks to the effect of cytokines on the central nervous system, might produce feelings of fatigue. Further investigation into this link still needs to be done.

An Inflammatory Theory

"Some researchers are beginning to suspect that some types of depression may be triggered by inflammatory reactions in the body," Dr. Wamboldt says.

"If you took certain substances called cytokines, which are released during an inflammatory reaction, and injected them into a person, it is thought that they would cause sickness behaviors such as poor concentration, wanting to be left alone, and depression. So that's one possible connection," she adds.

But this theory is far from proven, and for now, there is no single treatment that will relieve both allergies and depression, Dr. Marshall notes.

"All we can really do is treat the depression with therapy and/or antidepressant medications and treat the allergies with shots, antihistamines, and avoidance of the allergens," Dr. Marshall says. "We really don't have any other answers at this point."

HEADACHES

MORE THAN 40 MILLION Americans seek treatment annually for the most common type of pain—headaches. Headaches affect 90 percent of the U.S. population each year. A mere 1 percent of people report being headache-free for their lifetimes. That's a lot of pain, and we spend over $4 billion a year on pain relievers, just for headaches.

Some doctors believe that headaches are a common symptom of allergies. In fact, up to 15 percent of Americans who have allergies may endure headaches triggered by pollen, food, and other allergens, according to Dennis Gersten, M.D., who practices psychiatry and nutritional medicine in Solana Beach, California, and is the author of *Are You Getting Enlightened or Losing Your Mind?*

"If you look at the big picture, most headaches are related to tension, hormonal fluctuations, skipped meals, drops in blood sugar, vision difficulties, and nutritional deficiencies. But if all of those things have been ruled out, then I think allergies are a definite possibility," Dr. Gersten says.

Although headaches are seldom the sole symptom of an allergy, they are perhaps the most painful and debilitating, says Russell Roby, M.D., director of the Texan Allergy Center in Austin and founder of the Online Allergy Center. Dr. Roby spent several years in graduate school at the University of Texas studying for his Ph.D. in immunology. It was this research work that led to his interest in exploring the causes of headaches. "Headaches, like those caused by allergens, make people want to scream in agony. Even severe body pain seems more easily tolerated than severe headache pain," he notes. "When I was in a head-on car wreck in England a few years ago, my left lung was collapsed, my nose split in two, seven ribs and my breastbone were fractured, my leg was broken in three places, my kneecap was fractured, and my right thigh was driven out the back of my pelvis, which was shattered into several pieces. But did it hurt? Not much. I've had headaches that have hurt a lot worse.

"I think it has to do with limits. When I was in this car wreck, I could see the damage, assess the pain, and, with moderate medication, get myself on a plane a week later and make the 2-day trip home from Manchester to Austin for surgery," Dr. Roby says. "On the other hand, a headache, particularly when it is triggered by allergies, has no limits. There is no injury we can view and assess. When a headache begins, we never know where it will go, how severe it will be, or how long it will last."

What Is the Role of Allergies in Headaches?

Not all doctors agree about the connection between headaches—especially migraines—and allergies. In fact, according to the National Headache Foundation, which based its conclusion on several scientific studies: "The relationship between allergies and headache continues to be a controversial area. Many patients with migraine headache attribute their reactions to certain foods as being an allergic condition. In most cases, this is not correct."

Statements like this frustrate physicians like Dr. Roby, who believe there is evidence of just such a connection. When he was in his thirties, Dr. Roby developed flulike symptoms that wouldn't go away. Finally, he was hospitalized for tests. After 10 days of poking and prodding, his doctors came to a

Use Your Mind to Heal Your Headache

Imagery, a powerful mind/body technique, can help relieve headache pain caused by allergies, says Dennis Gersten, M.D., who practices psychiatry and nutritional medicine in Solana Beach, California.

To try it, take a couple of deep breaths. Then imagine that you are holding a ball of mercury (the silvery liquid found in thermometers) in your hands and that it can draw the pain out of your body like a magnet. Next imagine that any pain developing in your head—even if you don't feel it right now—is sucked into this magnetic ball of mercury, disappearing into the ball. Then let the ball, now full of pain, dribble onto the floor and flow out of sight.

Do this for 1 minute twice a day to help keep allergy-induced head pain at bay, Dr. Gersten suggests.

momentous conclusion: There was nothing wrong with him. Dr. Roby deduced his symptoms were due to allergic reactions and altered his diet. Within a few days, his symptoms were gone.

Thirty years later, physicians like Dr. Roby and Dr. Gersten are still fighting an uphill battle. "Traditional medicine," Dr. Roby notes, "refers to 'triggers' of headaches and includes things like hormones and foods. These triggers might just as well be considered to be causes of headache. If we treat these things as causes and either desensitize the patient to them or instruct the patient in avoidance techniques, then the condition can be prevented."

Allergies are rarely suspects in tension headaches, acknowledges Dr. Roby. These are almost invariably caused by stress or fatigue and often feel as if a tight band is wrapped around your head. But sinus and migraine headaches are a different story.

As you probably know, if you breathe in an allergen, such as ragweed, it can trigger swelling and obstruction of the nasal passages. As a result of this reaction, the sinuses are unable to drain, and this increases pressure throughout the skull, which triggers a headache, says Harold Nelson, M.D., senior staff physician at the National Jewish Medical and Research Center in Denver. In fact, this condition, known as sinusitis, may be one of the most frequent causes of headaches in people with allergies. Symptoms include pressure in the forehead, cheeks, and behind the eyes, along with tooth pain and yellow or green nasal discharge.

"There are two kinds of allergic response—immediate and delayed," Dr. Gersten explains. "Only about 5 percent of allergic response is the immediate kind. With these, you'll experience symptoms in less than 30 minutes after you eat the food to which you're allergic. Your body will react with sinus problems, or you might experience shortness of breath, hives, gastrointestinal distress, anaphylactic shock, or even death. On the other hand, with a delayed allergic response, our bodies take 6 to 72 hours to respond to the offending food. Remember, about 95 percent of allergic reactions are the delayed type."

Both immediate and delayed reactions can cause headaches and a host of other problems. "Blood testing done through a reputable lab can accurately test for allergies symptomized by delayed reaction. You can be tested for more than 90 foods," Dr. Gersten notes.

The relationship between allergies and migraine is a bit more complex, notes Dr. Nelson. But basically, researchers suspect that cells in the immune system, which are sensitive to particular allergens, release chemicals that encourage blood vessels in the head to swell, inciting a migraine. Certain foods, such as chocolate, red wine, and pickled herring, which contain a substance called tyramine, are notorious for triggering migraines in some people.

This swelling, which Dr. Roby refers to as

a "brain allergy," is a natural outgrowth of the immune system, which serves as the body's defense mechanism. "Most of the headaches I see in my allergy practice are from swelling, which leads to increased pressure on some areas of the brain. In fact, almost all allergy symptoms are to some extent related to swelling," he says. "Over the 500,000 years of human development, we have evolved a marvelous system of defense. Whether we are under attack from the outside, such as from bacteria or viruses, or from the inside, such as from cancers or toxins, we have defender cells that cause inflammation and localize the invader. But this very defense can cause swelling in un-

The Natural Approach to Migraine Relief

Migraines, believed by some doctors to be one of the most common headaches caused by allergies, often put people out of action for days at a time. In addition, they frustrate doctors who frequently find that their arsenal of medications doesn't do the job, says Andrew Weil, M.D., director of the program in integrative medicine and clinical professor of medicine at the University of Arizona College of Medicine in Tucson. But migraines can be short-circuited or even prevented with the following natural strategies.

As a preventive, take the herb feverfew, which is a little plant related to the chrysanthemum. You can either buy a plant at a local nursery—it's a common ornamental—and chew a few leaves daily, or you can buy a standardized extract at any health food store, Dr. Weil says. Do not use feverfew if you are pregnant or nursing. (If you choose to chew the leaves, be warned: They don't taste great. Also, some people develop mouth sores if they chew the leaves. If this occurs, discontinue use.) If you purchase the extract, read the label carefully in order to make sure that it contains the necessary active component—parthenolides. One or two tablets or capsules a day will significantly reduce the frequency of allergy-induced migraines in many people, he says. You can stay on feverfew indefinitely.

Eliminate both caffeinated and decaffeinated coffee (and other sources of caffeine). Once a person with allergies isn't consuming caffeine, coffee can be used as a treatment. Drink one or two cups of strong coffee at the first sign of a migraine attack, then lie down in a dark room, Dr. Weil suggests.

In addition, eliminate other dietary triggers like chocolate, red wine (sometimes white wine, too), strong-flavored cheeses, sardines, anchovies, pickled herring, and fermented foods such as soy sauce and miso.

Get Away from It All

How can you tell if an allergy is causing your headache? The simplest experiment is geographical, says Russell Roby, M.D., director of the Texan Allergy Center in Austin and founder of the Online Allergy Center. The next time you travel, note if your headache symptoms diminish when you're out of town or out of state.

"Most of my patients feel better when they go 50 miles, in any direction, away from home," reports Dr. Roby. "So the obvious question is, are the headaches caused by something in the house?" To test this notion out, spend a night or two at a nearby hotel in a smoke-free room. If you feel better in the hotel, the problem might be an allergen within your home. Once you realize this, you can take steps to isolate and then eliminate the allergen from your household or limit your exposure to it. (For specifics, see The Allergy-Free Home on page 73.)

intended ways that can lead to other problems including fatigue, loss of short-term memory, mood swings, depression, and yes, headaches."

Outsmarting Your Own Defenses

To muffle allergy-related headaches, you'll need to outwit your immune system's natural defenses. Here are some practical steps you can take to do just that.

Super-clean your house. To limit potential allergens, try using high-efficiency particulate air (HEPA) filters in your home. (For details, see The Allergy-Free Home on page 73.) Get new pillows; seal cracks in all walls, floors, and ceilings; and steam-clean your carpets and drapes, Dr. Roby suggests.

Begin the elimination diet. Once you've cleared the air around you, concentrate on

your diet. "I find that any time my patients are having allergy problems, food is often part of the problem. It is unusual for food to be the only cause of a problem like headaches, but it does happen," Dr. Roby says. "This 5-day plan does not require medical supervision in a healthy adult. If one has health problems, advice and consent from your physician is advised before trying these suggestions."

For at least 5 days, eliminate the following foods, which are common headache triggers, from your diet.

- Chocolate
- Citrus fruits and juices
- Dark-colored soft drinks, such as cola
- Eggs
- Grains (all except brown rice)
- Milk and milk products
- Sugar
- Tomatoes and tomato products

After 5 days, resume eating these foods one at a time and note your body's reaction to them. In particular, keep track of your weight.

"When patients eat something they are allergic to, they swell. This swelling is entirely due to water retention," Dr. Roby explains. "As a result, your best indication of an allergic reaction is a sudden weight gain of 2 to 10 pounds overnight. When my patients see this type of increase, they know this is their earliest warning sign of allergy. If it isn't dealt with, their allergy symptoms, including headaches, will begin in the next 24 to 48 hours. Some things one can do include beginning a very simple diet of chicken breast, lettuce, and water. Or, you might take an over-the-counter antihistamine, an antacid, or bicarbonate of soda. If swelling persists, a corticosteroid might be indicated. See your physician for advice."

Cut out your favorite foods. Eliminate any foods you typically crave, Dr. Roby urges. Paradoxically, the foods we are most emotionally attached to often are the ones causing the allergy. One of his patients, for instance, ate a large amount of peanuts daily. So in addition to the eight foods listed above, Dr. Roby had her stop chomping on peanuts for 5 days.

"I told her to eat whatever she missed the

When to See Your Doctor

The vast majority of headaches, even those caused by allergies, are merely annoying. But you should seek immediate medical attention if you develop any of the following symptoms, says Dennis Gersten, M.D., who practices psychiatry and nutritional medicine in Solana Beach, California, and is the author of *Are You Getting Enlightened or Losing Your Mind?*

• You've never had headaches before, but now you're getting them.

• Your headache persists for more than 72 hours or prevents you from doing normal activities.

• The headache awakens you from sleep or feels like a sudden "explosion" in your head.

• You are also experiencing vision problems, difficulty talking, problems with coordination, weakness in your arms and legs, or difficulty thinking clearly.

• You have a fever or stiff neck.

• You get a headache whenever you exert yourself.

• You're also vomiting but don't feel nauseated.

• Your headaches are becoming more frequent and severe.

most on the sixth day," Dr. Roby recalls. "Naturally, she chose peanuts. Within minutes, she developed one of the worst headaches she had ever had. Needless to say, she no longer eats peanuts."

After a round on the elimination diet, in most instances, Dr. Roby advises his patients to reintroduce whatever food they miss the most. "This is the most likely food to cause serious symptoms. I do this so that the patient gets a clear signal that the headaches are indeed related to foods, at least some of the time," he explains. "Once they feel symptoms beginning, usually within minutes of ingesting the food, I have them take an antidote to the reaction. The best antidotes are magnesium compounds like Epsom salts or buffered vitamin C powder. Alka-Seltzer and liquid antacids work fairly well. Once the patient understands the relationship of foods to symptoms, then we begin a long process of elimination and reintroduction to more carefully investigate which foods or drinks cause which symptoms."

Inflammatory Bowel DISEASE

SOME OF THE same chemicals that swell your sinuses when you have allergic rhinitis (hay fever) also inflame your intestines when you have inflammatory bowel disease (IBD).

IBD encompasses both Crohn's disease and ulcerative colitis. They share three symptoms during flare-ups: chronic diarrhea, abdominal pain, and bleeding. Fortunately, a fairly simple change in your diet may help you control IBD, says James Scala, Ph.D., a nutritionist in Lafayette, California; professional lecturer at Georgetown University School of Medicine in Washington, D.C., and the University of California, Berkeley; and author of *The New Eating Right for a Bad Gut*.

To take charge of your IBD symptoms, your doctor may recommend a dietary approach to reduce inflammation, which involves separating the good fats in your diet from the bad ones. In particular, you'll want to limit your intake of animal fats. At the same time, you should increase your intake of such good fats as those found in fish and flaxseed oils.

"Once you balance those fats, a number of things fall into place," says Dr. Scala. "By altering your dietary fat, you are reducing your sensitivity to foods that otherwise would bother you."

Why the need for such segregation in the world of fats? It all comes down to acids.

Know Your Omegas

The key to getting a grip on IBD is to know your sixes from your threes—your omega-6 fatty acids from your omega-3 fatty acids, that is. In general, the omega-6's are found in animal fats, and they should be limited in your diet as much as possible. Among the biggest offenders is red meat. Beef is the worst, so limit your intake to no more than one very lean steak a month, recommends

Dr. Scala. Poultry isn't as bad, but trim the skin and stick with the white meat. Omega-3's, on the other hand, should become your new best friends. As already mentioned, they can be found in fish, fish oil, and flaxseed oil.

What do these numerically named substances have to do with IBD? To understand that, you first need to be introduced to your mast cells.

The Mast Cell Connection

No one knows just what causes IBD, nor is there a cure. But scientists do know that mast cells and their chemical contents are a big part of the problem.

The mast cells produce histamine—infamous as the instigator of allergic rhinitis. But they also produce lesser-known chemicals—prostaglandins and leukotrienes—during an allergic response, which are even more powerful than histamine. These substances can cause chronic sinus inflammation and internal bleeding when you have an allergy for an extended time, says Raphael Kellman, M.D., founder and director of the Kellman Center for Progressive Medicine in New York City and author of *Eat with Your Brain, Think with Your Gut*. During an IBD flare-up, these same chemicals are released by the mast cells lining the intestines, triggering inflammation and bleeding that can result in obstructive scar tissue.

Scientists have discovered that these chemicals are made from arachidonic acid, a type of fat high in omega-6 fatty acids.

Inflammatory Bowel Disease at a Glance

Inflammatory bowel disease (IBD) is the umbrella term for several diseases that cause inflammation of the intestines. Following are descriptions of the more specific diseases within this category.

Crohn's disease. Typically consisting of inflammation of the small intestine, abdominal pain, and diarrhea, this disease sometimes causes rectal bleeding and weight loss as well. The inflammation can occur anywhere along the gastrointestinal tract, however, from the mouth to the anus. The intestines can become blocked from swelling and scar tissue, or an ulcer may form an opening in the intestinal wall, requiring surgery.

Ulcerative colitis. This condition is similar to Crohn's disease, but the inflammation occurs only in the intestines and in a single continuous area. Crohn's, in contrast, can consist of many patches of inflammation.

Irritable bowel syndrome. Sometimes considered a form of IBD, irritable bowel syndrome (IBS) takes two opposing forms: severe diarrhea in the morning or after eating, or painful constipation—and sometimes alternating bouts of both.

Fish Oil: Not a Magic Elixir

Though some doctors and researchers have concluded that reducing animal fat and increasing "good" fats such as those found in fish and flaxseed oils can significantly help people with inflammatory bowel disease (IBD), this idea is still controversial in the medical community. Not all doctors are seeing results in their patients.

For example, Gary R. Lichtenstein, M.D., associate professor of medicine and director of the inflammatory bowel disease program at the University of Pennsylvania in Philadelphia, reports some success using eicosapentaenoic acid (EPA) found in fish oils to calm flare-ups in patients with ulcerative colitis. He notes that it works modestly but cautions that it's not as potent as steroids.

Moreover, Dr. Lichtenstein says that EPA supplements appear safe, and they may help your cardiovascular system.

You can't, however, use EPA capsules like a prescription pill, expecting quick results, cautions James Scala, Ph.D., a nutritionist in Lafayette, California, and author of *The New Eating Right for a Bad Gut*. "Using the omega-3 oils to help control IBD requires a complete dietary commitment, and simply taking a few EPA capsules is probably like eating hair to cure baldness," he says.

Further, you have to stick with your new diet because the typical Westerner's fat cells are chock-full of arachidonic acid. "It takes about 3 months to shift your fat reserve's balance and begin to see results," says Dr. Scala.

Will the diet also help irritable bowel syndrome (IBS)? This is a less-studied area, but Dr. Scala says that it is worth a try.

And what's the biggest source of arachidonic acid in the typical modern diet?

Animal fat.

The Prime Suspect: Meat

Dr. Scala believes it's no coincidence that the occurrence of IBD has been on the rise in developed countries as meat consumption has increased. "IBD has become common only with the development of agriculture in the last couple of hundred years. And especially since the invention of the roller mill in 1897, animals are being fattened on corn, which increases the omega-6 oils in their fat," he says.

There's no need to go on a fat-free diet, though. People in Greenland eat plenty of fat but mostly ones low in omega-6 oils. The result? IBD is virtually nonexistent. But in Denmark, where the diet is high in omega-6 oils, IBD is common.

This connection to omega-6 fatty acids may be one reason that vegetarians seem to have less inflammation in general, Dr. Scala says. But you don't have to go vegetarian. In fact, the fat in cold-water fish like salmon can actually help reduce inflammation.

Natural Strategies: Up Your Intake of Good Fats

According to research, there are good versions of prostaglandins and leukotrienes that actually inhibit inflammation and tissue damage. These versions are made from good fats like eicosapentaenoic acid (EPA), found in fish oils, and alpha-linolenic acid (ALA), found in flaxseed oil.

EPA and ALA are both high in good omega-3 oils, unlike arachidonic acid's bad omega-6 oils. If you don't care to get these good fats from your diet, you can take them in capsules as supplements, Dr. Scala suggests.

A study conducted at the University of Bologna in Italy found that using an enteric-coated fish oil capsule for a year reduced the rate of relapses in Crohn's patients by more than half. These capsules released the oil directly into the small intestine, rather than the stomach.

IBD and Food Intolerances

IBD may act like an allergy, but it's important to remember that it's not. People sometimes assume that certain foods trigger flare-ups, much like an allergic reaction, says Gary R. Lichtenstein, M.D., associate professor of medicine and director of the inflammatory bowel disease program at the University of Pennsylvania in Philadelphia. But the problem is most often a food intolerance, in which the person simply has difficulty digesting something like lactose, the milk sugar found in dairy products.

These food intolerances add insult to injury in people with IBD, but they don't play a central role, notes Dr. Lichtenstein. Still, people with IBD should seek to identify these culinary culprits by keeping a diet diary or by avoiding a food for a week or two, Drs. Lichtenstein and Scala agree.

Foods that may cause symptoms indistinguishable from flare-ups and diarrhea include spicy foods, alcohol, coffee, chocolate, raw vegetables, stringy meats such as pot roast and Swiss steak, nuts and seeds, fatty red meats, diet beverages, unpeeled raw fruit, sugar, food additives, processed meats, dairy products, and shellfish.

The IBD Diet

If you have IBD, you probably find yourself scheduling your day so that you'll be near a bathroom when the telltale diarrhea and abdominal pain hit. But by keeping a diet diary to identify any food intolerances that you might have and by modifying your diet to increase your intake of the beneficial omega-3's and limit your intake of omega-6's, you can gain a feeling of control over your symptoms. Here are the specifics to follow, according to Dr. Scala.

• Increase your intake of omega-3 fatty acids by getting at least 2 grams of EPA a day from fish or capsules; 5 grams is better. Good food sources of omega-3 oils include salmon, mackerel, anchovies, cod, striped bass, snapper, trout, and tuna. A 3.5-ounce serving of salmon or mackerel or a 7-ounce serving of most other types of dark-skinned finfish such as tuna will supply 2 to 5 grams of EPA. Do not eat shellfish, Dr. Scala notes. Oils that provide omega-3's include walnut, flaxseed, sesame seed, soybean, cod liver, salmon, menhaden, rapeseed, avocado, and canola, as well as the Puritan brand of oil.

• Get some ALA each day by taking capsules or by drizzling 2 tablespoons of flaxseed oil on your food. If you are on a vegan diet, take 3 to 5 tablespoons daily.

• Eliminate red meat and the dark meat of poultry.

• Use olive oil or canola oil instead of corn oil.

• Use fat-free milk instead of whole milk.

Worms to the Rescue

Researchers at the University of Iowa are taking a page out of the caveman's cookbook to treat inflammatory bowel disease (IBD).

Observing that the rise in IBD in developed countries has coincided with the decline in intestinal worms, lead researcher Joel Weinstock, M.D., professor of internal medicine at the University of Iowa in Iowa City, reasoned that after three million years of intestinal infestation, maybe the human immune system had gotten used to the critters.

So he gave six IBD patients a worm-egg cocktail. After a few weeks, five of these patients, who were not helped by traditional drugs, were symptom-free.

Apparently, the worms quiet the overactive immune system, which is triggering the inflammation in people with Crohn's disease and ulcerative colitis, says Gary R. Lichtenstein, M.D., associate professor of medicine and director of the inflammatory bowel disease program at the University of Pennsylvania in Philadelphia.

The worm theory would explain why IBD rates are lower in countries with poor hygiene, Dr. Lichtenstein notes. Best of all, there are no side effects from the worm shake, he says. In fact, he believes a treatment for IBD may potentially come from the research.

But don't try this at home, Dr. Lichtenstein warns. The unusually polite parasites used in the experiment moved out after just a couple of months, whereas your garden-variety parasites usually move in permanently.

Multiple Chemical SENSITIVITY

EMILY'S SENSITIVITY TO ODORS and chemicals has not only made life frustrating for the teenager, it has actually threatened it. She once had an allergic reaction to some pancakes her mother made that was so severe she had trouble breathing and had to go to the emergency room.

According to her mom, "Emily goes crazy if someone smokes. In classes where people wear perfume, she feels bad physically, and her sinuses swell. Cleaning fluids, fumes of any kind, and animal dander all cause her discomfort."

Understandably, her sensitivity has been hard on Emily socially, since it can be difficult or embarrassing to ask her friends or teachers to stop wearing perfume.

Another incident occurred when Emily needed tutoring in math. The tutor she saw owned horses. Emily could "smell" the horse scent on the tutor, and despite the fact that it made her ill, she felt awkward about what she was going through and couldn't express it to her tutor. She suffered miserably—flushed, hot, and mentally confused.

Emily also has eczema, which appears as an itchy, ugly rash on her arms. And she can't wear jeans with metal buttons or any necklaces, earrings, belts, or rings. (She does cheat sometimes, but then she breaks out in huge red sores or welts.)

She occasionally takes something for her eczema, some vitamins, and sometimes Benadryl (an over-the-counter medicine) for itching. Emily also has exercise-induced asthma, for which she uses an inhaler.

Though her story sounds incredible, it is true. Further, she is not alone in her symptoms.

Imagine that you were a doctor and had to treat Emily as well as three patients like these: The first patient reports having headaches, mental confusion, memory loss, weakness, and fatigue. The second patient is bothered by odors at work. She says that she is working in an office that was newly carpeted and the smell makes her sick. She finds it difficult to concentrate because of these smells. They make her drowsy and irritable, and she is constantly sneezing and itching. Finally, a third patient reports that over the last few months she has had constant muscle and joint pain, nausea, and diarrhea.

You, of course, want to help your patients, so after taking a thorough medical history and performing laboratory tests, you give them medications to alleviate the symptoms while you await the results of the tests. But the test results are normal. None of the people have an infection, anemia, or diabetes. In fact, you can't find anything wrong with them. You call them with the results, and not only are they upset that you can't find out what is wrong with them, but they tell you they're feeling worse.

All of these patients had very different sets of symptoms. Yet some researchers believe that they all have the same problem, a syndrome called multiple chemical sensitivity (MCS). The condition is also known as idiopathic environmental intolerance, chemical AIDS, chemical hypersensitivity, total allergy, 20th-century illness, or environmental illness. Some who suffer with it refer to it as chemical injury.

A Controversial Diagnosis

There is no blood test to diagnose multiple chemical sensitivity. In fact, there aren't even agreed-upon criteria for the illness, as there are for chronic fatigue syndrome (CFS), which has many of the same symptoms as MCS. Even among physicians who treat MCS, the level of chemical exposure needed to initiate the condition is debated. And then there are some psychiatrists who believe that the causes are psychological.

"There is extreme polarization around the issue of MCS," says Richard Jackson, M.D., director of the National Center for Environmental Health at the Centers for Disease Control and Prevention (CDC). A government report he helped to draft said, in effect, that MCS is a label in search of scientific basis.

"MCS advocates believe that we have not adequately incorporated the literature that supports their position, and the critics have argued that we have been too willing to listen to the advocates," Dr. Jackson relates.

While critics of an MCS diagnosis argue that there is no medical basis for it, advocates charge that the chemical industry is thwarting a diagnosis in the fear that it would cost them billions of dollars.

One of the problems with diagnosing the condition is its broad range of symptoms. Over the years, diseases thought to be connected to MCS include memory disabilities and learning problems; physical problems including acne, arthritic pain, gastrointestinal discomfort, headaches, and hypertension; and behavioral disorders such as depression, hyperactivity, and schizophrenia.

Another problem with diagnosis is the lack of clear-cut cause-and-effect studies. Because of this, some members of the medical establishment do not believe that MCS is a disease. "In 1991, the American Medical Association (AMA) issued a report that found there were no well-controlled studies establishing a clear cause-and-effect mechanism. When the council met to consider looking at MCS again, no evidence was found to change our stance," says Myron Genel, M.D., associate dean at Yale

Beware the Hidden Dangers in Your Home

Although scientists and medical practitioners are still debating whether or not multiple chemical sensitivity truly exists, there is widespread agreement that certain individual chemicals can cause allergic reactions or other medical problems for people who are sensitive to them. Further, these chemicals can be found nearly anywhere. The homes we live in contain a myriad of contaminants, some of which come from such unlikely sources as carpeting, furniture, foam insulation, and particleboard.

One of the most pervasive of these chemicals is the preservative formaldehyde. Though the U.S. government now considers it to be a probable carcinogen, it is still used in some composite wood, such as particleboard and chipboard, that uses resin adhesives and in some plywood and wallboard. It may be present in cabinetry and furniture made with composite wood, too. Other sources of exposure include combustion from auto emissions, foam insulation, and the resin in rugs, fabrics, and papers.

Exposure to formaldehyde can cause conjunctivitis, corneal burns from exposure to the eyes, skin discoloration, and hives. If inhaled, it can cause breathing difficulties, headaches, weakness, and a rapid heartbeat. If ingested, it can cause dizziness and nausea. If you experience a severe reaction to formaldehyde, get immediate medical attention.

It's wise to limit your exposure to formaldehyde as much as possible by eliminating products that contain the chemical. Try to isolate or seal off the source, if possible. In addition, increase the ventilation in your home by opening windows, and vent space heaters and cooking appliances to the outside. It's also a good idea to buy a number of low-light houseplants, which research has shown

University School of Medicine and past chairperson of the AMA's Council on Scientific Affairs.

These people certainly feel ill, concedes Dr. Genel. There is a large difference, however, between having an illness and a specific disease. Further, people with MCS are not alone. "It is also hard for doctors to doc-ument chronic Lyme disease or chronic fatigue syndrome," he says.

Dr. Genel feels that patients expect more than medicine can deliver. "Sometimes, they expect too much. Medicine is both a science and an art," he says. "From all the anecdotes, I am convinced that something is going on with patients who claim to suffer from

can reduce the levels of formaldehyde in the home because they absorb the chemical as food. Helpful plants include philodendrons and spider plants.

Another potentially dangerous substance found in many homes is lead. Though lead was banned by the federal government in 1978 in consumer paints, it can still be found in homes older than that, and it's still used in most industrial and commercial building.

More than 90 percent of the lead we're exposed to accumulates in our bones, where it's stored. When it's released, it can affect the body's organs for years— even decades—after the original exposure. Lead toxicity can damage the cardiovascular and central nervous systems and cause kidney problems. It is also a suspected cause of miscarriages and stillbirths.

If you think that your home has high levels of lead, get your children tested for lead exposure, even if they seem healthy. If your house was built before 1978, and especially before 1950, have your home tested. You might also want to consider having it tested if the paint—exterior or interior—is peeling or otherwise deteriorating. Make a point of washing your children's hands often, as well as anything, such as bottles, pacifiers, and toys, that could come in contact with lead dust. In addition, be sure to clean the floors, window frames, windowsills, and other surfaces in your home weekly with a sponge, warm water, and an all-purpose cleaner or a cleaner made specifically for lead. Clean up and remove paint chips immediately. Finally, don't try to remove lead-based paint yourself. For guidelines on avoiding exposure to lead when you're remodeling or renovating, call the National Lead Information Center of the Environmental Protection Agency at (800) 424-LEAD.

MCS, but at this point, we don't know precisely what we are dealing with."

What Are the Criteria for a Diagnosis?

There are, of course, many individual doctors who believe that multiple chemical sensitivity is real. Few statements by mainstream medical groups have ever been issued, however.

In 1999, 34 researchers and clinicians with experience in the study, evaluation, or treatment of MCS published a consensus statement describing diagnostic criteria for the condition. The criteria to establish a diagnosis of MCS were:

• The symptoms are reproducible with repeated chemical exposure.

• The condition is chronic.

• Low levels of exposure (lower than previously or commonly tolerated) result in manifestations of the syndrome.

• The symptoms improve or resolve when the triggers are removed.

Another Reason to Banish the Butts

Unless you've been living in a cave for the past 20 years, you know about the harmful effects of smoking. But did you know that a link has been discovered between tobacco smoke and allergies and asthma?

Just as scientists are currently debating whether or not multiple chemical sensitivity truly exists as a distinct disease, they're also debating whether or not a direct allergy to nicotine actually exists. If it does, it is extremely rare. In general, what might appear to be an allergic reaction to breathing in smoke, such as asthma, is usually due to irritation of the lungs, says Charles H. Feldman, M.D., associate professor of pediatrics at Columbia University College of Physicians and Surgeons in New York City.

Tobacco smoke *has* been shown, however, to increase your risk of developing allergies and asthma or to intensify their symptoms if you already have an allergy. It seems that people who smoke are more easily sensitized to airborne and occupational allergens, and if they already have allergic rhinitis (hay fever), they'll probably be more sensitive to tobacco smoke, which may help trigger sneezing episodes.

Ironically, where allergies are concerned, smokers may do more harm to those around them than to themselves. One study found that secondhand smoke may be more likely to exacerbate an allergic response than puffing on a

• Responses occur to multiple chemically unrelated substances.

• Symptoms involve multiple organ systems.

These criteria, however, are not as widely accepted as the CDC's criteria for chronic fatigue syndrome. And although no government agency endorses any specific definition of MCS, more than 20 government agencies recognize it, and 9 have funded research on it. The closest that the MCS community has to federal acknowledgment are two consensus statements. The first one was issued in 1994 by the American Lung Association, the AMA, the U.S. Environmental Protection Agency, and the U.S. Consumer Product Safety Commission.

The 1994 statement recommended that a patient's complaints of multiple chemical sensitivity should not be dismissed as a psychological problem, but rather should warrant a thorough workup. The 1999 statement took it a step further and recommended that "MCS be diagnosed whenever all of the six consensus criteria are met, along with any other disorders that also may be present,

cigarette yourself. And the effects on children can be particularly troublesome: Exposure to environmental tobacco smoke, particularly in early childhood, is the best identified risk factor for the development of allergic disease, according to some experts.

And passive smoking in the home is even worse, especially for children who already have asthma. A recent study of New York City children with one or both parents who smoke showed an increase of respiratory infections and subsequent emergency room treatments for asthma.

Tobacco's effects begin while a child is still in the womb. A mother who smokes during pregnancy or exposes her child to smoke during the first 3 years significantly increases her child's risk of developing food allergies. One study found higher rates of allergies to milk, eggs, soybeans, or wheat in children so exposed.

In addition, children whose parents smoke have an earlier onset of allergy and wheezy bronchitis, higher rates of sensitization to airborne allergens, reduced lung function, and increased risk of developing asthma. All of this makes giving up cigarettes something you need to do for the people around you as much as for yourself.

such as asthma, allergy, migraine, chronic fatigue syndrome, and fibromyalgia." The reason? Researchers have found a "significant overlap" of people with MCS who also have chronic fatigue syndrome and fibromyalgia.

Who Gets Multiple Chemical Sensitivity?

Assuming that MCS as a disease entity really exists, who is at risk?

We all know someone who is allergic to cats or suffers from allergic rhinitis (hay fever). Our drugstores are full of over-the-counter allergy medicines, and advertising for prescription drugs for allergies can be found in most magazines and newspapers and are commonly seen on television.

Indeed, vast numbers of us—20 percent of adults—are allergic to something. Three groundbreaking surveys indicate that more than 16 percent of people with allergies report being sensitive to chemicals.

The first survey was done in 1996 among 1,000 rural adults and was published in the *Archives of Environmental Health*. The study authors found that one-third of the group reported chemical sensitivity, with the major irritants being perfumes, pesticides, cigarette smoke, and fresh paint.

In 1999, the Departments of Health in New Mexico and California reported other survey findings. In New Mexico, 16 percent of the population reported being sensitive

to chemicals, and 2 percent reported being diagnosed with MCS. Another 2 percent said they suffered a job loss due to their problem. In California, among a random study of adults, 15.9 percent reported being "allergic or unusually sensitive to chemicals." Slightly more than 6 percent had been diagnosed with MCS.

Causes of Multiple Chemical Sensitivity

So far, a clear-cut mechanism for why MCS happens has not been established. One possible link might have to do with blood pressure. Researchers at the Johns Hopkins University in Baltimore have found that some people have an imbalance in the regulation of their blood pressures, known as neurally mediated hypotension. This imbalance might be a factor in causing chronic fatigue syndrome. "No one knows why this happens to people. It is certainly a factor in people with chronic fatigue and may play a role in MCS as well," says David B. K. Golden, M.D., associate professor of medicine at the Johns Hopkins University.

Some studies suggest a link through the olfactory and limbic systems in the brain. The theory is that because of continuous, low-level exposures to chemicals in our environment, our olfactory systems become oversensitized to chemical stimulation. The olfactory nerve jars the limbic system, negatively impacting sleep, energy levels, and moods, which could account for many of the reported MCS symptoms.

There may be a gender gap in who gets MCS: In studies that consist of volunteer samples or medical cases, women report symptoms of MCS more often than men.

There are many theories about why women have been shown to be more sensitive to chemicals than men. One obvious reason is that the study samples consist largely of women. But there are other reasons as well. "Traditionally, women report that they suffer from chronic diseases, such as arthritis, fibromyalgia, and chronic fatigue syndrome, more than men," says Dr. Golden. He also notes that both MCS and CFS have correlations with panic disorder and depression, both illnesses that affect women more than men. The biological differences between men and women also may play a role. Women have a higher total percentage of body fat, which stores chemicals, than men. And since, on average, women are smaller than men, they may be slower to metabolize chemicals. Women also have less of the enzyme alcohol dehydrogenase, which makes them slower to metabolize alcohol and other chemicals.

In addition, women wear more cosmetics than men, exposing them to chemicals that they may become sensitive to later in life. (Complaints about perfumes are common among people with MCS.) Finally, despite all the talk of equality between men and women, most cleaning chores are done by women, which exposes them to more chemicals, according to Pamela Reed Gibson, Ph.D., associate professor of psychology at James Madison University in Harrisonburg, Virginia, and author of *Multiple Chemical Sensitivity: A Survival Guide*.

The Immune System Dysregulation Theory

The concept of "immune system dysregulation" was first suggested by Theron Randolph, M.D., in the 1940s. Dr. Randolph believed that allergies to common foods and substances could cause symptoms such as depression, fatigue, confusion, and irritability. In addition, he theorized that we weren't successfully adapting to modern synthetic chemicals.

Modern proponents of the theory have identified hypersensitivity to the following long list of items as causes underlying this dysregulation: air pollutants, chemicals in building materials, household cleaners, food additives, foods, synthetic fabrics, standard allergens including pollen and mold spores, perfumes and aftershave lotions, water from most sources, viral infections, and fungal infections including excess growth of *Candida albicans*. In addition, some people have posited that MCS might have something to do with the illnesses experienced by some women who have silicone implants and veterans who believe they have Gulf War syndrome. (For more information on this diagnosis, see "Gulf War Syndrome on page 492.")

When there is no single pathogen that

Quack Attack

Ever since the 16th century, people have used the word *quack* for the sound a duck makes. Perhaps because a duck's quack is so much empty noise, people also started to describe patent-medicine salesmen—who often made empty or even fraudulent claims about the "miraculous" properties of their potions—as quacks.

Hundreds of years later, we're still using the term, because there's no lack of quacks even today. But, unlike the web-footed quacks, health care quacks aren't so easy to spot. Here are some tips from the FDA and Federal Trade Commission that should raise a red flag about the truthfulness of the claim, efficacy of the product, or credentials of the advocate.

Be skeptical of products that promise quick relief or cures. Be especially cautious if the claims are made for serious conditions like cancer or for controversial ones like multiple chemical sensitivity. If the product sounds too good to be true, it probably is.

Don't be fooled by the term *natural*. In health fraud, it's often used as an attention-grabber and to suggest that the product is safer than conventional treatments. But "natural" doesn't necessarily mean it's safe.

Be wary of products that claim to be century- or decades-old remedies. These claims suggest that the product's longevity proves it is safe and effective, but that isn't necessarily the case if it's not backed by science.

Be careful of strong promises such as a money-back guarantee. Many credible companies offer guarantees because their products are so reliable. Marketers of fraudulent products, however, offer them because they rarely stay in one place for long, so customers aren't likely to find them to ask for their money back.

Be suspicious of products advertised to be effective for many ailments. No product can treat every disease and condition.

Be wary of "breakthrough products" developed in other countries but not yet for sale in drugstores in the United States. Other countries often don't test their products as rigorously as the United States does.

can be shown to cause an illness, there are likely to be many theories about what causes the illness. The position of the American College of Allergy, Asthma, and Immunology is: "There is no evidence that these patients have any immunologic or neurological abnormalities. In addition, no form of therapy has yet been shown to

Sometimes quackery results only in money wasted, but it can be a serious problem if it prevents you from seeking professional medical care. Also, because quacks operate on the fringe of science, the products they peddle are unlikely to have been properly tested or proven medicinally effective, and they could be dangerous.

The first way to protect yourself is to carefully question what you see or hear in ads. Although there are a few exceptions, the editors of newspapers, magazines, radio, and TV do not regularly screen their ads for truth or accuracy.

Second, if you have any doubts about a product someone is trying to sell you that promises the relief you have been looking for, discuss it first with your family doctor or other informed health professional.

Third, if you have been victimized by a health fraud scheme, report your experience to one of the following agencies:

- FDA. The FDA answers questions about medical devices, medicines, and food supplements that are mislabeled, misrepresented, or in some way harmful. Write to them at HFD250, Room 1765, 5600 Fishers Lane, Rockville, MD 20857, or call them at (888) INFO-FDA.

- U.S. Postal Service, Office of Criminal Investigation. The Postal Service monitors quack products purchased by mail. Call them toll-free at (800) 372-8347, go to their Web site at www.usps.com/postalinspectors, or visit your local post office to file a complaint.

- Council of Better Business Bureaus. Contact your local better business bureau via the Web at www.bbb.org, or call them for information on companies and products or to file a complaint.

- Federal Trade Commission. This agency looks into charges of false advertising wherever products are sold—in print, radio, TV, or the Internet. Write to them at Federal Trade Commission Consumer Response Center, Room 130, 600 Pennsylvania Avenue NW, Washington DC 20580, call toll-free at (877) FTC-HELP (382-4357), or go online to www.ftc.gov.

THE HIDDEN CONNECTION

Breast Implants and Allergies?

You might not keep it in a shaker on your kitchen table, but chances are, you ingest silicon in some way, shape, or form almost every day. This element, which combines with oxygen to form glasses, sands, and 75 percent of the Earth's crust, is one of the most abundant on the planet. As a result, silicon appears quite frequently as an ingredient in cosmetics, foods, and other products we use on a daily basis. Something as common in our lives as silicon couldn't possibly provoke allergic reactions . . . could it?

The answer to this medical dilemma is a definitive . . . maybe. A possible allergy to silicone was among the many concerns of women with silicone gel–filled breast implants when the FDA removed them from the open market in 1992. But now that the furor, attention, and the flood of lawsuits against implant manufacturers have subsided, the most recent medical research has indicated no link between breast implants and allergies.

Stuart Bondurant, M.D., professor of medicine and dean emeritus at the University of North Carolina at Chapel Hill, was the chairperson of the Institute of Medicine's study of breast implants, which was published in 1999. The study found that implants cause some problems in the breast area, such as infection, rupture, or capsular contracture (hardening of the scar tissue around the implant). Claims of allergy, cancer, connective tissue disease, neurologic disease, or problems with breastfeeding, however, could not be linked to breast implants. "There was a lot of evidence of local complications, but we were unable to find any reports that fit even the minimum standards of having an allergic basis," says Dr. Bondurant.

alter the patient's illness in a favorable way. A causal connection between environmental chemicals, foods, and/or drugs and the patient's symptoms continues to be speculative and cannot be based on the results of currently published studies."

The Mind-Body Theory

Many psychiatrists believe that MCS is a psychological problem. They assert that people who think that they have it do indeed have physical symptoms, which they believe are caused by many factors.

While the connection between breast implants and allergies seems unlikely, ongoing studies are looking at the link between breast implants and conditions similar to allergies—autoimmune disorders. Whereas an allergic condition occurs when the body produces antibodies against a substance foreign to the body, an autoimmune condition occurs when the body produces antibodies against its own cells and tissues. Arthur Dale Ericsson, M.D., founder and director of the Institute of Biologic Research in Houston, has been studying how breast implants may cause autoimmune disorders such as fibromyalgia and rheumatoid arthritis. "What we find when we start looking at these sick people is that they tend develop autoimmune diseases at a much higher rate than the population at large would be expected to," he says.

The medical community may be up in arms over what is and what is not caused by breast implants, but meanwhile, a lot of women have developed symptoms such as muscle aches and pains, weakness, numbness, muscle fatigue, and burning in their lower extremities after getting implants. In many of these cases, nothing else but breast implants seems to be a logical cause of the symptoms.

If you feel like you fit into this category, you may want to sit down and have a serious discussion with your doctor about getting the implants removed. And if you're considering breast implants, definitely have a chat with your doctor about the risks involved. "I would simply raise the questions, 'Am I going to react, or am I not going to react?' 'How can I protect myself in the best possible way?'" says Dr. Ericsson.

According to these psychiatrists, however, these patients are in reality suffering from a mental disorder, and most of them will respond in time.

These psychiatrists cite the fact that when patients who believe they are being poisoned by environmental chemicals are monitored, they rarely ever show an unusually high level of exposure to chemicals. In a study published in 2000, doctors contacted 120 patients who had come to an outpatient clinic in Germany complaining of MCS in years past. They found that only 39 percent of the patients were still convinced that the environmental poisons had been responsible for their complaints, 44 percent had accepted other reasons, and 17 percent had accepted a psychological origin. They concluded, "About half of the patients with MCS accept some sort of psychotherapy. Improvement does not depend on 'detoxification' or changing their lifestyles. In most patients, the belief that they are poisoned disappears with time."

Gulf War Syndrome

From 1990 to 1991, America and its allied forces fought the army of Iraq, which had invaded Kuwait. Many soldiers returned home to both the United States and Great Britain reporting symptoms of multiple chemical sensitivity (MCS), chronic fatigue syndrome (CFS), fibromyalgia, nausea, light-headedness, fatigue, headaches, and sensitivity to vehicle exhaust, pesticides, bleach, certain disinfectants, paint thinner, and perfume. Clusters of these symptoms became known as Gulf War syndrome.

One member of the Department of Veterans Affairs expert panel that studied Gulf War veterans' medical problems was Claudia S. Miller, M.D., associate professor of environmental and occupational medicine at the University of Texas Health Science Center at San Antonio. Dr. Miller, who has evaluated hundreds of Gulf War veterans and has been asked to testify before a congressional committee on this subject, believes that they are suffering from problems resembling MCS, and she has postulated a two-step disease process called TILT (toxicant-induced loss of tolerance) that causes the symptoms of MCS, chronic fatigue, migraines, and Gulf War syndrome. It's a theory that parallels the germ and immune theories of disease.

Unlike most government and university researchers, who tend to see such health problems as originating from mental or emotional conflict or being stress-induced, Dr. Miller feels that the exposure of the soldiers to the agents of war may explain many of their symptoms. To date, most studies have failed to find an explanation, or dismissed it as a psychiatric illness. A panel of experts from the Institute of Medicine (IOM) reviewed soldiers' exposures to poison gas, uranium, drugs, and vaccines. They concluded that there was not enough data to determine whether exposure to any of these agents had caused the illnesses experienced by veterans. The committee's conclusion echoes the findings by both the Department of Defense and the Department of Veterans Affairs.

Where to Go for Help

People with documented chemical allergies (such as factory workers exposed to toxins in the workplace) can turn to the American College of Occupational and Environmental Medicine for help. This group represents more than 7,000 physicians who specialize in occupational and environmental medicine. According to the organization's Web

Under a congressional mandate, the IOM must look at 33 agents to determine whether they might be responsible for the veterans' symptoms. To date, 4 agents have been studied: sarin, a potent nerve toxin used in chemical weapons; vaccines against anthrax and botulinum toxin, which the soldiers received before serving in the war; pyridostigmine bromide, a drug that many soldiers received that was meant to counteract the effects of nerve gas; and depleted uranium, a low-level emitting form of uranium that was used in some ammunition and as a layer of armor for tanks.

The IOM committee also plans to study further the effects of sarin and vaccinations but thus far concludes that there is little evidence that exposures during the war had any adverse effects.

British researchers have reached similar conclusions. A statement published by the British Ministry of Defense in 2000 concluded: "There is no evidence that Iraq used chemical weapons against British troops in the Gulf conflict."

There are approximately 700,000 veterans of the Gulf War. More than 68,000 have become members of the Veteran Affairs' Gulf War Registry. Of those surveyed, nearly 16 percent qualified for the officially recognized diagnosis of CFS, and about 13 percent qualified for MCS; slightly more than 3 percent reported having both conditions. According to the survey authors, "There were no effects of gender, race, branch, duty status (active or reserve), or rank, although multiple chemical sensitivities was somewhat more prevalent in women and African-Americans." They concluded that there was an increased prevalence of CFS and MCS among the registry veterans, and they said that further investigation into these complaints is warranted.

site, about 2,200 physicians are board-certified in occupational medicine in the United States. This group does not believe in MCS; however, there are some occupational physicians who may champion your cause. There are other, mostly nonprofit, organizations that offer referrals, support, and resources. (See "For More Information.")

Given the fact that many occupational-medicine doctors, the official body of allergists, and many psychiatrists don't believe in MCS, it should come as no surprise that most people who believe they have the disease have turned away from mainstream physicians. Many turn to environmental-medicine physicians who base their treatments on the theories of Dr. Randolph.

Treatments used by environmental-medicine physicians include advising the patient to eliminate foods that are believed to cause reactions and avoid irritants (everything from detergents to car fumes to newsprint to new building materials).

Two other therapies include provoca-

For More Information

Since the diagnosis and treatment of multiple chemical sensitivity (MCS) is controversial, you may feel alone with your symptoms. Finding out all you can about your condition can help you feel empowered. Contact the following groups for help or further information.

- MCS Referral and Resources. This group is engaged in professional outreach and public advocacy devoted to the diagnosis, treatment, accommodation, and prevention of MCS disorders. They also provide a referral service for people who think they might have MCS. You can write to them at 508 Westgate Road, Baltimore, MD 21229, or contact them on the Internet at www.mcsrr.org.
- MCS Survivors. This online support group contains legal information, research, bulletin boards, and more. Visit their Web site at www.mcsurvivors.com.
- Chemical Injury Information Network. This nonprofit educational and advocacy group is a resource for the negative health effects of chemicals and the publisher of a monthly newsletter, "Our Toxic Times." You can write to them at PO Box 301, White Sulphur Springs, MT 59645, or contact them at their Web site, www.ciin.org.
- National Gulf War Resource Center. This international coalition of advocates and organizations provides a resource for information, support, and referrals for all those concerned with Persian Gulf War issues, especially Gulf War illnesses. Contact them at their Web site, www.ngwrc.org, or write to them at 8605 Cameron Street, Suite 400, Silver Spring, MD 20910.

tion/neutralization therapy and serial dilution. In provocation/neutralization, samples of the suspected allergen or chemical irritant are administered under the skin surface or under the tongue to determine reactivity; in serial dilution, an allergen injection is used. These therapies work under the assumption that an individual has an end point at which he ceases to react to an allergen. The end-point dosage, then, can be administered to stave off future reactions.

What Should You Do If You Have Symptoms?

While doctors and researchers argue about the cause and even the existence of MCS, everyone agrees that the symptoms are real and people who have them feel miserable.

People who have these symptoms become incredibly desperate, says Dr. Gibson. "I have seen people completely deplete themselves of their financial resources, yet try to borrow $1,000 to try a treatment they 'know' will work." She cites the case of one patient who was $40,000 in debt but wanted to spend $700 on yet another treatment, which the seller promised would be a total cure. "The truth is that there is not one surefire way to cure MCS. But there are many sensible things you can do."

Dr. Gibson wants doctors and the public to know that people with MCS are coping with real physical problems and need to be listened to and supported. "People with MCS seen by researchers and doctors want to get better. They want to work," she says. "They don't want to stay home and be dependent on other people. The perception that these people want to live in total isolation in their houses is a myth."

She suggests the following coping strategies.

Avoid your chemical triggers. Clean up your home and work environment as much as possible. The best thing that you can do is to educate yourself about environmentally safer alternatives to toxic products. Get rid of pesticides in your lawn, home, and garden. Use safer personal-care products. Commercial soaps, shampoos, and fragrances expose you to hundreds of chemicals. Avoid dry-cleaning your clothes. Learn about safe ways of renovating and redecorating that involve paints with lower levels of volatile organics and petrochemical solvents. (See "For More Information.")

Express yourself. It's important to let people know your needs. If you're having company, ask them to arrive fragrance-free if that will help you. If your loved one wears a new perfume that is bothering you, for example, speak up.

Ask for accommodations. Getting your employer to change your work environment can be difficult, and it's often not practical to change jobs. But don't think that your situation is hopeless. Although a diagnosis of MCS does not guarantee coverage by the Americans with Disabilities Act, you may be covered under an individual basis, depending on the nature of your problem.

Ask to change offices if you are near a copier and the smell bothers you. You might also ask for an air filter. If your boss won't buy one, it might be worth the investment for you to get one. In addition, try to work near a window if you can handle fresh air. You might even consider asking if you can work flexible hours so you will be exposed less to perfumes and deodorants that people wear.

Seek counseling. Find a counselor who is sympathetic to your cause and has some understanding of your condition. It might be a good way to explore the many issues that face you, such as dealing with your loved ones, boss, and coworkers.

Counseling also gives you a safe outlet where you can express your feelings about having MCS. Since this condition is stressful, any kind of supportive environment is welcome.

Resource GUIDE

Organizations

American Academy of Allergy, Asthma, and Immunology
611 East Wells Street
Milwaukee, WI 53202
(414) 272-6071
www.aaaai.org

American Academy of Environmental Medicine
7701 East Kellogg, Suite 625
Wichita, KS 67207
(316) 684-5500
www.aaem.com

American College of Allergy, Asthma, and Immunology
85 West Algonquin Road, Suite 550
Arlington Heights, IL 60005
(847) 427-1200
(800) 842-7777
www.allergy.mcg.edu

American Lung Association
1740 Broadway
New York, NY 10019
(212) 315-8700
(800) LUNG-USA
www.lungusa.org

Asthma and Allergy Foundation of America
1233 20th Street N.W., Suite 402
Washington, DC 20036
(800) 727-8462
(202) 466-7643
www.aafa.org

National Institute of Allergy and Infectious Diseases of the National Institutes of Health
Office of Communications and Public Liaison
Building 31, Room 7A-50
31 Center Drive MSC 2520
Bethesda, MD 20892-2520
(301) 496-5717
e-mail: ocpostoffice@niaid.nih.gov
www.niaid.nih.gov

Resources for Children

Asthma and Allergy Information—produced by the Asthma and Allergy Foundation of America—offers asthma and allergy information for kids and teens as well as information about educational support groups. It also provides a forum for children and teens with asthma and allergies to discuss their management strategies.
www.aafa.org/kidsandteens

Food Allergy News for Kids offers practical advice to help children and teens manage their food allergies. Their Web site even includes science fair projects children can do to learn more about their allergies.
www.fankids.org

Healthlines SAY is a bimonthly publication from the Asthma and Allergy Foundation of America for teens with asthma and allergies. For a free subscription, call (202) 466-7643, ext. 230.

Resources for Parents

The Allergy and Asthma Network/Mothers of Asthmatics offers information and support for parents, including product recall information and the latest news about asthma and allergy medications.
(703) 641-9595
(800) 878-4403
www.aanma.org

The Food Allergy and Anaphylaxis Network offers resources for helping children and teens take responsibility for managing their allergies. It's also a source for breaking news in the field of food allergies.
(703) 691-3179
(800) 929-4040
www.foodallergy.org

Products

Many drugstores now carry various supplies for people with asthma and allergies, such as peak-flow meters, dust mite–proof pillows, and even attractively colored carrying cases for EpiPens. If you're unable to find the products you need at your local stores, however, you will likely find them online. Here is just a sampling of some of the companies that offer allergy and asthma products on the Internet.

The Allergy Buyers Club
Carries large array of products for people with allergies, asthma, and sinus problems, including air purifiers, water purifiers, carpet cleaners, bedding, and air conditioners. Their Web site also includes consumer reviews and ratings of products.
160 Pine Street, Suite 10
Newton, MA 02466
(617) 969-3148
www.allergybuyersclub.com

Allergy Control Products, Inc.
Offers a full line of products to reduce allergen exposure, including allergen-proof pillow and mattress encasings, HEPA filters, HEPA filter vacuum cleaners, mold-control products, and carpet treatments.
96 Danbury Road
Ridgefield, CT 06877
(203) 438-9580
www.allergycontrol.com

Allergy Store

Online store offering a full range of allergy products, including supplements such as grape seed extract, sinus irrigators, and personal steam inhalers.

1841 S.W. 94th Avenue

Miami, FL 33165

www.allergystore.net

Comfortliving.com

A source for numerous allergy and asthma products, including hypoallergenic down-alternative comforters, pillows, and mattress covers; HEPA filters; and nebulizers.

2924 Telstar Court

Falls Church, VA 22042

(877) 378-4411

www.comfortliving.com

Med-Systems, Inc.

This company manufactures the Sinu-Cleanse system, which includes a plastic version of a neti pot and packets of dry ingredients for a nasal irrigation solution. This system was developed by Diane Heatley, M.D., associate professor of pediatric otolaryngology at the University of Wisconsin in Madison.

PO Box 45634

Madison, WI 53744

(888) 547-5492

www.sinucleanse.com

National Allergy Supply, Inc.

This company offers a wide variety of allergy products, including dustless vacuum bags, disposable dust and pollen masks, skin-care products, and bedding designed for people with sensitive skin.

1620 Satellite Boulevard, Suite D

Duluth, GA 30097

e-mail: info@nationalallergy.com

(770) 623-3237

www.nationalallergy.com

Stopallergy.com

Offers products ranging from soaps and shampoos designed for people who can't tolerate strong fragrances and other additives to dehumidifiers and air purifiers.

Crossings of Blue Ash

9525 Kenwood Road, Suite 7

Cincinnati, OH 45242

(513) 936-0224

(877) 566-3786

www.stopallergy.com

In addition to various other products, you can also obtain Breathe-Ease, the salt mix developed by Murray Grossan, M.D., an otolaryngologist at Cedars Sinai Hospital in Los Angeles, for nasal rinsing; the special pulsatile nasal irrigator he developed; and Clear-Ease enzyme formula from his Web site, www.sinus-relief.com.

You can obtain Sinus Survival Botanical Nasal Spray at www.sinussurvival.com. It is also available at some health food stores.

If you have trouble finding freeze-dried nettle, the Eclectic Institute may be able to help. Call their toll-free number, (888) 799-4372, and they can tell you where to buy the capsules in your area or ship them to you directly. Their address is 36350 S. E. Industrial Way, Sandy, OR 97055.

Allergen Testing

The Johns Hopkins University Dermatology, Allergy, and Clinical Immunology (DACI) Reference Laboratory does reservoir dust testing for environmental allergens, produced by dust mites, cats, dogs, mice, and cockroaches. For a $10 fee, they'll provide a special filter for your vacuum cleaner that you can use to collect house dust for testing. They charge $25 for each specific allergen tested, and can be contacted at (800) 344-3224, or you can visit their Web site at www.hopkins-allergy.org/services.

Guidelines for Safe Use of Herbs, Essential Oils, and Supplements

Herbs

Although herbs are generally safe and cause few, if any, side effects, researchers and specialists in natural medicine caution that you should use them responsibly. First and foremost, if you are under a doctor's care for any health condition or are taking any medication, you should not take any kind of herb without your doctor's knowledge. Certain natural substances can change the way your body absorbs and processes certain medications. Also, if you are pregnant, do not treat yourself with any natural remedy without the consent of your obstetrician or midwife. The same goes for nursing mothers and women trying to conceive.

Every product has the potential to cause adverse reactions. Following are cautions for the herbs mentioned in this book that may be more likely than others to cause adverse reactions in some people. Though such occurrences are rare, you should be aware of what they are and discontinue use of the herb if you experience an unusual reaction. Also, do not exceed the recommended dosages—more is *not* better.

Herb	Safe Use Guidelines and Possible Side Effects
Aloe (*Aloe vera*)	May delay wound healing; do not use gel externally on any surgical incision. Do not ingest the dried leaf gel, as it is a habit-forming laxative.
Chamomile (*Matricaria recutita*)	Very rarely, can cause an allergic reaction when ingested. People allergic to closely related plants such as ragweed, asters, and chrysanthemums should drink the tea with caution.
Curcumin	See Turmeric entry.
Echinacea (*Echinacea*, various species)	Do not use if allergic to closely related plants such as ragweed, asters, and chrysanthemums. Do not use if you have tuberculosis or an autoimmune condition such as lupus or multiple sclerosis because echinacea stimulates the immune system.
Feverfew (*Tanacetum parthenium*)	Fresh leaves, if chewed, can cause mouth sores in some people.
Ginger (*Zingiber officinale*)	May increase bile secretion, so if you have gallstones, do not use therapeutic amounts of the dried root or powder without guidance from a health care practitioner.
Ginkgo (*Ginkgo biloba*)	Do not use with antidepressant MAO-inhibitor drugs such as phenelzine (Nardil) or tranylcypromine (Parnate), aspirin, or other non-steroidal anti-inflammatory medications, or blood-thinning medications such as warfarin (Coumadin). Can cause dermatitis, diarrhea, and vomiting in doses higher than 240 mg of concentrated extract.
Ginseng, American (*Panax quinquefolius*) and Korean (*P. ginseng*)	May cause irritability if taken with caffeine or other stimulants. Do not take if you have high blood pressure.
Goldenseal (*Hydrastis canadensis*)	Do not use if you have high blood pressure.
Jewelweed (*Impatiens capensis*)	Do not use internally without the guidance of a qualified practitioner.
Licorice (*Glycyrrhiza glabra*)	Do not use if you have diabetes, high blood pressure, liver or kidney disorders, or low potassium levels. Do not use daily for more than 4 to 6 weeks because overuse can lead to water retention, high blood pressure caused by potassium loss, or impaired heart and kidney function.
Lobelia (*Lobelia inflata*)	Can cause nausea and vomiting in large doses.
Marshmallow (*Althaea officinalis*)	May slow the absorption of medications taken at the same time.
Nettle (*Urtica dioica*)	If you have allergies, your symptoms may worsen, so take only one dose a day for the first few days.
Turmeric (*Curcuma domestica*)	Do not use as a home remedy if you have high stomach acid or ulcers, gallstones, or bile duct obstruction.

Essential Oils

Essential oils are inhaled or applied topically to the skin, but with few exceptions, they are never taken internally.

Of the most common essential oils, lavender, tea tree, lemon, sandalwood, and rose can be used undiluted. The rest should be diluted in a carrier base—which can be an oil (such as almond), a cream, or a gel—before being applied to the skin.

Many essential oils may cause irritation or allergic reactions in people with sensitive skin. Before applying any new oil to your skin, always do a patch test. Put a few drops of the essential oil, mixed with the carrier, on the back of your wrist and wait for an hour or more. If irritation or redness occurs, wash the area with cold water. In the future, use half the amount of essential oil or avoid it altogether.

Do not use essential oils at home for serious medical problems. During pregnancy, do not use essential oils unless they're approved by your doctor. Essential oils are not appropriate for children of any age.

Store essential oils in dark bottles, away from light and heat and out of the reach of children and pets.

Essential Oil	Safe Use Guidelines and Possible Side Effects
Eucalyptus (*Eucalyptus globulus*)	Do not use for more than 2 weeks without the guidance of a qualified practitioner. Do not use more than 3 drops in the bath. Do not use at the same time as homeopathic remedies. Do not apply externally to the faces of infants and young children. Can be used undiluted for dental pain.
Lemon (*Citrus limon*)	Do not use more than 3 drops in the bath. Avoid direct sunlight because this oil can cause skin sensitivity.
Lime (*Citrus aurantifolia*)	Avoid direct sunlight because this oil can cause skin sensitivity.
Peppermint (*Mentha piperita*)	Do not use more than 3 drops in the bath. Do not use at the same time as homeopathic remedies. Do not get it near your eyes. Do not use it on the faces of infants and small children. Peppermint oil can be used internally, with this caution: Ingestion of peppermint essential oil may lead to stomach upset in sensitive individuals. If you have gallbladder or liver disease, do not use without medical supervision. Can be used undiluted for dental pain.
Rosemary (*Rosmarinus officinalis*)	Do not use if you have hypertension. Do not use if you have epilepsy, due to the powerful action on the nervous system.
Sage (*Salvia sclarea*)	Do not use with alcohol because it can cause lethargy and exaggerate drunkenness.
Thyme, white, common (*Thymus*, various species)	This oil may irritate the skin if used in high concentration. If it irritates your skin, use more carrier base to further dilute it. Do not use more than 3 drops in the bath. Do not use if you have hypertension.

Flower essences are not essential oils, but they aren't recommended for use in the eyes, on mucous membranes, or on broken or abraded skin. Most contain alcohol as a preservative, so if you're sensitive to alcohol, check with your doctor before using them.

Vitamin and Mineral Supplements

Although serious side effects from vitamin and mineral supplements are not common, they can happen. The guidelines presented here are designed to help you use the supplements mentioned in this book safely and wisely.

Be sure to talk to your doctor before using any supplement if you have a chronic illness requiring medical supervision or medication. In fact, if you have any type of health problem, your doctor or pharmacist needs to know about any supplements you're taking before treating you with a prescription or over-the-counter medicine. If

Nutrient	Daily Value (DV) or *Suggested Daily Intake*	Safe Upper Limit
Calcium	1,000 mg; *1,200 mg if over age 50*	2,500 mg
Magnesium	400 mg	350 mg from supplements only
Pantothenic acid	10 mg	1,000 mg
Selenium	70 mcg	400 mcg
Vitamin B$_6$ (pyridoxine)	2 mg	100 mg
Vitamin C	60 mg; *100 to 500 mg*	2,000 mg
Vitamin D	400 IU *up to 600 IU if over age 70*	2,000 IU (50 mcg)
Vitamin E	30 IU; *100 to 400 IU*	1,500 IU (natural form, d-alpha-tocopherol) or 1,100 IU (synthetic form, dl-alpha-tocopherol) from supplements only
Zinc	15 mg	40 mg

you are a woman who is pregnant, nursing, or attempting to conceive, do not use supplements unless under the supervision of your physician.

The vitamin and mineral doses listed below are the Daily Values or the suggested daily intakes (noted in italics). Also given below are the safe upper limits for adults, above which harmful side effects can occur. These amounts are the total from both food and supplements. Do not take more than the safe upper limit of any vitamin or mineral without first consulting your physician. (*Note:* mg = milligrams; mcg = micrograms; IU = international units)

Emerging Supplements

Reports of adverse effects from emerging supplements are rare, especially when compared to prescription drugs, and supplement manufacturers are required by law to provide information on labels about reasonably

Cautions and Other Information

Taking more than 2,500 mg a day can cause serious side effects such as kidney damage. For best absorption, avoid taking more than 500 mg at one time. If you are over age 50, look for a formula that contains vitamin D as well as calcium, since you may need more vitamin D than is supplied by a multivitamin alone. Some natural sources of calcium, such as bonemeal and dolomite, may be contaminated with lead and other dangerous or undesirable metals.

Check with your doctor before beginning supplementation in any amount if you have heart or kidney problems. Doses exceeding 350 mg a day can cause diarrhea in some people.

A healthy, balanced diet provides enough of this nutrient to meet your body's needs.

Taking more than 400 mcg a day can cause dizziness, nausea, hair or nail loss, or a garlic odor on the breath or skin.

Taking more than 100 mg a day can cause reversible nerve damage. When selecting a B-complex supplement, check the label for the amount of each ingredient to help you determine its safe use.

Taking more than 2,000 mg a day can cause diarrhea in some people. To help maintain levels of vitamin C throughout the day, take half of the recommended dose in the morning and half at night.

Because it acts like a blood thinner, consult your doctor before taking vitamin E if you are already taking aspirin or a blood-thinning medication, such as warfarin (Coumadin).

Taking more than 2,000 IU a day can cause headache, fatigue, nausea, diarrhea, or loss of appetite.

Taking more than 40 mg a day can cause nausea, dizziness, or vomiting. When levels of zinc are elevated, the absorption of copper can become impaired.

safe recommended dosages for healthy individuals. Be aware that the potency and dosing strategy can very significantly among products.

You should note, however, that little scientific research exists to assess the safety or long-term effects of many emerging supplements, and some supplements can complicate existing conditions or cause allergic reactions in some people. For these reasons, you should always check with your doctor before taking any supplements.

We recommend that you take supplements with food for best absorption and to avoid stomach irritation, unless otherwise directed. Never take them as a substitute for a healthy diet, since they do not provide all the nutritional benefits of whole foods.

And, if you are pregnant, nursing, or attempting to conceive, do not supplement without the supervision of a doctor.

Supplement	Safe Use Guidelines and Possible Side Effects
Acidophilus	If you have any serious gastrointestinal problems that require medical attention, check with your doctor before supplementing. Amounts exceeding 10 billion viable *Lactobacillus acidophilus* organisms daily may cause mild gastrointestinal distress. If you are taking antibiotics, take them at least 2 hours before supplementing.
Bee pollen	May cause stomach pain, diarrhea, irritation and itching in the mouth and throat, and, less commonly, headache, malaise, fatigue, and asthma attacks. If you have asthma or diabetes, check with your doctor before taking; pollen contains allergens that can worsen asthma, and it contains natural sugars. Rarely, may cause life-threatening anaphylactic shock in sensitive people; do not take if you have a history of anaphylactic reactions.
Bromelain	May cause nausea, vomiting, diarrhea, skin rash, and heavy menstrual bleeding. Can also increase the risk of bleeding in people taking aspirin or anticoagulants (blood thinners). Do not take if you are allergic to pineapple.
Creatine	One person reported side effects including gastrointestinal distress, nausea, dehydration and muscle cramping, and muscle pulls. May also cause stress on the kidneys. There are no long-term studies of impact on human health.
EPA (fish oil)	Do not take if any of the following apply: bleeding disorder, uncontrolled high blood pressure, anticoagulants (blood thinners) or regular aspirin use, allergy to any kind of fish. People with diabetes should not take fish oil because of its high fat content. Increases bleeding time, possibly resulting in nosebleeds and easy bruising, and may cause upset stomach. Take fish oil, not fish liver oil, because fish liver oil is high in vitamins A and D—toxic in high amounts.

Supplement	Safe Use Guidelines and Possible Side Effects
Gamma-linolenic acid (borage and black currant)	May cause headaches, indigestion, nausea, and softening of stools. Take under the supervision of a knowledgeable medical doctor if you take aspirin or anticoagulants (blood thinners) regularly, have a seizure disorder, or are taking epilepsy medication such as phenothiazines.
MSM (methylsulfonyl-methane)	Do not use if you are allergic or sensitive to sulfur-containing drugs.
Proanthocyanidin (bioflavonoid)	In some people, may reduce blood-clotting ability and result in bleeding or, in extreme instances, lead to hemorrhages.
Quercetin (bioflavonoid)	Doses above 100 mg may dilate blood vessels and cause blood thinning in some people. Should be avoided by individuals at risk for low blood pressure or problems with blood clotting.
Spirulina (blue-green algae)	To avoid possible heavy-metal contamination, buy spirulina only from reputable sources. Check the label for an indication that it's been analyzed for heavy-metal content, or for an 800 number for consumer questions.

INDEX

Underscored page references indicate boxed text and tables. **Boldface** references indicate illustrations.

A

Acaricides, avoiding, for reducing dust mites, 274
Accolate, for treating
  asthma, 201, 372
  pet allergies, 365, 366
ACE inhibitors, allergies from, 265
Acidophilus
  for preventing yeast infections, 454
  for treating
    allergies, 148, 154, 279
    candidiasis hypersensitivity, 454, 455
    intestinal problems, 460
Acrivastine, for allergic rhinitis, 315
Acupuncture
  in alternative medicine, 52
  for asthma, 256
Addictions, linked to allergies, 45
Additives, food, hidden sources of, 304–5
ADHD. *See* Attention-deficit hyperactivity disorder
Adolescence, asthma in, 203
Adrenal glands, supplements strengthening, 156–58
AeroBid, for asthma, 51
Air conditioners, cleaning, 79, 346

Air filters. *See also* HEPA filters
  in bedroom, 77, 87–88
  for controlling
    dust mites, 274
    mold, 346
    pet allergies, 77, 364–65
  maintaining, 84
  natural, 51
  selecting, 86–87
  over vents, 88
Air travel, allergy-free, 126–27
Albuterol, for treating
  anaphylaxis, 339
  asthma, 372
ALCAT, in environmental medicine, 42
Alcohol, for poison plant allergy, 379
Alcoholic beverages, avoiding, in allergy-free diet, 141, 143
Allegra, for treating
  allergic rhinitis, 196, 309, 315, 315
  eye allergies, 430
Allergen detective kits, 79
Allergens, 19, 20, 21. *See also specific allergens*
Allergic dermatitis, from latex allergy, 328, 338–39
Allergic march. *See* Atopic march

Allergic rhinitis
  action plan for, 325–26
  anatomy of, 309–12
  asthma and, 238, 314
  best medication for, 317
  in children, 18, 194–97, 195, 202
  with chronic fatigue syndrome, 461–62
  conditions associated with, 18, 307–9,
    313–14
  with fibromyalgia, 459
  incidence of, 18
  loss of smell from, 318
  natural gas and, 320
  vs. nonallergic rhinitis, 310–11
  occupational, 115
    diagnosis of, 118–19
  oral allergy syndrome with, 308
  ozone affecting, 370
  perennial, 312
  seasonal, 312
  sinusitis from, 382–83
  vs. sinusitis, 383
  symptoms of, 18, 313, **313**, 383
  treating, with
    anticholinergic drugs, 319–20
    antihistamines, 57, 196, 309, 314–16,
      325, 459
    antioxidants, 323–24
    avoidance strategy, 320
    cromolyn, 319, 325
    decongestants, 196, 319, 325
    fatty acids, 323
    homeopathy, 324
    honey, 324, 326
    immunotherapy, 24, 32, 312, 325–26
    nasal corticosteroids, 196–97, 316–17,
      319, 325
    NasalCrom, 51
    nasal rinsing, 320–23, 321, 322, 325
    nettle, 54, 57, 323, 326
    quercetin, 54, 323, 326
    stress reduction, 323
Allergists
  organizations representing, 33
  treatment approach of, 26–27
  when to see, 26–27
Allergy shots. *See* Immunotherapy
Allergy sinus solution, for asthma, 255
AllerMax, for treatment in alternative
  medicine, 55
Aloe, for skin conditions, 416

Alpha-linolenic acid (ALA), for inflammatory
  bowel disease, 478, 479
Alrex, for eye allergies, 430
Alternative medicine, 13
  benefiting conventional medicine, 58–59
  diagnosis of allergies in, 49–50
  exploring best therapies in, 61–63
  increasing popularity of, 47–48
  risk of combining conventional medicine
    with, 62–63
  similarity of, to conventional and
    environmental medicine, 56–58
  therapies used in, 48
  treatment strategies in, 48, 50–51
    acupuncture, 52
    aromatherapy, 52
    Ayurveda, 52
    breathing exercises, 52
    chiropractic, 52
    cranial therapy, 52
    detoxification, 52–53
    dietary changes, 53
    herbs and spices, 54, 55, 64
    homeopathy, 53, 64–66
    manipulative work, 53
    mind-body techniques, 53, 66–67
    sinus irrigation, 53
    steam inhalation, 53–54
    supplements, 54–55, 150–52
    Traditional Chinese Medicine, 67–68
    vitamins and minerals, 68
  view of allergies by, 48–49
Americans with Disabilities Act (ADA), for
  help with workplace allergies, 119,
  496
Anaphylaxis
  action plan for, 217, 220–21
  vs. anaphylactoid reactions, 216
  causes of, 216, 218–19
    drug allergy, 262
    exercise, 159–60
    food allergies, 19, 192, 279, 283
    insect stings, 393–94, 394, 398, 399,
     402
    latex allergy, 339
  conditions mimicking, 220
  preventing, 214, 215–16
  symptoms of, 27, 211–14, 212, 217, 410,
    424
  treating, 213, 214–15, 217, 220, 221, 339,
    393–94, 402

Angioedema
  action plan for, 419
  symptoms of, 411–12
Angiotensin-converting enzyme (ACE)
    inhibitors, allergies from, 265
Animal skins, allergies from, <u>366</u>
Anosmia, <u>324</u>
  from allergic rhinitis, <u>318</u>
  symptoms of, **407**
Antibiotics
  allergic reaction to, 261
  allergy risk from, 23, 284–85
  drawbacks of, 10
  for treating
    otitis media, 436, 437
    sinusitis, 385, 391, <u>459</u>
  yeast infections from, 451, <u>454</u>
Anticholinergic drugs, for allergic rhinitis,
    319–20
Antigen leukocyte cellular antibody test
    (ALCAT), in environmental medicine,
    <u>42</u>
Antihistamines
  alternative medicine view of, 51
  avoiding, with chronic fatigue syndrome,
    463
  sedating effects of, 314, <u>315</u>
  for treating
    allergic rhinitis, 57, 196, 309, 314–16,
      325, <u>459</u>
    contact dermatitis, 422
    eye allergies, 430
    food allergies, 291
    hives, 371–72, 419
    hormone allergy, <u>415</u>
    latex allergy, 339
    sinusitis, 386, 391–92
Anti-inflammatory drugs, allergies from, 265
Antioxidants, for treating
  allergic rhinitis, 323–24
  asthma, 248, 259
Ants, stinging
  fire ants, 395–96, 398–99, <u>399</u>
  harvester ants, <u>399</u>
Apples, for treating
  allergies, <u>142</u>
  asthma, 248
Aromatherapy, as treatment strategy in
    alternative medicine, 52
Arthritis, rheumatoid, linked to allergies,
    46

Asian pyramid, for allergy-free diet, 137–38,
    137
Aspartame allergy, 304
Aspirin
  allergies from, 265, 419
  as asthma cause, 239
  for food allergies, 291
  food allergy associated with, <u>282</u>
Astelin, for allergic rhinitis, 316, <u>459</u>
Asthma
  action plan for, 259–60
    developing, 236–38, <u>237</u>
  in adolescence, 203
  age of onset of, 227
  allergic rhinitis and, 238, 314
  anatomy of, 222–24, **223**
  avoiding air travel with, 126–27
  categories of, 226–27, 243
  in children, <u>18</u>, 197–202, 202, 203
    medications for, 200, <u>200–201</u>
  conditions mimicking, <u>230</u>
  cough-variant, 232
  deaths from, 18, 223, 224
  diagnosing, 25, 199–200, 229–31
  early intervention for, 225–27
  exercise-induced
    medications for, 259
    overview of, 159–60, 232
    preventing, 246
    school considerations for, 160, 203
    syndromes mimicking, <u>162–63</u>
  exercising with, 9, 159–60, 162–66, 198
  facts about, 224–25
  famous people with, <u>226</u>
  fatty foods aggravating, 9
  former remedies for, <u>225–26</u>
  incidence of, 18
  increase in, 4, 6–7
  induced by exercise and cold air, 369–70,
    372
  lifestyle affecting, 228
  mountains affecting, 128
  obesity and, 160–61, 198
  occupational, 111, 112–14, 231–32
    diagnosis of, 117
  Olympic athletes with, <u>161</u>, <u>164–65</u>, 197
  ozone affecting, <u>370</u>
  during pregnancy, <u>188</u>
  preventing, similarities between disciplines
    in, 57
  risk factors for, 227

Asthma *(cont.)*
scuba diving with, 128
similarities between disciplines in treating, 57–58
smoking and, <u>484–85</u>
symptoms of, 228–29, **408**, **409**
treating, with
AeroBid, 51
conventional medicine, 63, 200–201, 235–36
dietary supplements, 251–52
drugs, 27, 30–31, 201, 224, <u>240–41</u>, 242–43, 246, 259, 372
environmental control, 238–39, 259
herbs, 54, 252–56, <u>253</u>
hypnosis, 178
immunotherapy, 201, 246, 259
inhalers, <u>200–201</u>, 243–46, <u>244</u>, 259, 372
integrated approach, 236
lung-friendly foods, 248–49
massage, 180–81, **181**
mind-body interventions, 256–58, <u>257</u>, <u>258</u>
peak-flow meters, 117, 200–201, 239, 242, 259
sinus remedies, <u>255</u>
steam inhalation, <u>247</u>
vitamins and minerals, 68, 250–51, <u>250</u>, 260
triggers of, 233–35, <u>233</u>, <u>234</u>
vegetable oil affecting, 138–39
warning signs of, 237–38
when to see an allergist about, <u>26</u>
Astragalus, for treating
asthma, 254
sinusitis, 389, 392
Atopic dermatitis. *See* Eczema
Atopic keratoconjunctivitis, 427
Atopic march, <u>18</u>, 189, 283
Attention-deficit hyperactivity disorder (ADHD)
hidden allergy connection with, 45, 443, 446–47, 448, 449
incidence of, 445
signs of, 445
treating, with
elimination diet, <u>448</u>, 449
environmental control, <u>448</u>
Ritalin, 445–46

Aveeno Daily Moisturizing Bath, for physical allergy, 371
Aveeno Soothing Bath Treatment, for treating
eczema, 420
hives, 419
Avoidance strategy
in conventional medicine, 30
for delaying allergy in infants, <u>186</u>
in environmental medicine, 33
for treating
allergic rhinitis, 320
food allergies, 191, 290–91
sinusitis, 388
Ayurveda, as treatment strategy in alternative medicine, 52
Azelastine, for allergic rhinitis, 316, <u>459</u>

B

Bacterial infection, food allergies and, 284–85
Baking soda, for food allergies, <u>295</u>
Basements, allergy-proofing, 95–96
Bat feces, as allergen, <u>77</u>
Bathrooms, allergy-proofing, 93, **93**, <u>94</u>
Bedding
encasing, 85–86, 346, 363
selecting, 88
washing, 87
Bedrooms, allergy-proofing, 30, 77, 85–89, **85**, 273, 275
Bee pollen, for respiratory allergy symptoms, 151–52
Bees
identifying, **397**
stings from, 397, 400
Behavioral changes, for treating asthma, 256
Benadryl
avoiding, as premedication for food allergies, <u>290</u>
for treating
allergic rhinitis, 196, 314, <u>315</u>
anaphylaxis, 215, 221, 339
Benzoates, sources of, 304
Berberine, for sinusitis, 389, 392
Beta$_2$-agonists, for preventing exercise-induced asthma, 246, 259
Beta-blockers, as asthma cause, 239
BHA/BHT, sources of, 304–5
Biofeedback, for stress reduction, 174–75
in asthma treatment, 256–57

Bioflavonoids, as treatment strategy in alternative medicine, 55

Birds, allergies to, 358

Biting insects. *See also* Insect allergies
allergies from, 394, 395

Black currant seed oil, for treating
allergic rhinitis, 326
asthma, 252

Blended medicine, benefits of, 61

Blood tests
in alternative medicine, 50
for diagnosis of
allergies, 25
asthma, 231
food allergies, 289

Body piercings, record for, 353

Borage oil, for treating
allergies, 142, 155, 326
asthma, 252

Boric acid, for roach control, 91, 277

Boswellia, for asthma, 254

Breakfast, foods recommended for, 147

Breastfeeding, for allergy prevention, 9, 187–88

Breast implants, allergies and, 490–91

Breath-actuated metered-dose inhaler, 244

Breathe Right strips, for allergic rhinitis, 458

Breathing exercises, 166–67
for asthma, 257, 257
as treatment strategy in alternative medicine, 52

Bromelain, combined with quercetin, 150

Bronchitis, chronic asthmatic, 232–33
symptoms of, **409**

Bronchodilators, for asthma, 200

Burdock, for skin conditions, 417

Bus travel, allergy-free, 129

C

Caffeinated beverages, avoiding, in allergy-free diet, 141

Calamine lotion, for treating
contact dermatitis, 422
poison plant allergy, 380

Calcium, for preventing corticosteroid side effects, 68, 250

Calendula, for skin conditions, 416

Camping, allergy-free, 128

Candidiasis hypersensitivity
causes of, 451
consulting doctor about, 452–53
controversy about, 450–51, 452–53
diet for treating, 453–55
hidden allergy connection with, 45, 443
from poor diet, 143
symptoms of, 143, 451–52

Canola oil, for allergies, 142

Carbon monoxide poisoning, 97

Carmine, sources of, 305

Carpeting
allergens in, 73
avoiding mite killers on, 83
choosing, 94
mold growth in, 346
removing, to reduce dust mites, 273, 275
vacuuming, 82–83, 365
washing, 81–82, 82

Car travel, allergy-free, 125–26

Cat allergies. *See* Pet allergies

Cataracts, from corticosteroid use, preventing, 68, 250

Cat dander, 358, 359

Caterpillars, allergy to, 396

Celiac disease, 281

Cereal grains, causing allergies, 292

Cetirizine, for treating
allergic rhinitis, 196, 315
eye allergies, 430

CFS. *See* Chronic fatigue syndrome

Chamomile, for chronic fatigue syndrome, 464

Chemical exposure, increasing allergy risk, 34, 37

Chemicals
avoiding, in home, 79, 84
safe use of, 97
storing, 97

Chest tightness, as asthma symptom, 229

Chicken soup, for sinusitis, 390, 392

Children
allergies in
allergic rhinitis, 194–97, 195
delaying, 186, 187–88
eczema, 18, 192–94, 193
food allergies, 189–92
increased incidence of, 185
natural remedies for, 202
onset of, 18
origin of, 186–87, 187

Children *(cont.)*
  allergies in *(cont.)*
    risk of developing, <u>187</u>
    at school, 202–3
    unique aspects of, 189
  asthma in, 197–98
    managing, 198–202
    medications for, 200, <u>200–201</u>
    school considerations for, 203
  atopic march in, <u>18</u>, 189, 283
  passive smoking affecting, 83, 187, 438,
    <u>485</u>
  resources for, 497–98
Chiropractic, as treatment strategy in
    alternative medicine, 52
Chlorpheniramine, for allergic rhinitis, 196
Chlor-Trimeton, for allergic rhinitis, 196
Chronic asthmatic bronchitis, 232–33, **409**
Chronic fatigue syndrome (CFS)
  fibromyalgia with, 457
  in Gulf War veterans, <u>492</u>, <u>493</u>
  hidden allergy connection with, 45–46,
    443–44, 457–59, 461
  role of cytokines in, 462–63, <u>462</u>
  role of histamine in, 462–63
  symptoms of, 456
  treating, <u>458–59</u>, 463–64, <u>463</u>
Cinnamon, for allergies and asthma, 64
Claritin, for treating
  allergic rhinitis, 57, 150, 196, 309, 315,
    <u>315</u>
  eye allergies, 430
Cleaners, household
  avoiding, with sinusitis, 390
  for kitchen, 92
  limiting, 79
  natural alternatives to, <u>90</u>
Cleanliness, allergies and, 9–10
Clear-Ease, for sinusitis, 390
Clinical titration, for allergy diagnosis, 42–43
Clobetasol, for nickel allergy, 355
Closets, allergy-proofing, **93**, 95
Clotrimazole, for eczema, 194
Cockroach allergies. *See also* Cockroaches
  action plan for, 277
  genetics and, 271
Cockroaches. *See also* Cockroach allergies
  allergens from, 74
    prevalence of, 268
  controlling, 79, 274, 277
    in kitchen, 90–91
  hiding places of, 269–70
  killing, 91–92, 277
Coffee, for treating
  asthma, 248–49, 254
  migraines, <u>469</u>
Cognitive reframing, for stress reduction,
    175–76
Cold air, affecting asthma, 369–70, 372
Colds
  vs. allergic rhinitis, <u>195</u>
  limiting childhood exposure to, 188
Coleus, for asthma, 64, 254
Combination remedies, as treatment strategy
    in alternative medicine, 55
Comforters, selecting, 88
Comprehensive environmental control
    program, as diagnostic test in
    environmental medicine, 43
Compresses, for treating
  contact dermatitis, 422
  eye allergies, 429
  hives, 419
  sinusitis, 389, 392
Concomitant food allergy, 286–87,
    <u>287</u>
Condoms, latex allergy from, 330–31
Conjunctivitis
  atopic keratoconjunctivitis, 427
  vs. dry-eye syndrome, <u>427</u>
  giant papillary, 428, 430–31
  identifying symptoms of, **432–33**
  nonallergic, 428
  seasonal and perennial, 426, 429–30
  vernal keratoconjunctivitis, 427, 430
Contact dermatitis
  action plan for, 422
  affecting eyes, 428, 431, **432**
  from latex allergy, 328, 338
  from nickel allergy, 349
  occupational, 114–15
  photoallergic, <u>368</u>, **425**
  preventing, 418
  symptoms of, **424**
  types of, 418
Contact lenses, with eye allergies, 430–31
Conventional medicine
  alternative medicine concepts adopted in,
    <u>58–59</u>
  diagnosis of allergies by, 24–25
  risk of combining alternative medicine with,
    <u>62–63</u>

similarity of, to environmental and
    alternative medicine, 56–58
treatment strategies in, 13, 26–27
    allergy drugs, <u>28–29</u>, 30–31
    avoidance, 30
    immunotherapy, 24, 32
    view of allergies by
    allergy-related conditions, 18–19
    allergy risk factors, 21–23
    origin of allergies, 14–18, **15**
    role of allergens, 19, <u>20</u>, 21
Corticosteroid cream. *See* Steroid cream
Corticosteroid eyedrops, for eye allergies, 430
Corticosteroid(s)
    inhaled
        alternative medicine view of, 51
        for asthma, 31, 57, <u>200</u>, <u>240–41</u>, 242
        preventing osteoporosis from, 68
    licorice root combined with, <u>57</u>
    nasal spray, for treating
        allergic rhinitis, 196–97, 316–17, 319,
            325
        sinusitis, 386, 391
    oral, for treating
        allergic rhinitis, 197
        asthma, 27, 31
    preventing side effects from, 68, <u>250</u>
    for treating
        contact dermatitis, 422
        food allergies, 291
Coughing
    asthma-related, 228–29
    determining cause of, **408–10**
Counseling, for multiple chemical sensitivity,
    496
Cow's milk
    allergy to, 9, <u>18</u>, 189, 284, 285
    anaphylaxis from, <u>218</u>
Cranial therapy, as treatment strategy in
    alternative medicine, 52
Crawl spaces, allergy-proofing, 96
Creatine, for chronic fatigue syndrome, <u>459</u>
Crohn's disease, <u>476.</u> *See also* Inflammatory
    bowel disease (IBD)
Crolom, for eye allergies, 430
Cromolyn
    for preventing exercise-induced asthma,
        246, 259
    for treating
        allergic rhinitis, 197, 319, 325
        asthma, <u>240–41</u>, 242–43, 372

food allergies, 291
latex allergy, 339
Cromolyn-based inhalers, for asthma, <u>200</u>
Cruises, allergy-free, 128–29
Curcumin, for asthma, 254
Currant seed oil, for fighting allergies, <u>142</u>
Cytokines
    allergies from, 265
    role of, in
        chronic fatigue syndrome, <u>462</u>
        depression, 467
Cytotoxic testing, in environmental medicine,
    <u>42</u>

D

Dairy products
    avoiding
        in allergy-free diet, 140, <u>141</u>
        for sinusitis, 389–90, 392
    causing allergies, <u>292</u>
    milk (*see* Milk)
Dandelion root, for food allergies, 298
Decongestants, for treating
    allergic rhinitis, 196, 319, 325
    sinusitis, 386, 391
Dehumidifier
    for basement, 95
    cleaning, 81
Depression
    hidden allergy connection with, 46, 444,
        465–66, <u>467</u>
    from inflammatory reactions, 467
    major, symptoms of, <u>466</u>
Dermatitis
    atopic (*see* Eczema)
    contact (*see* Contact dermatitis)
    from dietary nickel, <u>350</u>
    from latex allergy, 328, 338–39
Dermographism
    incidence of, <u>369</u>
    as physical allergy, 368
Detoxification, as treatment strategy in
    alternative medicine, 52–53
DHEA supplements, strengthening adrenals,
    158
Diagnosis of allergies, in conventional
    medicine, 24–25
Diary, food, for diagnosis of food allergies,
    288

Diet
  allergy-proofing, with
    apples, 142
    Asian pyramid, 137–38, **137**
    black currant seed oil, 142
    borage oil, 142
    canola oil, 142
    cold-water fish, 142
    evening primrose oil, 142
    fiber, 146
    fruits, 143, 145
    gamma-linolenic acid, 144–45
    juices, 145–46
    magnesium-rich foods, 143
    meal-by-meal plan, 147
    natural decongestants, 148
    olive oil, 143
    omega-3 fatty acids, 144–45
    regular meals, 148
    spices, 143
    spirulina, 143
    veganism, 148
    vegetables, 143, 145
    water drinking, 139
    yogurt, 143, 146–48
    zinc-rich foods, 143
  best choices for, 145
  influencing allergic response, 134,
      135–36
  poor
    as allergy trigger, 9
    health effects of, 142–44
  substances to avoid in
    alcoholic beverages, 141
    caffeinated beverages, 141
    meat and poultry, 141
    milk and dairy products, 140, 140
    omega-6 fatty acids, 138–40, 140
    protein, 140
    saturated fat, 136, 140
    sugar, 140–41, 141
    sulfites, 141–42
    trans fats, 140–41
  as treatment strategy in
    alternative medicine, 53
    environmental medicine, 44
Digestive tract problems, allergies linked to,
    460
Dining out
  with food allergies, 302–3
  latex allergy affecting, 337

Dining rooms, allergy-proofing, **89**, 90–92
Dinner, foods recommended for, 147
Diphenhydramine, for treating
  allergic rhinitis, 196, 314, 315
  anaphylaxis, 215, 221, 339
Dog allergies. *See* Pet allergies
Domeboro Astringent Solution, for treating
  contact dermatitis, 422
  poison plant allergy, 380
Down, goose, allergies from, 366
Doxepin, for chronic fatigue syndrome,
    459
Drug allergies
  action plan for, 266–67
  anaphylaxis from, 218–19, 262
  drugs causing, 261, 264–65
  vs. nonallergic drug reactions, 262–63
  as noninherited, 262
  prevalence of, 267
  symptoms of, 261–62
  types of, 263–64
Drugs. *See also specific drugs*
  allergy, 30–31
    pros and cons of, 28–29, 30–31
  anaphylaxis from, 218–19
  asthma, 27, 30, 31
    pros and cons of, 28–29, 240–41
  dosage-related response to, 263
  hospital errors with, 264
  idiosyncratic reaction to, 263
  intolerance to, 263
  rhinitis from, 311
  side effects of, 262–63
  when to take, 104
Dry-cleaned clothes, airing out, 95
Dryer, venting of, 95
Dry-eye syndrome, 427
Dry-powder inhalers, for asthma, 200–201,
    244–45
Duct cleaning, 74–75, 76
Dust mite allergies. *See also* Dust mites
  action plan for, 275–76
  genetics and, 271
  snail allergy with, 276
  symptoms of, **407**
Dust mites. *See also* Dust mite allergies
  as allergy triggers, **20**
  as asthma triggers, 234
  environmental control for, 272–74,
      275–76
  hiding places of, 269

killing
   in carpets, 81–82
   with chemicals, 83
   with hot water, <u>82</u>
   prevalence of, 268–69
Dust removal, 84
Dyes, radiology
   allergy to, 265, 267
   anaphylaxis from, <u>218–19</u>

E

Ear disease, allergies and, 196
Ear problems
   identifying symptoms of, **439**
   infections (*see* Otitis media)
   Ménière's disease, <u>435</u>
East Germany, allergies in, 4, 5, 22, 23
Echinacea
   allergic reactions to, 252
   for sinusitis, 389, 392
Eczema
   action plan for, 420–21
   causes of, 413, 415
   in children, <u>18</u>, 192–94, <u>193</u>
   diagnosis of, 25
   from dietary nickel, <u>350</u>
   incidence of, 19
   managing, 413–15, <u>413</u>
   migrating to eyes, 427
   probiotics for, <u>279</u>
   skin conditions occurring with, 115
   sun protection with, 128, 129
   symptoms of, **423**
Eggs
   allergy to, 9, 189, <u>292</u>
   anaphylaxis from, <u>218</u>
   hidden sources of, <u>199</u>, 304
Eicosapentaenoic acid (EPA) supplements, for inflammatory bowel disease, <u>477</u>, 478, 479
Electro-dermal testing, for diagnosis
   in alternative medicine, 50
   of food allergies, 290
Elimination diet
   in alternative medicine, 50
   for diagnosis of food allergies, 43
   for treating
      attention-deficit hyperactivity disorder, <u>448</u>

food allergies, 291, 295–96
   headaches, 472–74
Environment, as allergy risk factor, 6–10, <u>7</u>, 21, 22–23, 37
Environmental control
   at home (*see* Home, allergy-proofing areas of)
   for treating
      asthma, 238–39, 259
      attention-deficit hyperactivity disorder, <u>448</u>
      dust mite allergy, 272–74, 275–76
      headaches, 472
      mold allergy, 345–47
      multiple chemical sensitivity, 495
      pet allergies, 363–66
Environmental medicine
   allergy-linked conditions defined by, 45–46
   basics of, 13, <u>36</u>
   causes of allergies defined by, 37, 39–40
   choosing practitioner of, <u>35</u>
   vs. conventional medicine, 33
   diagnostic process in
      medical history, 40–41
      tests, 41–43, <u>42</u>
   founding of, 34
   incidence of allergies defined by, 37–39
   similarity of, to conventional and alternative medicine, 56–58
   treatment strategies in
      dietary changes, 44
      exercise, 44
      immunotherapy, 33, <u>35</u>, 43–44
      sauna therapy, 44
      stress reduction, 44–45
      supplements, 45
   view of allergies by, 34–37
Enzyme-potentiated desensitization
   in environmental medicine, 44
   for treating
      chronic fatigue syndrome, <u>463</u>
      food allergies, 298
Enzymes, for treating
   food allergies, 298
   sinusitis, 390, 392
EPA supplements, for inflammatory bowel disease, <u>477</u>, 478, 479
Ephedra, for respiratory allergy symptoms, 54, 58, 152
Ephedrine, for asthma, 57

Epinephrine. *See also* EpiPen
  for treating
    anaphylaxis, <u>213</u>, 214–15, 221, 339
    hives or angioedema, 419
EpiPen. *See also* Epinephrine
  for anaphylaxis, <u>213</u>, 217, 220, 221, 339,
    393–94, 402
  for travel, 124
Essential fatty acids. *See also* Gamma-linolenic
    acid (GLA); Omega-3 fatty acids;
    Omega-6 fatty acids
  as supplements, 144–45, 155–56
Essential oils, guidelines for safe use of, 503,
    <u>503</u>, 504
Ethylene gas, latex allergy and, <u>329</u>
Eucalyptus oil, for killing mites, 81–82
Evening primrose oil, for allergies, <u>142</u>,
    155
Exercise(s)
  with allergies, 159, 160
  allergy-free plan for, 134, <u>171</u>
  for allergy treatment, 8–9, 159
  anaphylaxis from, 159–60, <u>219</u>
  with asthma, 160, 162–66, 198
  asthma induced by, 159, 232, 246,
    369–70
  best and worst sports for, <u>168–69</u>
  breathing, <u>166–67</u>
  choosing, 167–68
  chronic fatigue syndrome and, 458–59,
    <u>459</u>
  indoor, 168–72
  lack of, as allergy trigger, 8
  medical approval of, 161–62
  outdoor, <u>170</u>, 172
  premedication for, <u>160</u>, 168, 170
  questions about starting, 166–67
  swimming, <u>160</u>, 167, <u>168</u>, 198
  as treatment strategy in environmental
    medicine, 44
  walking, <u>160</u>
Exercise-induced allergy, food-dependent,
    287–88, <u>288</u>, **410**, **425**
Exercise-induced asthma. *See* Asthma,
    exercise-induced
Exercise-induced hyperventilation, <u>162</u>
Exercise-induced vocal-cord dysfunction,
    <u>162–63</u>
Extermination, cockroach, 91–92
Eyedrops, for eye allergies, 429, 430,
    430

Eye problems
  atopic keratoconjunctivitis, 427
  contact dermatitis, 428, 431
  giant papillary conjunctivitis, 428,
    430–31
  identifying symptoms of, **432–33**
  nonallergic conjunctivitis, 428
  seasonal and perennial allergic
    conjunctivitis, 426, 429–30
  vernal keratoconjunctivitis, 427, 430

F

Fall allergies, concomitant food allergy with,
    <u>38</u>
Fast food, promoting allergies, 9
Fasting, for diagnosing food allergies, <u>297</u>
Fat, saturated, avoiding in allergy-free diet,
    136, <u>140</u>
Fatigue
  chronic (*see* Chronic fatigue syndrome)
  nasal congestion and, 461–62
Fatty acids, essential. *See* Essential fatty
    acids
Feeding tests, for diagnosis of food allergy, 41,
    42–43
Feverfew
  for preventing migraines, <u>469</u>
  for treating
    allergic rhinitis, <u>459</u>
    chronic fatigue syndrome, 464
Fexofenadine, for treating
  allergic rhinitis, 309, 315, <u>315</u>
  eye allergies, 430
Fiber, in allergy-free diet, 146, 154–55
Fibromyalgia
  allergic rhinitis with, 459
  mold sensitivity with, 457–58
  sleep disturbances with, 461
  symptoms of, 457, 461
  treating, <u>458–59</u>
Filters. *See* Air filters; HEPA filters
Fire ants
  anaphylaxis from, 398, 399
  identifying, **399**
  stings from, 395–96
Fireplace, safe use of, 92
Fish
  allergy to, <u>292</u>, 305–6
  anaphylaxis from, <u>218</u>

for treating
  allergies, <u>142</u>
  asthma, 249, 260
Fish oil, for treating
  allergies, 155, 156
  asthma, 251
  inflammatory bowel disease, <u>477</u>, 478
Flaxseed oil, for treating
  allergies, 155, 156
  inflammatory bowel disease, 478, 479
Fleabites, hives from, 394
Flonase, for allergic rhinitis, <u>458</u>
Flovent, for asthma prevention, 57
Flunisolide, for asthma, 51
Fluocin, for nickel allergy, 355
Fluocinonide, for nickel allergy, 355
Fluticasone
  for allergic rhinitis, <u>458</u>
  for asthma prevention, 57
Food additives, hidden sources of, 304–5
Food allergens, families of, <u>292–94</u>
Food allergies
  action plan for
    deciphering food labels, 300–301
    in home food preparation, 301–2
    identifying hidden sources of trouble,
      303–6
    with shopping guidelines, 301
    when eating out, 302–3
  adult onset of, 285–86
  alternative medicine view of, 282–83, 284,
    285
  anaphylaxis from, 279, <u>283</u>
  aspirin sensitivity and, <u>282</u>
  attention-deficit hyperactivity disorder
    linked to, 447–49
  avoiding premedication for, <u>290</u>
  causes of
    leaky-gut syndrome, 279
    proteins, 278
  in children, <u>18</u>, 203
    managing, 190–92
    symptoms of, 189–90
  chronic fatigue syndrome and, 457
  chronic illness associated with, 282–83
  concomitant, 286–87, <u>287</u>
  conventional medicine view of, 19,
    282
  diagnosis of
    in alternative medicine, 289–90
    with conventional procedures, 288–89

  in environmental medicine, 38, 41,
    42–43, 289–90
  environmental medicine view of, 34, 39–40,
    282–83, 284, 285
  food-dependent exercise-induced allergy,
    287–88, <u>288</u>, **410**, **425**
  vs. food intolerance, 280
  foods causing, **280**
  immediate and delayed reactions with,
    281–82
  incidence of, 38
  latex allergy and, <u>336</u>, <u>337</u>
  oral allergy syndrome, 286, <u>308</u>
  persons susceptible to, 283
  ragweed allergy coexisting with, 38–39, <u>38</u>
  risk factors for, 284–86
  symptoms of, 278, **407**, **425**
  testing for, 281
  during travel, avoiding, 127, 129–30
  treating, with
    animal enzymes, 298
    antihistamines, 291
    aspirin and NSAIDs, 291
    avoidance, 290–91
    baking soda, <u>295</u>
    corticosteroids, 291
    cromolyn, 291
    digestive herbs, 298
    elimination diet, 295–96
    enzyme-potentiated densensitization,
      298
    fasting, <u>297</u>
    homeopathy, 298–99
    immunotherapy, 291, 294, 297
    leukotriene inhibitors, 291
    microbial enzymes, 298
    plant enzymes, 298
    probiotics, <u>279</u>
    rotary diversified diet, 296–97
    therapeutic elimination diet, 291
    vitamins, minerals, and nutrients, <u>296</u>
  unusual, <u>289</u>
  when to see the doctor about, <u>283</u>
Food challenge test, for diagnosis of food
  allergies, 281, 289
Food-dependent exercise-induced allergy,
  287–88, <u>288</u>, **410**, **425**
Food diary, for diagnosis of food allergies, 288
Food intolerances
  vs. food allergies, 280
  inflammatory bowel disease and, 478

Food labels, for identifying food allergens, 300–301

Food preparation, with food allergies, 301–2

Food sensitivity, alternative medicine view of, 49, 50

Formaldehyde
allergic reactions from, 482–83
in permanent-press clothes, 95
in pressed-wood products, 94

Formulas, infant, hypoallergenic, 188

Fragrances
as asthma trigger, 234
avoiding, with sinusitis, 390

Fruits
causing allergies, 38, 292–93
for treating allergies, 143

Fungi, causing allergies, 293, 348

G

Gamma-linolenic acid (GLA)
anti-inflammatory properties of, 144–45
sources of, 142, 144–45
for treating
allergic rhinitis, 323, 326
allergies, 155
skin conditions, 417

Gamma oryzanol, for allergies, 155

Garages, allergy-proofing, 96, 97

Garlic, for treating
allergies, 64
asthma, 64, 253–54
sinusitis, 389, 392
yeast infections, 454

Garlic oil, for otitis media, 437–38

Gas stoves, respiratory irritation from, 92

Gastrocrom, for food allergies, 291

Gastroesophageal reflux disease (GERD), asthma from, 238

Gender, as risk factor for
allergies, 37, 187
asthma, 228

Genetics
as allergy risk factor, 4–5, 21, 22, 37, 186–87, 187
food allergies and, 284
insect allergies and, 271

Gentian root, for food allergies, 298

GERD, asthma from, 238

Germany, allergies in, 3–5, 22, 23

Giant papillary conjunctivitis, 428
action plan for, 430–31

Ginger, for treating
allergies, 143
asthma, 254
food allergies, 298

Ginkgo, for respiratory allergy symptoms, 64, 152–53, 254

Ginseng, for strengthening adrenals, 157

GLA. *See* Gamma-linolenic acid

Gloves, latex, allergy from, 329–30, 337
preventing, 333–35

Glycerin, allergy to, 40

Gold allergy, 351

Goldenseal, for sinusitis, 389, 392

Goose down, allergy to, 366

Grains, cereal, causing allergies, 292

Grapefruit seed extract, for killing dust mites, 82

Grape seed extract, for allergic rhinitis, 326

Grass pollen
affecting outdoor exercise, 170
season of, **123**

Guaifenesin, for sinusitis, 386

Guayule latex, as hypoallergenic alternative, 334

Guided imagery
for stress reduction, 176–77
for treating
asthma, 257, 258
headaches, 469

Gulf War syndrome, 492–93

H

Harvester ants, stings from, 399

Hay fever. *See* Allergic rhinitis

Headaches
detecting allergens causing, 472
linked to allergies, 46, 444, 468–72
migraine, 469
sinus, massage for, 181, **181**, **182**
treating, with
elimination diet, 472–74
imagery, 469
when to see the doctor about, 473

Health fraud schemes, protection from, 488–89

Heat depuration therapy, as treatment strategy in environmental medicine, 44

HEPA filters, for removing allergens, 51, 88, 274, 276, 346, 347, 365, 472
Herbs. *See also specific herbs*
  allergic reactions to, 63, 252, 293, 299
  guidelines for safe use of, 501, 502
  risks associated with, 252
  for treating
    allergic skin conditions, 416–17
    asthma, 252–56, 253
    food allergies, 298
    sinusitis, 389, 392
  as treatment strategy in alternative medicine, 54, 55, 64
Histamine
  discovery of, 15
  role of, in chronic fatigue syndrome, 462–63
History of allergies, 14–15, 16–17
Hitting the wall, 163
Hives
  action plan for, 419
  acute, 412
  causes of, 367
  cholinergic urticaria, 369
  chronic, 412
  cold urticaria, 369, 412
  vs. eczema, 193
  from fleabites, 394
  incidence of, 369
  occupational, 115, 117
  physical urticaria, 412
  rare forms of, 369
  symptoms of, **423**
  when to see an allergist about, 27
Hobby rooms, allergy-proofing, 97
Home
  allergens in, 73–75
    inspecting for, 80
  allergy-proofing areas of, 51, 72, 78
    basement, 95–96
    bathroom, 93, **93**
    bedroom, 77, 85–89, **85**,
    closets, **93**, 95
    consulting allergist about, 76
    crawl space, 96
    filters for (*see* Air filters)
    garage, **96**, 97
    general tips for, 77–79, 81–84
    hobby room or workshop, 97
    with humidity control, 77, 81, 92, 275, 345, 346
    kitchen and dining room, 89, 90–92
    laundry room, **93**, 94–95
    living room, 92
    outside, 79–81
    problems with products for, 76
    starting, 76–79
  duct cleaning in, 74–75
  new, allergy-proofing, 94
Homeopathy
  adverse reactions from, 63
  study results on, 65–66
  for treating
    allergic rhinitis, 324
    asthma, 255
    food allergies, 298–99
  as treatment strategy in alternative medicine, 53, 64–66
Honey, for allergic rhinitis, 324, 326
Hormonal supplements, as treatment strategy in alternative medicine, 55
Hormone allergy, 414–15
Hornets
  identifying, **398**
  stings from, 397, 398
Hotels, allergy protection in, 127
Household cleaners. *See* Cleaners, household
Houseplants
  allergies to, 51
  mold spores from, 84, 346
  as natural air filters, 51
Humidity control
  for dust mite allergy, 77, 81, 92, 275
  for mold allergy, 92, 345, 346
Humor therapy, for stress reduction, 177–78
Hydrocortisone cream. *See* Steroid cream
Hygiene hypothesis, explaining allergies, 9–10, 23, 60, 186, 285
Hypersensitivity pneumonitis, 358
Hyperventilation
  as asthma symptom, 229
  exercise-induced, 162
Hypnosis
  for asthma, 257
  for stress reduction, 178–79
Hyposmia, 324
  from allergic rhinitis, 318

I

IBD. *See* Inflammatory bowel disease
IgE. *See* Immunoglobulin E

IgG blood tests, for diagnosis of food allergies, 289

Imagery, guided. *See* Guided imagery

Immune system, overactive, in allergies, 15, 21

Immune system dysregulation theory, concerning multiple chemical sensitivity, 487–90

Immunoglobulin E (IgE)
 blood tests for detecting, 25
 in food allergies, 282
 in penicillin allergy, 261
 role of, in allergic reactions, 15–18, **15**
 viewed by environmental medicine, 33, 36

Immunoglobulin G (IgG) blood tests, for diagnosis of food allergies, 289

Immunotherapy
 in conventional medicine, 24, 32
 in environmental medicine, 33, <u>35</u>, 43–44
 for treating
  allergic rhinitis, 197, <u>312</u>, 325–26
  asthma, 201, 246, 259
  chronic fatigue syndrome, 463–64
  cockroach allergy, 277
  dust mite allergy, 276
  food allergies, 291, 294, 297
  mold allergy, 348
 venom, for preventing insect sting anaphylaxis, 215–16, 394, 402

Indian tobacco, for asthma, 54, 256

Indoor allergies, symptoms of, 76

Infants
 delaying allergies in, <u>186</u>, 187–88
 introducing solid foods to, <u>190–91</u>

Infections
 bacterial, food allergies and, 284–85
 ear (*see* Otitis media)
 increasing allergy risk, 37
 mold causing, 341
 respiratory, as asthma cause, 238
 yeast (*see* Yeast infections)

Infectious rhinitis, <u>310</u>

Inflammatory bowel disease (IBD)
 cause of, 476–77
 food intolerances and, 478
 linked to allergies, 46, 444
 treating, with
  balancing dietary fat, 444, 475–76, 477–78, <u>477</u>, 479
  diet, 478–79
  intestinal worms, <u>479</u>

Inhalers, asthma
 correct use of, <u>244</u>
 technique for using, 245–46
 types of, <u>200–201</u>, 243–45, 372

Insect allergies
 action plan for
  prevention, 400–401
  treatment, 401–2
 development of, 396–97
 EpiPen for treating, 393–94
 insects causing, 394–96
  bees, 397
  caterpillars, <u>396</u>
  fire ants, 398–99
  wasps, 397–98
 skeeter syndrome, <u>395</u>
 symptoms of, **408**
 venom immunotherapy for preventing, 215–16, 394

Insect stings
 anaphylaxis from, <u>218</u>, 393–94
  deaths from, <u>394</u>
 myths about, <u>401</u>

Insulin
 allergy to, 265
 anaphylaxis from, <u>218–19</u>

Insurance, travel, 124

Intal. *See* Cromolyn

Integrative medicine, benefits of, 61

Interleukin-4, in allergic reactions, 22

Intestinal problems, allergies linked to, <u>460</u>. *See also* Inflammatory bowel disease (IBD)

Intracutaneous one-to-five serial dilution titration, used in environmental medicine, 42

Irritable bowel syndrome, <u>476</u>

Itraconzole, for mold allergy, 348

IvyBlock, for preventing poison plant allergy, 378

J

Jewelry
 allergy from (*see* Nickel allergy)
 hypoallergenic, 351, 354

Jewelweed, for poison plant allergy, 380

Journaling
 for asthma, 257
 for stress reduction, 179–80

Joyner-Kersee, Jackie, <u>164–65</u>
Juice fast, for diagnosing food allergies, <u>297</u>
Juices, selecting, 145–46
Junk food, avoiding, with asthma, 249

K

Keratoconjunctivitis
  atopic, 427
  vernal, 427, 430
Ketotifen, for eye allergies, 430
Kinesiology testing, in alternative medicine,
  50
Kitchens, allergy-proofing, **89**, 90–92

L

Labels, food, for identifying food allergens,
  300–301
Lactobacillus acidophilus. See Acidophilus
Lactose intolerance, 280
Lady beetle allergies, <u>270</u>
Latex. *See also* Latex allergy
  alternatives to, <u>332</u>
  anaphylaxis from, <u>219</u>
  hypoallergenic, <u>334</u>
Latex allergy. *See also* Latex
  action plan for
    preparing for emergency, 335
    prevention, 333–35
    treatment, 338–39
    when to call the doctor, 339
  from condoms, 330–31
  food allergies and, <u>336</u>, <u>337</u>
  food handling affecting, <u>337</u>
  gas-treated food and, <u>329</u>
  from gloves, 329–30, <u>337</u>
  prevalence of, <u>328</u>
  products causing, 327–28
  steps to eliminate, 331–32
  symptoms of, 339, **406**, **407**, **425**
Latex sensitization, 328–29
  occupations at risk for, <u>331</u>
Laundry rooms, allergy-proofing, **93**, 94–95
Lead exposure, <u>483</u>
Leaky-gut syndrome, 9, 39–40
  causes of
    alcoholic beverages, <u>141</u>, 143
    caffeinated beverages, <u>141</u>

poor diet, 142
  sugar, <u>141</u>
  food allergies from, 279
Legumes, causing allergies, <u>293</u>
Leukotriene antagonists, for asthma, 201
Leukotriene inhibitors, for food allergies, 291
Leukotriene modifiers, for preventing
    exercise-induced asthma, 246, 259
Licorice root
  combined with corticosteroids, <u>57</u>
  for treating
    allergies, 64
    asthma, 57, 64, <u>253</u>
Lifestyle
  as allergy risk factor, <u>7</u>, 21, 23
  Western, promoting allergy and asthma,
    3–5, 23, 60, 228
Living rooms, allergy-proofing, 92
Lobelia, for asthma, 54, 256
Loratadine, for treating
  allergic rhinitis, 57, 150, 196, 309, 315,
    <u>315</u>
  eye allergies, 430
Loteprednol, for eye allergies, 430
Lotrisone, for eczema, 194
Lunch, foods recommended for, <u>147</u>
Lung function tests, for diagnosis of asthma,
  231

M

Magnesium, for treating
  allergies, <u>143</u>
  asthma, 68, 250–51, 260
Ma huang, for asthma, 54. *See also* Ephedra
Manipulative work, as treatment strategy in
    alternative medicine, 53
Marshmallow, for treating
  latex allergy rashes, 338
  skin conditions, <u>416</u>
Masks
  for air pollution, 124–25
  for yard work, <u>108</u>
Massage
  for asthma, 257–58
  for stress reduction, 180–81, <u>180</u>, **181**, **182**
Material safety data sheets, for diagnosis of
    workplace allergies, 117
Mattress, encasing, 85–86, 89, 346, 363
MCS. *See* Multiple chemical sensitivity

Meat
  allergies from, <u>293–94</u>
  avoiding, in allergy-free diet, <u>141</u>
Medical errors, deaths from, <u>264</u>
MedicAlert bracelet, 125, 221, 267, 335, 402
Medical history
  for diagnosis in
    conventional medicine, 24–25
    environmental medicine, 40–41
    workplace allergies, 116–17
  for diagnosis of
    asthma, 230
    food allergies, 288
Medication errors, <u>264</u>
Medications. *See* Drugs
Meditation, for stress reduction, 182–83
Melons, allergy to, <u>38</u>
Ménière's disease, <u>435</u>
  identifying symptoms of, **439**
Metered-dose inhalers, for asthma, <u>201</u>,
    243–44, 259
Methylene chloride, safe use of, 97
Methylphenidate, for attention-deficit
    hyperactivity disorder, 445–46, <u>446</u>,
    <u>448</u>
Methylsulfonylmethane (MSM), for allergies,
  153
Microbial enzymes, for treating food allergies,
  298
Migraines, preventing and treating, <u>469</u>
Milk
  anaphylaxis from, <u>218</u>
  avoiding, in allergy-free diet, 140, <u>140</u>
  cow's, allergy to, 9, <u>18</u>, 189
  hidden sources of, <u>199</u>, 302, 303–4
Milk substitutes, 304
Mind-body techniques
  for treating asthma, 256–58, <u>257</u>, <u>258</u>
  as treatment strategy in alternative
    medicine, 53, 66–67
Mold. *See also* Mold allergy
  affecting outdoor exercise, <u>170</u>
  as allergy trigger, **20**, 98, 99, 340–41
  avoiding, with candidiasis hypersensitivity,
    454
  basement, 95–96
  bathroom, 92
  conditions for growth of, 342–43, <u>342</u>
  detecting odor of, 84
  harmful effects of, 341–42
  outdoor, 98, 99, 104, 109–10, 347

  prevalence of, 104, 342, 343–44, <u>347</u>
  preventing, 79
  refrigerator, 92
  removing, <u>344</u>
    gadgets ineffective for, <u>346</u>
Mold allergy. *See also* Mold
  action plan for
    indoor prevention, 345–47
    indoor treatment, 347
    medical treatment, 348
    outdoor prevention, 347–48
  chronic fatigue syndrome and, 457–58
  foods to avoid with, <u>341</u>, 348
  symptoms of, 341, **406**, **407**
Mometasone, for allergic rhinitis, <u>458</u>
Monosodium glutamate (MSG), sources of,
  305
Montelukast, for asthma, 201, 372
Mosquito bites
  preventing, 401
  skeeter syndrome from, <u>395</u>
MSG, sources of, 305
MSM, for allergies, 153
Mucolytics, for sinusitis, 386
Mullein oil, for otitis media, 437–38
Multiple chemical sensitivity (MCS)
  alternative medicine view of, 50
  causes of, 486
  controversy about, 481–84
  coping strategies for, 495–96
  diagnostic criteria for, 484–86
  difficulty diagnosing, 481–83
  in Gulf War veterans, <u>492</u>, <u>493</u>
  hidden allergy connection with, 46, 444
  immune system dysregulation theory and,
    487–90
  persons at risk for, 486
  as psychological problem, 490–92
  resources on, <u>494</u>
  substances causing, <u>482–83</u>
  symptoms of, 480–81, 482
  treating, 493–95
Multivitamins, 149–50, 326

N

N-acetylcysteine (NAC), for asthma, 252
NARES, <u>311</u>
Nasal challenge, for diagnosis of allergic
  rhinitis, 118

NasalCrom, for allergic rhinitis, 51, 197, 319

Nasal rinsing, for treating
allergic rhinitis, 53, 320–23, <u>321</u>, <u>322</u>, 325, <u>458</u>
asthma, <u>255</u>
sinusitis, 387–88, <u>388</u>, 391

Nasal sprays, corticosteroid
for allergic rhinitis, 196–97, 316–17, 319, 325
for sinusitis, 386, 391

Nasonex, for allergic rhinitis, <u>458</u>

Nebulizers, for asthma, 126, <u>201</u>, 245, **245**, 258

Neck tightness, as asthma symptom, 229

Nedocromil, for treating
asthma, 242, 246, 259, 372
latex allergy, 339

Nettle, 54, 150–51
for treating
allergic rhinitis, 54, 150–51, 323, 326
food allergies, <u>296</u>
skin conditions, <u>417</u>

Nickel, objects containing, 351, <u>351</u>

Nickel allergy
action plan for, 354–55
causes of, 349, 351
chronic fatigue syndrome and, 457
diet and, <u>350</u>
predisposition to, 352–53
prevalence of, <u>352</u>
symptoms of, 351–52, **425**
tongue piercing immune to, <u>355</u>

Nitrates and nitrites, sources of, 305

Nolvadex, for hormone allergy, <u>415</u>

Nonallergic conjunctivitis, 428

Nonallergic rhinitis
with eosinophilia syndrome, <u>311</u>
types of, <u>310–11</u>

Nonsteroidal anti-inflammatory drugs (NSAIDs), for food allergies, 291

Nose-blowing, with sinusitis, 389

NSAIDs, for food allergies, 291

Nutrition. *See also* Diet
increasing allergy risk, 37

Nuts
peanuts (*see* Peanuts)
tree
allergy to, 189, <u>294</u>
anaphylaxis from, <u>218</u>
hidden sources of, 303, 306

O

Obesity, asthma linked to, 160–61, 198

Obstructive sleep apnea, as asthma cause, 238

Occupational allergies. *See* Workplace allergies

Olbas Analgesic Oil, for treatment in alternative medicine, 55

Olive leaf extract, for sinusitis, 388–89, 392

Olive oil, for treating
allergies, <u>143</u>
asthma, 249
otitis media, 438

Olopatadine, for eye allergies, 430

Omega-3 fatty acids, 155
anti-inflammatory properties of, 144–45
sources of, <u>142</u>, 144
for treating
allergies, 155
asthma, 249, 260
inflammatory bowel disease, 476, 478, 479

Omega-6 fatty acids
avoiding, 138–40, <u>140</u>
with inflammatory bowel disease, 475–76, 477–78
sources of, 155, 156

Optimal-dose immunotherapy, in environmental medicine, 44

Oral allergy syndrome, 286, 294, <u>308</u>

Oregon grape, for treating
latex allergy rashes, 338
skin conditions, <u>416–17</u>

OSHA standards, on workplace allergies, 119, 120

Osteoporosis, from corticosteroid use, preventing, 68, <u>250</u>

Otitis media, 434, **434**
action plan for, 437–38
causes of, 435
identifying symptoms of, **439**
linked to allergies, 19, 195–96, 308, 436
treatment of, 436, <u>436</u>

Outdoors
allergy-free travel in, 127–28
exercising in, <u>170</u>, 172

Ozone, affecting allergies and asthma, <u>103</u>, <u>370</u>

P

Pantothenic acid
  for asthma, 251, 260
  for strengthening adrenals, 157
Papaya and pineapple enzymes, for sinusitis,
    390, 392
Paper wasps
  identifying, **398**
  stings from, 397, 398
Parasites, intestinal, <u>460</u>, <u>479</u>
Patanol, for eye allergies, 430
Patch tests, for allergy diagnosis, 25
Peak-flow meter, for managing asthma, 117,
    239, 242, 259
  in children, 200–201
Peanuts
  allergy to, 6, 9, 189
  anaphylaxis from, <u>218</u>
  avoiding, in pregnancy, 187
  hidden sources of, 302, 306
Penicillin allergy
  anaphylaxis from, <u>218–19</u>
  detecting, 267
  as IgE-mediated, 261
  mold allergy and, 348
  as noninherited, 262
  prevalence of, <u>267</u>
Perilla seed oil, for asthma, 252
Pest control, chemical-free, in yard,
    <u>100–101</u>
Pet allergens, 73, 74
  controlling, 78–79, 85, 125–26, 169–70
  removing, <u>360</u>
  verifying, 360, 362
Pet allergies
  action plan for
    prevention, 363–66
    treatment, 366
  breeds preventing, 362
  causes of, 356–58, <u>359</u>
    bird allergens, <u>358</u>
    dark-haired cats, <u>361</u>
    leftover pet allergens, 358–59
  symptoms of, 359–60, **406**, **409**
  treating, with
    removal of pet from household, <u>357</u>
    zafirlukast, <u>365</u>
Pet ownership, prevalence of, <u>359</u>
Photoallergic contact dermatitis, <u>368</u>,
    425

Physical allergy
  action plan for, 371–72
  asthma induced by exercise and cold air,
    369–70, 372
  definition of, 367
  photoallergic contact dermatitis, <u>368</u>, **425**
  symptoms of, **423**
  urticaria, 367–69, 412
Physical examination
  for diagnosis of asthma, 231
  before starting exercise, 162
Piercing
  body, record for, <u>353</u>
  tongue, immune to nickel allergy, <u>355</u>
Pigeon breeder's disease, <u>358</u>
Pillows, selecting, 88
Plane travel, allergy-free, 126–27
Plantain, for poison plant allergy, 380
Plant enzymes, for treating food allergies, 298
Poison bait trays, for roach control, 91
Poison ivy
  growth locations of, 374, **374**
  identifying, 375, **375**
Poison oak
  growth locations of, 374, **374**
  identifying, 375, **375**
Poisonous plants
  facts about, <u>379</u>
  prevalence of, 374, **374**
Poison plant allergy
  action plan for
    prevention, 378
    treatment, 378–80
  identifying plants causing, 374–75, **375**
  persons susceptible to, 376–77
  rash from, 373, 376, 377
  symptoms of, **424**
  topical skin protectant for, <u>376</u>
Poison sumac
  growth locations of, 374, **374**
  identifying, 375, **375**
Pollen
  allergic reactions to, 104–5
    symptoms of, **406**, **407**
  foods cross-reacting with, 286, 287, <u>287</u>,
    308
  on laundry hung outside, 80–81
  plants producing, <u>108–9</u>
  prevalence of, <u>99</u>
  production of, 98, 99–104
  protecting self from, <u>108–9</u>

screens blocking, 83–84
sources of, **20**
tracking, during travel, 123, **123**
washing away, 89
Pollen counts, <u>102–3</u>
Pollution
  indoor, as allergy trigger, 7–8
  outdoor, as allergy trigger, 6–7
Polyps, nasal
  from allergic rhinitis, 314
  sinusitis and, 384, **384**
  surgery to remove, 386–87
Poultry, avoiding, in allergy-free diet,
  <u>141</u>
Prebiotics, for digestive health, 154–55
Pregnancy
  allergens to avoid in, 187
  allergies and asthma during, <u>188</u>
Pregnancy rhinitis, <u>311</u>
Primrose oil, for allergies, 155
Proanthocyanidins, for asthma, 251
Probiotics, for treating
  allergies, 154
  eczema, <u>279</u>
  food allergies, <u>279</u>
Products, allergy and asthma, sources of,
  498–500
Protein, avoiding, in allergy-free diet, 140
Protopic, for eczema, 194, <u>413</u>, 420
Proventil, for treating
  anaphylaxis, 339
  asthma, 372
Provocation/neutralization test, for diagnosis
  of food allergies, 289
Provocation/neutralization therapy, for
  multiple chemical sensitivity, 495
Provocation tests, for allergy diagnosis, 25
Psoriasis, symptoms of, **424**
Pulmonary function tests, for allergy diagnosis,
  25
Pyrethrins, avoiding, in yard, <u>101</u>

Q

Quackery, protection from, <u>488–89</u>
Quercetin, for treating
  allergic rhinitis, 54, 323, 326
  asthma, 251
  eye allergies, 429
  food allergies, <u>296</u>

physical allergy, 371
respiratory allergy symptoms, 150
Quiz, for identifying allergic tendency, 207–8

R

Radioallergosorbent test (RAST)
  for diagnosis of
    eczema, 421
    food allergies, 289
  in environmental medicine, 41–42
Radiology dyes
  allergy to, 265, 267
  anaphylaxis from, <u>218–19</u>
Ragweed allergy
  affecting outdoor exercise, <u>170</u>
  environmental medicine view of, 38–39,
    38
  pyrethrin sensitivity with, <u>101</u>
  season for, **123**
Raja's Cup, for treatment in alternative
  medicine, 55
Rashes
  from latex allergy, 338–39
  poison plant, 376, 377
  when to see an allergist about, <u>27</u>
RAST. *See* Radioallergosorbent test
Reishi mushroom concentrate, for asthma,
  252
Relaxation, for sinusitis, 390
Research, on allergy treatments, 60–61
Resources
  for children, 497–98
  on multiple chemical sensitivity, <u>494</u>
  organizations as, 497
  for parents, 498
  on products, 498–500
Respiratory infections, as asthma cause, 238
Restaurant dining
  with food allergies, 302–3
  latex allergy affecting, <u>337</u>
Rheumatoid arthritis, linked to allergies, 46
Rhinitis medicamentosa, <u>311</u>, 319
Rhinosinusitis, 18, 238
Risk factors
  for allergies, 21, 22–23
  for asthma, 227
Ritalin, for attention-deficit hyperactivity
  disorder, 445–46, <u>446</u>, <u>448</u>
Roaches. *See* Cockroach allergies; Cockroaches

Rodent allergies, <u>364</u>
  symptoms of, **407**, **408**
Rotary-diversified diet, for food allergies, 43, 296–97
Runny nose, determining cause of, **406–7**

S

Saiboku-to, for allergies and asthma, 64
Saline irrigation. *See* Nasal rinsing
Saline sprays
  preservatives in, <u>323</u>, 325
  for sinusitis, 392
Salmeterol, for asthma, 235, 372
Salt water, for nasal rinsing, 320–22, <u>321</u>
Saturated fat, avoiding, in allergy-free diet, 136, <u>140</u>
Sauna therapy, as treatment strategy in environmental medicine, 44
Screens, pollen-proof, 83–84
Scuba diving, with asthma, 128
Seafood. *See* Fish; Shellfish
Selenium, for allergic rhinitis, 326
Self-help strategies, 11, 12
Self-treatment, dangers of, <u>60</u>
Semprex-D, for allergic rhinitis, <u>315</u>
Sensitivities, vs. allergies, 17
Serevent
  for treating, asthma, 235, 372
Shellfish
  allergy to, 9, <u>292</u>, 305–6
  anaphylaxis from, <u>218</u>
Shopping, with food allergies, 301
Siberian ginseng, for treating
  allergic rhinitis, <u>459</u>
  chronic fatigue syndrome, 464
Sick building syndrome, <u>118</u>
Silicone breast implants, allergies and, <u>490–91</u>
Similasan, for eye allergies, 429
Singulair, for asthma, 201, 372
Sinuses
  allergic rhinitis affecting, 313
  anatomy of, 381–82, **382**
Sinus headaches, massage for, 181, **181**, **182**
Sinus irrigation. *See* Nasal rinsing
Sinusitis
  action plan for, 391–92
  acute vs. chronic, 384
  causes of, 382–84
    allergic rhinitis, 308

complications from, 384
specific sinus affected by, <u>382</u>
symptoms of, <u>383</u>, 384, **410**
treating, with
  allergen avoidance, 388
  antibiotics, 385, 391
  antihistamines, 386, 391–92
  chicken soup, 390, 392
  dairy avoidance, 389–90
  decongestants, 386, 391
  herbs, 389, 392
  irritant avoidance, 390
  mucolytics, 386
  nasal corticosteroids, 386, 391
  nasal washing, 387–88, <u>388</u>, 391
  olive leaf extract, 388–89, 392
  papaya and pineapple enzymes, 390, 392
  proper nose-blowing, 389
  relaxation, 390
  Sinus Survival Botanical Nasal Spray, 389, 392
  steam, 389, 392
  surgery, 386–87, 392
  warm compresses, 389, 392
  water drinking, 390, 392
Sinusol, for improving asthma, <u>255</u>
Sinus Survival Botanical Nasal Spray, for sinusitis, 389, 392
Skeeter syndrome, from mosquito bites, <u>395</u>
Skin conditions, contact dermatitis, 418
Skin-prick tests
  allergic reaction to, <u>40</u>
  for diagnosis of
    allergies, 25, 38
    asthma, 231
    drug allergies, 266–67
    eczema, 421
    food allergies, 289
    occupational asthma, 117
Skin problems
  angioedema, 411–12
    action plan for, 419
  atopic dermatitis (*see also* Eczema)
    action plan for, 420–21
    causes of, 413, 415
    managing, 413–15, <u>413</u>
  in children, 202
  contact dermatitis, 418, 422 (*see also* Contact dermatitis)
  herbs for treating, <u>416–17</u>
  hives, 411–12, 419 (*see also* Hives)

from hormone allergy, 414–15
occupational, 114–15
    diagnosis of, 117
symptom solver for identifying, **423–25**
Sleep disturbances, with fibromyalgia, 461
Smell
    loss of, with allergic rhinitis, 318
    testing sense of, 324
Smoking
    allergy and asthma risk from, 484–85
    avoiding
        in home, 83
        during pregnancy, 187
        with sinusitis, 390
        during travel, 125, 126
    passive
        affecting children, 83, 187, 438, 485
        food allergies and, 284
Snacks
    foods recommended for, 147
    hidden milk and eggs in, 199
Snail allergy, with dust mite allergy, 276
Sneezing, determining cause of, **406–7**
Social involvement, for stress reduction,
    183
Sodium bicarbonate, for food allergies, 298
Sodium cromolyn, for eye allergies, 430
Soy
    allergy to, 9, 189
    anaphylaxis from, 218
    sources of, 306
Spacers, for asthma, 201
Spices
    causing allergies, 293
    as treatment in alternative medicine, 64
Spirulina, for treating
    allergies, 143
    asthma, 251–52
Sporanox, for mold allergy, 348
Sports, best and worst, for allergy sufferers,
    168–69
Status asthmaticus, 227
Steam inhalation
    for asthma, pros and cons of, 247
    for sinusitis, 389, 392
    as treatment strategy in alternative
        medicine, 53–54
Steroid cream, for treating
    atopic dermatitis, 413–14
    eczema, 194
    eye allergies, 431

latex allergy rashes, 338
nickel allergy, 355
Steroids. *See* Corticosteroid(s)
Stinging ants, varieties of, 399
Stinging insects. *See also* Insect allergies
    allergies from, 394–95
    bees, 397, **397**, 401
    fire ants, 395–96, 398–99, **399**
    wasps, 397–98, **398**, 401
Stinging nettle. *See* Nettle
Stress, increasing risk of
    allergies, 9, 37, 134, 173–74
    asthma, 198
Stress reduction
    methods of
        biofeedback, 174–75
        cognitive reframing, 175–76
        guided visualization, 176–77
        humor therapy, 177–78
        hypnosis, 178–79
        journaling, 179–80
        massage, 180–81, 180, **181**, **182**
        meditation, 182–83
        social involvement, 183
        yoga, 183–84, 183, **184**
    for treating
        allergic rhinitis, 323, 325
        asthma, 258, 260
        eczema, 421
        hives, 371, 419
    as treatment strategy in environmental
        medicine, 44–45
Stuffed animals, washing, 89
Sugar
    avoiding
        in allergy-free diet, 140–41, 141
        for candidiasis hypersensitivity, 454, 455
    statistics on consumption of, 453
Sulfites
    anaphylaxis from, 218
    as asthma trigger, 234, 239
    avoiding, in allergy-free diet, 141–42
    sources of, 305
Sun protection, with atopic dermatitis, 128,
    129
Sunscreen, dermatitis from, 368
Supplementation schedule, allergy-free, 134
Supplements. *See also specific supplements*
    dietary, for asthma, 251–52
    emerging, guidelines for safe use of, 505–6,
        506–7

Supplements *(cont.)*
  hormonal, 55
  multivitamins, 149–50, 326
  for respiratory allergy symptoms
    bee pollen, 151–52
    ephedra, 152
    ginkgo, 152–53
    methylsulfonylmethane, 153
    nettle, 150–51
    quercetin, 150
    schedule for, <u>151</u>
    vitamin C, 152
    vitamin E, 152
  strengthening adrenal glands, 156–57.
    DHEA, 158
    ginseng, 157
    pantothenic acid, 157
  supporting digestive health
    essential fatty acids, 155–56, <u>156</u>
    gamma oryzanol, 155
    prebiotics, 154–55
    probiotics, 154
  as treatment strategy in environmental
    medicine, 45
  vitamin and mineral *(see* Vitamins and
    minerals)
Surgery, for treating
  otitis media, <u>436</u>
  sinusitis, 386–87, 392
Sweet wormword, for intestinal parasites,
  <u>460</u>
Swimming, <u>160</u>, 167, <u>168</u>, 198
Symptom solver charts, for identifying cause
  of
  coughing and wheezing, **408–10**
  ear problems, **439**
  eye problems, **432–33**
  runny nose and sneezing, **406–7**
  skin problems, **423–25**

T

Tacrolimus, for eczema, 194, <u>413</u>,
  420
Tamoxifen, for hormone allergy, <u>415</u>
Tartrazine. *See* Yellow dye no. 5
Tecnu Oak-N-Ivy Brand Outdoor Skin
    Cleanser, for preventing poison plant
    allergy, 378
Temovate, for nickel allergy, 355

Tests
  diagnostic
    in alternative medicine, 50
    for asthma diagnosis, 231
    in conventional medicine, 25
    in environmental medicine, 41–43,
      <u>42</u>
    before starting exercise, 161
  laboratory, for identifying allergens, <u>272</u>,
    500
Tilade. *See* Nedocromil
Tocopherol, for allergic rhinitis, 326
Tongue piercing, immune to nickel allergy,
  <u>355</u>
Traditional Chinese Medicine
    as alternative treatment strategy, 67–68
    for asthma, 254–56
Train travel, allergy-free, 129
Trans fats, avoiding
  in allergy-free diet, <u>140–41</u>
  with asthma, 198, 249, 260
Travel, allergy-free, 72
  in another person's home, 130
  avoiding food allergies for, 129–30
  on bus, 129
  in car, 125–26
  on cruises, 128–29
  general guidelines for, 122–25
  in hotels, 127
  in outdoors, 127–28
  in plane, 126–27
  on train, 129
Tree pollen season, **123**
Turmeric, for allergies, <u>143</u>
Tylophora indica, for allergies and asthma,
  64
Tympanostomy with tube placement, for
  otitis media, <u>436</u>

U

Ulcerative colitis, <u>476.</u> *See also* Inflammatory
    bowel disease (IBD)
UltraClear fast, for diagnosing food allergies,
  <u>297</u>
Urticaria. *See* Hives
Urushiol
  facts about, <u>377</u>
  poison plant rashes from, 373–74, 377,
    378

V

Vacuum(ing)
  carpets, 82–83, 365
  for dust mite control, 276
  filters for, 77, 82, 276, 365
  selecting, 86
Vaginitis. *See* Yeast infections
Vasocon-A, for eye allergies, 429
Vasomotor rhinitis, 310
Vegan diet, for allergies, 148
Vegetable oil, health effects from, 138–40
Vegetables
  causing allergies, 294
  for treating allergies, 143
Vegetarianism, for asthma, 249
Venom immunotherapy, for preventing insect
    allergies, 215–16, 394, 402
Ventilation
  basement, 95
  house, 83–84
Vernal keratoconjunctivitis, 427
  action plan for, 430
  identifying symptoms of, **433**
Viruses, limiting childhood exposure to, 188
Visine-A, for eye allergies, 429
Visualization, guided. *See* Guided imagery
Vitamin B$_6$, for asthma, 251, 260
Vitamin C
  for preventing corticosteroid side effects,
      250
  for treating
    allergic rhinitis, 326
    asthma, 68
    eye allergies, 429
    respiratory allergy symptoms, 152
Vitamin D, for preventing corticosteroid side
    effects, 250
Vitamin E, for treating
  asthma, 248, 259
  respiratory allergy symptoms, 152
Vitamin E complex, for allergic rhinitis, 326
Vitamins and minerals. *See also specific
    vitamins and minerals*
  guidelines for safe use of, 504–5, 504–5
  for treating, asthma, 250–51, 250
  as treatment strategy in alternative
      medicine, 55, 68
Viva-Drops, for eye allergies, 429
Vocal-cord dysfunction, exercise-induced,
    162–63

W

Walking, 160
Washing machine, water temperature for, 82,
    87, 94–95
Wasps
  identifying, **398**
  stings from, 397–98
Water drinking
  importance of, 139
  for treating
    asthma, 249, 260
    sinusitis, 390, 392
Water temperature, washer, 82, 87, 94–95
Weed pollen season, **123**
Western lifestyle, promoting
  allergies, 3–5, 23, 60
  asthma, 228
West Germany, allergies in, 4, 5, 22
Wheat
  allergy to, 9, 189
  anaphylaxis from, 218
  hidden sources of, 302–3, 306
Wheat grass juice, as potential allergy fighter,
    62
Wheezing
  with asthma, 229
  determining cause of, **408–10**
Witch hazel, for poison plant allergy, 379
Woodstove, safe use of, 92
Workers' compensation, for workplace
    allergies, 120–21
Workplace allergies, 72
  allergic rhinitis, 115
  asthma, 112–14
  consulting doctors about, 116–19
  employer's role in solving, 119–20,
      495–96
  multiple chemical sensitivity and,
      495–96
  nickel allergy, 353
  from sick building syndrome, 118
  skin problems, 114–15
  substances causing, 111–12, 113
  workers' compensation for, 120–21
Workshops, allergy-proofing, 97

X

Xylitol gum, for preventing otitis media, 437

Y

Yard
  chemical-free pest control in, 100–101
  minimizing allergens in, 72, 105, 108–10, **110**
  pollen production in, 98, 99–104
  protection from allergens in, 108–9
  troublesome vs. trouble-free plants for, 106–7
Yeast infections. *See also* Candidiasis hypersensitivity
  from antibiotics, 451, 454
  incidence of, 453
  preventing, 454
  treating, 453, 454
Yellow dye no. 5
  hives from, 419
  sources of, 305
Yellow jackets
  identifying, **398**
  stings from, 397, 398, 400

Yoga, for stress reduction, 183–84, 183, **184**
Yogurt
  for digestive health, 153, 154
  for treating
    allergies, 143, 146–48
    asthma, 248
    candidiasis hypersensitivity, 454

Z

Zaditor, for eye allergies, 430
Zafirlukast, for treating
  asthma, 201, 372
  pet allergies, 365, 366
Zinc, for treating
  allergic rhinitis, 326
  asthma, 143
Zyrtec, for treating
  allergic rhinitis, 196, 315
  eye allergies, 430

MOSAICS

FOCUSING ON ESSAYS

SECOND EDITION

KIM FLACHMANN

Prentice
Hall

Upper Saddle River, New Jersey 07458

Library of Congress Cataloging-in-Publication Data

Flachmann, Kim.
    Mosaics, focusing on essays in context / Kim Flachmann.—2nd ed.
        p. cm.—(Mosaics)
    Rev. ed. of: Mosaics, focusing on essays / Kim Flachmann … [et al.]. c1998.
    Includes bibliographical references and index.
    ISBN 0-13-016311-2
        1. English language—Rhetoric. 2. English language—Grammar. 3. Report writing.
    I. Title: Focusing on essays in context. II. Mosaics, focusing on essays. III. Title.
    IV. Mosaics (Upper Saddle River, N.J.)

    PE1408 .F469 2001
    808'.042—dc21

2001050090

Editor in Chief: Leah Jewell
Acquisitions Editor: Craig Campanella
Editorial Assistant: Joan Polk
VP/Director of Production and Manufacturing: Barbara Kittle
Senior Managing Editor: Mary Rottino
Project Manager: Maureen Richardson
Copyeditor: Bruce Emmer
Proofreader: Rainbow Graphics

Prepress and Manufacturing Manager: Nick Sklitsis
Prepress and Manufacturing Buyer: Ben Smith
Marketing Director: Beth Mejia
Marketing Manager: Rachel Falk
Creative Design Director: Leslie Osher
Interior and Cover Designer: Kathryn Foot
Cover Art: Wolfgang Kachler Photography
Development Editor in Chief: Susanna Lesan
Development Editor: Harriett Prentiss

This book was set in 11/13 Goudy by Interactive Composition Corp. and was printed and bound by R R Donnelly & Sons Co. (Harrisonburg). Covers were printed by Phoenix Color Corp.

For permission to use copyrighted material, grateful acknowledgment is made to the copyright holders listed on pages 841–843, which is considered an extension of this copyright page.

© 2002, 1999 by Pearson Education, Inc.
Upper Saddle River, New Jersey 07458

For Michael

Printed in the United States of America
10 9 8 7 6 5 4 3 2 1

ISBN 0-13-016311-2 (Student Edition)
ISBN 0-13-094214-6 (Annotated Instructor's Edition)

Pearson Education LTD., *London*
Pearson Education Australia PTY, Limited, *Sydney*
Pearson Education Singapore, Pte. Ltd
Pearson Education North Asia Ltd, *Hong Kong*
Pearson Education Canada, Ltd., *Toronto*
Pearson Educaión de Mexico, S. A. de C. V.
Pearson Education–Japan, *Tokyo*
Pearson Education Malaysia, Pte. Ltd
Pearson Education, *Upper Saddle River, New Jersey*